Modern Medical Education

John Sandars • Shabih Zaidi • Ali N. Zaidi
Editors

Modern Medical Education

Preparing for the Future

Springer

Editors
John Sandars
Edge Hill University Medical School
Edge Hill University
Ormskirk, Lancashire, UK

Shabih Zaidi
al- Sadiq International Virtual University
London, UK

Ali N. Zaidi
Mount Sinai Adult Congenital Heart
Disease Center
Mount Sinai Hospital
New York, NY, USA

ISBN 978-3-032-27957-6 ISBN 978-3-032-27958-3 (eBook)
https://doi.org/10.1007/978-3-032-27958-3

This Springer imprint is published by the registered company Springer Nature Switzerland AG
The registered company address is: Gewerbestrasse 11, 6330 Cham, Switzerland

Contents

Undergraduate Medical Education 1

Mohammed Saeed Abdulzahra, Mulazim Hussain Bukhari, and Azim Mirzazadah

Key Points

- Competency-based medical education (CBME) is the dominant global paradigm, shifting focus from time spent to the measurable mastery of entrustable professional activities (EPAs).
- The implementation of EPAs requires robust faculty development in sophisticated assessment techniques and substantial investment in data-tracking LMS systems for programmatic assessment.
- The global proliferation of medical schools necessitates a robust focus on accreditation and quality standards to safeguard the competency of graduates and public health outcomes.
- Technological tools such as AI offer powerful pathways for personalized learning and virtual simulation but demand concurrent investment in faculty development and clear ethical frameworks.
- Future structural innovations, including longitudinal integrated clerkships (LICs) and mandated scholarly activity, are essential for cultivating well-rounded physicians who are also leaders and health advocates.

M. S. Abdulzahra (✉)
Department of Internal Medicine, University of Kufa College of Medicine, Najaf, Iraq
e-mail: mohammed.alnaseri@uokufa.edu.iq

M. H. Bukhari
al Sadiq International Virtual University, Lahore, Pakistan

A. Mirzazadah
Department of Medical Education, Tehran University of Medical Sciences, Tehran, Iran

J. Sandars et al. (eds.), *Modern Medical Education*,
https://doi.org/10.1007/978-3-032-27958-3_1

1.1 Introduction and Definition

Undergraduate medical education (UME) is the first phase of the continuum of training and practice in medicine. The other phases include postgraduate medical education (PGME) and continuing medical education/continuous professional development (CME/CPD). UME is also called basic medical education (BME), underscoring its role as the basis of training in medicine.

Although it is one of the three phases of training in medicine, UME is arguably the most important. It represents the student's first encounter with the profession, plays a major role in developing their identity as a doctor, and includes the foundational courses that shape a physician's core knowledge and skills. It is the necessary phase without which pursuing a career in medicine is impossible. Furthermore, in many countries, UME provides the human resources required for the general practitioner role, who often serve as the gatekeepers of the country's healthcare systems.

UME programs are usually provided by a medical school/college and include several phases, traditionally preclinical and clinical. In its most classic model, the preclinical phase includes basic science and pathophysiology, while the clinical phase encompasses clerkship and internship. Based on the curriculum, variations exist, including the integration of basic science and pathophysiology and the lack of an internship in programs (MBBS and MDs) where graduates must complete postgraduate training before being licensed for independent practice.

1.1.1 Global Variations in UME

Despite commonalities in core content, several differences exist between UME programs globally concerning entry requirements, degree titles, and length.

Entry Requirements: While many countries admit students to medical school directly after high school, others require applicants to hold a bachelor's degree as an admission prerequisite. These are termed Graduate Medical Entry (GME) programs and are the unique path to medical training in countries like the USA and Canada. In other nations, such as the UK and Australia, both types of programs are available.

Title of the Degree: Different UME program titles carry varying implications. In many countries, predominantly those in the Commonwealth, the degree is MBBS or its equivalents (MBBCh, MbChB, BMBS, MBBCh, MBChB), meaning Bachelor of Medicine and Bachelor of Surgery. Graduates typically need postgraduate training to receive a license to practice. In other countries like the USA and Canada, the degree is entitled "MD" (Medical Doctor), but graduates, similar to those with an MBBS, must complete postgraduate training (usually residency) to receive a license as independent practitioners. There are also countries, such as Iran, where the MD degree includes an internship and graduates are licensed to practice independently as general practitioners.

Program Length: Program duration varies significantly across different countries, heavily dependent on the intended role of the graduates. MBBS programs typically last 4–6 years. MD programs in countries like the USA and Canada, where graduates are not licensed for independent practice immediately, are usually 4 years. Conversely, in countries like Iran, where graduates will practice independently, the MD program includes an internship and is usually around 7 years in length.

1.2 Historical Evolution of Undergraduate Medical Education

The history of medical education traces back to ancient times, with roots in diverse civilizations including Egypt, India, Iran, and Greece. The most recognized early model for training was the "master-student" or "apprenticeship model," where an aspiring physician sought out an expert master and followed him during an undefined period to learn the required skills and attitudes.

In the medieval age, the first medical education institution, established in Salerno (currently in Northern Italy) in the tenth century, played a major role in shaping medical schools across Europe.

In the late nineteenth century, developments such as the mandatory linkage of medical schools to universities and the expansion of the mandatory knowledge base of basic sciences led to a new training model: the discipline-based model. The tradition of European universities, which had discipline-specific departments, led to greater involvement of basic scientists in medical student education through discipline-based courses. The length of medical education extended from 1 year to 2 and finally 4 years in many medical schools.

1.2.1 The Flexner Report and Curricular Reforms

Despite the existence of a few elite medical schools in the USA, there was a rapid proliferation of for-profit medical schools characterized by limited resources and low quality of education. In the beginning of the twentieth century, the American Medical Association (AMA) and the Association of American Medical Colleges (AAMC) requested the Carnegie Foundation to review medical schools.

In 1910, the resulting Flexner Report, based on Abraham Flexner's visits to all North American medical schools, revolutionized medical education globally. Many North American medical schools were closed, and the model of "2 + 2" (2 years of basic sciences and 2 years of clinical training) was established. The report emphasized basic sciences to strengthen the scientific foundation of medicine, allowing students to subsequently apply this knowledge to solve clinical problems during their clinical years.

By the 1930s and 1940s, critiques of the discipline-based model highlighted shortcomings: postponing student exposure to real medical practice, the total authority of departments leading to an overloaded curriculum, and the fragmented nature of knowledge that students were expected to integrate themselves.

In the 1950s, the integrated model was developed at Western Reserve School of Medicine and disseminated extensively worldwide. This model sought to resolve the challenges of the discipline-based model through horizontal integration (between disciplines in the same phase, e.g., anatomy and physiology) and vertical integration (between basic and clinical subjects). Topic committees based on life phases, organ systems, or specific topics were established to develop integrated courses, providing a platform for faculty discussion to find the most relevant and organized content.

In the 1970s, medical schools like McMaster in Canada and Maastricht in the Netherlands established problem-based learning (PBL). PBL represented a major shift: instead of students receiving information and then applying it, they confront a problem first, defining learning issues and studying to acquire the necessary knowledge to solve it. This group-based approach fosters knowledge acquisition, problem-solving, teamwork, communication, and leadership. While evidence supports PBL's effectiveness, its widespread use is constrained by being resource-intensive, which limits implementation in programs with high student numbers.

The most recent major change, initiated by the ACGME in the USA and the Royal College of Physicians and Surgeons of Canada at the beginning of the twenty-first century, is competency-based medical education (CBME). CBME, now revolutionizing UME, involves defining competencies, providing learning opportunities to achieve them, and using assessment and feedback for trainee development.

1.3 Current State and Global Challenges

While UME is crucial to providing healthcare with a competent workforce, despite improvements from integrated, competency-based reforms, critical challenges must be addressed by policymakers and stakeholders to maintain the quality of graduates and healthcare.

1.3.1 The Global Scale and Quality Challenge

The number of medical schools has dramatically increased in the last 50 years, from nearly 1000 to approximately 3785 by 2020. This tremendous increase presents challenges related to adequate staffing and potential poor quality. Establishing good quality standards before authorizing an institution to admit students and continuous monitoring of performance are crucial to ensuring quality education and fit-for-purpose outcomes.

1.3.2 The Challenge of Admission and Selection

Admission policy is variable across countries, ranging from centralized systems (e.g., in Iraq, based on secondary school grades) to decentralized processes where each college utilizes its own authority and admission team to review student attributes. Admitting students based solely on recall ability and high marks may expose them to stress and an inability to adapt to the high cognitive demands of a medical program. Certain countries, like the UK, use multiple parameters including GPA, the UK Clinical Aptitude Test (UKAT), and the Multiple Mini-Interview (MMI). Furthermore, many countries, including the USA, UK, and Australia, utilize Graduate Medical Entry (GME) programs.

1.3.3 Curriculum and Transformative Learning

There is a clear global movement toward systems-based integrated curricula, driven by recommendations from regulatory bodies like the World Federation for Medical Education (WFME), the General Medical Council (GMC), and the Association of American Medical Colleges (AAMC). These organizations advocate for the integration of basic and clinical sciences, a response partly aligned with adult learning theory, which posits that adults seek clinically relevant and applied knowledge.

The 2010 Lancet Commissions Report by Julio Frenk and Lincoln Chen explicitly stated that the old Flexner discipline-based model was no longer effective for complex healthcare challenges. It called for transformative learning where students must be equipped with critical thinking, leadership, interprofessional teamwork skills, and professional values. Furthermore, the 2020 follow-up report noted a disconnection between educational institutes and healthcare delivery, negatively impacting the quality of both.

1.3.4 Competency-Based Education and EPAs

The newest move is toward CBME, which focuses on the competency attained rather than the time spent. This shift has been accompanied by the move to define Entrustable Professional Activities (EPAs). An EPA combines multiple competencies into a single, observable, key unit of work that, when performed successfully, merits entrustment.

Methods of Defining and Assessing EPAs

EPAs are typically defined by faculty groups as core activities that must be performed unsupervised by a graduating physician (e.g., diagnose and manage a patient with pneumonia).

These activities are crucial, combining the skills of history taking, communication, physical exam, and management into one observable unit of work that is fit for purpose.

The essential component of CBME and the EPA framework is the entrustment decision. This decision is not derived from a single test score but rather from a holistic, programmatic judgment made by supervisors based on cumulative evidence collected from multiple observations over an extended period. This system moves away from a simple pass/fail judgment toward a continuous assessment of a trainee's readiness to execute a specific professional activity autonomously.

The assessment tools are meticulously mapped to the EPA; they are designed not only to test knowledge but also to collect performance data on the component competencies within the EPA in real clinical settings. Tools frequently used include Mini-CEX (mini-clinical evaluation exercise), DOPS (direct observation of procedural skills), and case-based discussions (CBD). The value of these tools lies in their ability to provide agile, formative assessment alongside targeted, immediate feedback within authentic, live clinical contexts. This constant feedback loop is nonnegotiable for students to move through the stages of skill acquisition and ultimately achieve entrustment.

The EPA framework utilizes a supervision scale to track progress, often ranging from level 1 (requires full supervision) to level 5 (can perform independently or fully entrusted). This scale provides granularity for both the student and the supervising faculty, clearly illustrating the developmental trajectory, for example, a student might be level 2 ("performing with direct supervision") for a common EPA like "performing a basic history and physical exam" early in their clinical years and level 4 ("performing unsupervised, indirectly supervised") for the same EPA by graduation. This visual and documented progression is what provides stakeholders—including patients and licensing bodies—the confidence that a graduate is truly fit for purpose.

However, the implementation of EPAs carries several organizational challenges: Firstly, it demands substantial faculty development. Educators must be trained not only in their clinical roles but also in sophisticated assessment methodologies, how to define and operationalize EPAs, and how to deliver high-quality, actionable feedback tied to the entrustment scale. Secondly, effective EPA tracking necessitates robust learning management systems (LMS) capable of collecting and integrating heterogeneous data points from multiple assessors and methods into a single, coherent student profile for programmatic assessment decisions. Failure to address these logistical and training challenges can result in the superficial adoption of CBME, where EPAs are merely used as new headings for old curricula, rather than fundamentally transforming assessment and learning.

1.3.5 The Clinical Learning Environment

The question of where students learn clinically is crucial. While hospitals have remained the main site for decades, offering exposure to severe, complex, and specialized illnesses, their pedagogical value is increasingly contested due to competing demands on faculty time, shortened patient stays, and a focus on high-acuity care that may not reflect the breadth of general practice.

In response, there is an increasing use of primary care centers and community-based medical education (CBME). Systematic reviews show that students often receive more teaching and examine more patients in general practices (GP) than in traditional hospitals. This is due to the different case mix—a higher prevalence of undifferentiated, common, and chronic illnesses—which provides a more accurate representation of the health challenges faced by the population. Primary care settings allow students to follow patients over time, observing the natural history of disease and the impact of social determinants on health, which is often difficult in the acute, episodic environment of a hospital.

Furthermore, other potential sites, such as community services at rural sites or private clinics, can provide students with a greater volume and mix of cases, enhancing their clinical exposure. These longitudinal placements foster sustained relationships between students, preceptors, and patients (a model known as longitudinal integrated clerkships), which is shown to enhance clinical educational depth and professional formation. The shift toward community settings also reinforces the essential role of the physician as a health advocate and promotes a focus on preventive medicine, aligning perfectly with the transformative learning called for by the Lancet Commissions. Policymakers should be aware of the critical situation of integrated planning between education and health institutes to optimize these diverse clinical placements, ensuring that community sites are adequately resourced and faculty are protected for teaching.

1.3.6 Evolving Assessment Paradigms

Since assessment drives learning, it is a crucial component of medical programs. Assessment for learning (formative assessment), paired with appropriate feedback, has become vital. Furthermore, standard setting and blueprinting (as a sign of exam validity) have become a standard practice. Workplace-based assessment (WBA) is increasingly implemented, and the objective structured clinical examination (OSCE) has become the norm, replacing older clinical exam formats.

Recently, the move toward programmatic assessment has been a cornerstone of successful CBME implementation. Programmatic assessment requires the continuous collection of data about students during formative and summative assessments by multiple assessors and using multiple methods. Critically, it ensures a clear separation between the moment of assessment and the high-stake decision moments. This holistic evaluative framework, crucial for ensuring the genuine preparedness of students, relies on mechanisms such as reflective practice exercises, the systematic compilation of portfolios, and structured peer-review components.

1.4 Future Directions and Technological Integration

The future of medical education is driven by evidence-based strategy, structural reform, and the accelerating integration of technology.

1.4.1 Strategic Curricular Reform

The evolutionary trajectory toward CBME has been rigorously informed by evidence-based educational strategies that prioritize active learning modalities and engagement with community health contexts. Through applying clinical problematics and synthesizing interdisciplinary approaches, contemporary medical education fosters a model that accurately mirrors the complex reality of medical practice. Issues deemed essential, such as infectious disease control and critical care interventions, have become deeply ingrained, indeed, almost axiomatic, elements within the final-year curricula.

The transformation in Pakistan, for example, reflects the response to regulatory requirements (WFME) and future healthcare needs. A new curriculum emphasizes an integrated, student-centered approach, alongside community-based medical education and a mandatory 1-year "house job" training. Yet, this transition presents a paradox: the heightened emphasis on modern, formalized curricula has sometimes coincided with a perceived erosion of traditional, informal bedside education. This shift is a symptomatic response to systemic pressures, including augmented patient throughput, heightened concerns for patient privacy, increased administrative documentation burdens, and a paucity of faculty with dual clinical and pedagogical expertise. This erosion highlights the imperative of strategic faculty development, necessitating rigorous training schema to adequately empower our cadre of educators to both teach and critically evaluate these newly emphasized skills with demonstrable efficiency.

1.4.2 Harnessing Technology and Digital Tools

The full fruition of technological capabilities, undeniably accelerated by the recent global exigencies of the COVID-19 pandemic, has dramatically reconfigured the very landscape of educational provision. Learning management systems (LMS), such as Moodle or Google Classroom, have undergone significant enhancements. They now underpin, and indeed facilitate, highly flexible and often hybrid learning ecologies.

Artificial intelligence (AI) tools, such as specialized software like ChatGPT, are actively reshaping the didactic landscape. Their contributions are manifold. The most transformative application of AI lies in its ability to enable personalized learning pathways by analyzing student performance data gathered via the LMS and programmatic assessment systems. AI algorithms can identify individual knowledge gaps, predict areas where a student might struggle, and dynamically curate specific learning modules (e.g., interactive 3D anatomical displays or virtual patient scenarios) to address that weakness. This shifts education from a one-size-fits-all approach to a truly tailored experience.

Furthermore, AI is instrumental in constructing detailed virtual patient scenarios for honing decision-making prowess, providing a safe learning environment similar to simulation but on a vast and cost-effective scale. Pioneering investigative efforts by preeminent institutions such as Stanford, for instance, convincingly underscore the immense prospective utility of AI-based computational models as integral assets, both in the quotidian reality of clinical practice and, naturally, within the sphere of medical education itself. This assistance extends to sophisticated assistance in diagnostics and the interpretation of medical imaging during active clinical rotations, effectively teaching the student how to interact with the next generation of clinical tools.

Assessment methodologies must commensurately evolve with these profound curricular adjustments. Web-facilitated tools are demonstrably improving efficiency and providing immediate feedback loops. Examples abound, with Google Forms and various proctoring solutions leveraging AI, which exemplify novel approaches to ensuring assessment security. Concurrently, however, they introduce substantial systemic challenges. These pertain to digital equity, ensuring all students have fair access to the required technology and bandwidth; unimpeachable academic honesty, as sophisticated AI tools challenge traditional definitions of student-produced work; and, an increasingly paramount concern, the inviolability of data privacy, as sensitive student performance data is collected and analyzed. Institutions, therefore, must engage in rigorous critical introspection regarding these dimensions of fairness and security to uphold the fundamental validity of online assessments and must establish clear, well-articulated institutional mandates to guide student and faculty use of these resources.

1.4.3 Structural Innovations

Projecting forward, the overarching telos, the fundamental objective, remains the cultivation of genuinely well-rounded physicians. These individuals must, by necessity, excel not merely as direct providers of care but also as proactive leaders, articulate communicators, rigorous scholars, and impassioned health advocates. The realization of this rather comprehensive vision necessitates a strategic transcendence of conventional curricula:

- Longitudinal Integrated Clerkships (LICs): This involves strategically embedding students in enduring, sustained relationships, both with their preceptors and with their patients, over extended temporal durations. This structure is precisely intended to markedly enhance both clinical educational depth and professional formation by allowing students to observe health, illness, and recovery as continuous processes.

- Dedicated Scholarly Activity: We must actively integrate mandatory research projects and substantive quality improvement initiatives directly into the fabric of the curriculum. This instills the habit of critical inquiry and ensures graduates are equipped to contribute to the evidence base of medicine.
- Formalized Skill Development: This necessitates the proactive establishment of structured educational modules explicitly addressing core competencies such as health systems science, advanced communication strategies, robust interprofessional collaboration, and effective leadership. These areas, often neglected in the traditional focus on biomedical facts, are essential for navigating the complex contemporary healthcare delivery system.
- Strategic Faculty Development: It is absolutely imperative that we invest substantially in rigorous training schema to adequately empower our cadre of educators. This ensures they possess the requisite competence to both teach and critically evaluate these newly emphasized skills with demonstrable efficiency, particularly within the context of CBME and advanced technological integration.

1.5 Conclusion

The prevailing climate of undergraduate medical education is, indisputably, in a state of continuous, dynamic metamorphosis, catalyzed by the intricate, interlinked forces of competency-based systemic restructuring, the strategic deployment of evidence-based learning paradigms, and the relentless march of technological innovation. The deliberate pivot toward CBME and progressively advanced assessment strategies endeavors to construct an educational system that is both inherently more accountable and demonstrably responsive to evolving needs. Concomitantly, technology presents an almost unprecedented array of learning and simulation tools, though these inevitably introduce novel ethical and equity-related superintendence challenges. As the variegated landscape of medical education continues its inexorable evolution, one fundamental mission remains constant and inviolable: to judiciously equip succeeding generations of medical professionals with the competencies, the acute critical thinking faculties, and the unwavering ethical foundation indispensable for the provision of truly outstanding patient care within the intricately complex contemporary healthcare delivery system. This will, without a shadow of a doubt, demand continuous critical self-reflection, agile accommodation to emergent realities, and an unwavering commitment to rigorously evidence-based innovation.

Postgraduate Curriculum of the Future: Toward a Flexible, Competency-Based, and Lifelong Learning-Oriented Model

2

Süleyman Yıldız, Cemre Yaşöz, and Sena Ece Ilgin

Key Points

- Postgraduate medical education must shift from rigid, time-based structures to flexible, modular, and individualized pathways that recognize diverse learner trajectories and evolving career goals.
- Competency-Based Medical Education (CBME) provides a more valid and transparent model of learner development, supported by milestones, entrustable professional activities (EPAs), and programmatic assessment.
- Artificial intelligence will be a central driver of the curriculum of the future, enabling adaptive learning, real-time analytics, and continuous curricular renewal while freeing educators to focus on mentorship and professional identity formation.
- Lifelong learning is no longer optional but a core professional competency, requiring systems that support self-regulation, reflective practice, e-portfolios, and continuous professional development (CPD).
- Global trends—from pandemics to migration and climate-related health challenges—require curricula that emphasize resilience, interprofessional collaboration, and preparation for unpredictable health system demands.

S. Yıldız (✉)
Department of General Pediatrics and Adolescent Health, Marmara University School of Medicine, Istanbul, Turkey
e-mail: email@yildizsuleyman.com

C. Yaşöz
Department of Child and Adolescent Psychiatry, Erenköy Mental Health and Neurological Disorders, Istanbul, Turkey

S. E. Ilgin
Department of Psychiatry, Marmara University School of Medicine, Istanbul, Turkey

J. Sandars et al. (eds.), *Modern Medical Education*,
https://doi.org/10.1007/978-3-032-27958-3_2

2.1 Introduction

Medical education, particularly at the postgraduate level, is more than the transmission of professional knowledge; it is a process that shapes the essence and spirit of the medical profession [1]. For this reason, the curriculum is regarded as the "heart and soul" of a medical school, serving as the fundamental structure that determines which values, attitudes, and competencies students and residents will acquire [2].

Yet, many postgraduate training programs today remain time-based, rigid, and lacking in interdisciplinary integration, making them insufficient to address the rapidly changing challenges of modern health systems [3]. Especially in the face of shifting health policies, the rapid entry of AI-supported technologies into clinical practice, increasing expectations for patient safety, global crises, and forced migration, the inadequacy of traditional educational models has become increasingly evident [4, 5].

In this new context, flexibility, competency-based approaches, and a culture of lifelong learning have emerged as indispensable principles for the curriculum of the future [6]. Competency-Based Medical Education (CBME) lies at the core of this transformation. It offers a model that is independent of time and outcome-oriented, aiming for learners to progress not simply at the end of a fixed training period but once they have demonstrably acquired the required skills and professional behaviors [7]. The essential tools of CBME include programmatic assessment, entrustable professional activities (EPAs), and portfolio systems [8].

At the same time, a modern curriculum must go beyond technical proficiency to encompass the development of professional identity, ethical reasoning, communication skills, and personal growth. Thus, the postgraduate curriculum of the future must be redesigned as a flexible, competency-based framework that actively supports lifelong learning.

2.2 Keeping Pace with Medical Education Through Artificial Intelligence

In the aftermath of the pandemic, medical education faced a profound disruption, revealing that the traditional model—centered on transferring established knowledge—was no longer sufficient for preparing learners for an unpredictable future marked by continual crises. As highlighted by global education leaders, the next generation of physicians must be equipped for professional roles, technologies, and societal challenges that have not yet emerged. In a time when information circulates at extraordinary speed, medical educators must reconsider long-held assumptions and design systems that respond to these new demands. With the rapid growth of computer- and AI-enhanced knowledge, human cognition is being pushed to evolve in ways not previously encountered. Decades ago, futurists emphasized that success in the twenty-first century would depend not on basic literacy alone but on the capacity to continually adapt—learning new concepts, letting go of outdated ones, and reshaping understanding as contexts change [9, 10]. The driving factor here is the exponential acceleration of knowledge. According to the Knowledge Doubling Curve, the doubling time of human knowledge was about 100 years in the early 1900s, but today in medicine, it has shortened to as little as 2 months [11]. This exponential growth means that fixed, time-bound curricula may already be outdated by the time students graduate, pushing medical education into a cycle of "learn, unlearn, and relearn."

Historically, every major societal transformation has reshaped education. The first industrial revolution, driven by steam power in the 1700s, expanded the geographic reach of production. The second, fueled by electricity in the 1800s, exponentially increased the scale and diversity of industrial output. The computer revolution of the 1990s represented the third major transformation, placing data processing at the center of discovery and innovation. Today, we are experiencing the fourth revolution, the era of artificial intelligence, which is redefining not only access to information but also our capacity to process, predict, and personalize knowledge [12].

Medical education, long caught in the cycle of static curricula and outdated content, may overcome these challenges through the very tool that is becoming ubiquitous: artificial intelligence. In this new era shaped by AI, medical education must go beyond producing physicians who simply master a body of knowledge; it must prepare professionals who can continually update their learning, respond effectively to global crises, and help shape the future of humanity.

2.3 Limitations of Traditional Postgraduate Curricula

Traditional postgraduate medical education has long been built upon a time-based model. Defining residency training by a fixed number of years overlooks the wide variation in individual learning trajectories [3, 7]. While some trainees may acquire certain competencies earlier, others may need more time; yet, the current system does not flexibly accommodate this diversity.

Another limitation is the frequent embedding of education within service delivery. Residents' heavy clinical workload often overshadows their educational goals [4]. This imbalance produces variability in training quality; in some institutions, service demands dominate, while education becomes secondary. Classical curricula are also often fragmented across disciplines. Although clinical rotations expose students to specific specialties, true interdisciplinary integration and systems-based perspectives are frequently lacking [3]. Given today's health systems—complex, with high burdens of chronic disease and a demand for multidimensional care—these deficiencies have become increasingly evident. Traditional assessment methods present further limitations. High-stakes, single examinations, or subjective evaluations by senior faculty often fail to capture a trainee's real progress and continuous performance [6]. This can lead to superficial learning and reinforce a "study to pass" culture. Finally, classical postgraduate curricula often fail to systematically promote a culture of lifelong learning. The assumption that a trainee is a "finished specialist" upon completion of training is no longer realistic in an era of rapidly expanding knowledge [3, 11].

2.4 Flexibility: Individualized and Modular Approaches

In place of the traditional time-based curriculum, flexibility and individualized learning pathways are gaining increasing importance. Because trainees differ in pace, interests, and career goals, rigid and standardized programs may restrict their potential. Modular curriculum structures allow learners, after achieving core competencies, to pursue elective rotations, research blocks, or clinical experiences tailored to their interests. This ensures both mastery of foundational skills and deeper exploration of future specialty areas. Similarly, portfolio-based approaches make a learner's developmental journey more visible. Portfolios record clinical experiences, feedback, and self-reflections, creating a continuous feedback loop for both learner and educator [7, 13]. This reinforces a stronger sense of ownership over learning, while technology further enhances flexibility by enabling learners to progress at their own pace through online modules, micro-credentials, and simulation-based training [14]. These methods became particularly prominent during the pandemic, laying the foundation for hybrid and remote models that have since become permanent in many contexts.

In conclusion, the principle of flexibility is not merely a pedagogical preference but a necessary feature for postgraduate medical education to respond effectively to the evolving demands of modern health systems [12].

2.5 Competency-Based Medical Education (CBME) and Programmatic Assessment

One of the most significant paradigm shifts shaping the future of postgraduate medical education is the Competency-Based Medical Education (CBME) approach. CBME emphasizes the acquisition of predefined competencies rather than the duration of training [7]. In this model, success is not measured by the number of years completed but by the trainee's ability to safely demonstrate the required knowledge, skills, and professional behaviors.

Two essential tools of CBME are the concepts of milestones and entrustable professional activities (EPAs). Milestones define the expected levels of performance at different stages of a trainee's development. EPAs, in contrast, determine the degree to which a learner can be entrusted to perform a professional task independently [13]. Together, these frameworks make a trainee's developmental progression more transparent, observable, and structured.

This approach has also brought forward the concept of programmatic assessment. Unlike single high-stakes examinations, programmatic assessment relies on frequent, low-stakes feedback and the use of multiple complementary assessment tools to monitor progress [8, 14]. This shifts the focus from "passing an exam" to sustained professional growth.

Implementing CBME is not without challenges. Developing new curricular structures, training faculty, and ensuring the reliability of assessment instruments demand significant resources and time. Nonetheless, the complexity of modern health systems, the imperatives of patient safety, and the need for alignment with international standards demonstrate that CBME is not an option but a necessity [7, 13].

2.6 Lifelong Learning Orientation

Postgraduate medical education should not be confined to the acquisition of knowledge and skills during residency. Given the exponential pace at which medical knowledge and technologies evolve, the capacity for continuous learning throughout a physician's career has become essential [3, 11]. Lifelong learning extends beyond keeping up with scientific updates; it also encompasses self-regulation, reflection, and the ability to plan and monitor professional development [3, 13]. Accordingly, postgraduate curricula should provide tools that enable learners to design and evaluate their own learning pathways.

E-portfolio systems make the learner's educational journey visible and transform lifelong learning into a tangible practice. Portfolios can be updated not only during training but also throughout continuing professional development (CPD), thereby integrating postgraduate experiences with career-long growth [3]. In addition, learning analytics and AI-supported tracking systems can identify individual strengths and weaknesses, offering personalized learning plans. This not only enhances motivation but also reinforces the perception of oneself as a "lifelong learner." The orientation toward lifelong learning is an essential component of resilience, encompassing not only the continual renewal of knowledge but also the ability to adapt to changing health systems, emerging technologies, and unforeseen crises [5].

2.7 Global Perspectives and Innovative Practices

Postgraduate medical education reforms are being implemented at different paces and through diverse models across the world. The Netherlands has been pioneer of CBME, with residency programs restructured around competencies and entrustable professional activities (EPAs). The United States, on the other hand, has emphasized accelerated medical programs and early specialization pathways as strategies to enhance flexibility [15]. In Europe, modular approaches have gained traction. While maintaining a fixed core curriculum, several countries have added flexible blocks that allow learners to make choices [15, 16]. This design not only accommodates diverse career trajectories but also reinforces a culture of lifelong learning.

Several Asian countries stand out for their interprofessional education models. By bringing together students of medicine, nursing, pharmacy, and allied health fields, these initiatives promote not only collaborative practice but also early development of systems-based thinking. In lower-resource settings, countries such as Somaliland have sought to improve quality by implementing harmonized national curricula. Such efforts demonstrate that CBME principles can be applied even under conditions of crisis and scarcity [17].

Global crises have also necessitated innovative practices. The COVID-19 pandemic catalyzed the integration of hybrid and online learning models, which have now become a permanent feature of medical education [2]. Similarly, migration, war, and climate change-related health challenges have underscored the need for curricula to incorporate global health and resilience training [18].

2.8 Conclusion

Postgraduate medical education is standing at a decisive crossroads. The complexity of modern health systems, the accelerating pace of scientific discovery, and the succession of global crises—from pandemics to climate change and forced migration—have all highlighted the inadequacies of time-bound, rigid curricula. At the same time, advances in technology, particularly the rise of artificial intelligence, are reshaping not only clinical practice but also the very foundations of how future doctors must learn.

In this context, the curriculum of the future cannot be a static roadmap. It must be a dynamic, flexible, and adaptive framework that prepares doctors not only for the knowledge and skills of today but also for the uncertainties of tomorrow. Flexibility will allow learners to pursue individualized trajectories, balancing shared core competencies with opportunities for deeper exploration. Competency-based models will ensure that progression depends on demonstrated performance rather than elapsed time, reinforcing both patient safety and educational fairness. Lifelong learning will become a professional identity rather than an optional activity, sustaining doctors across decades of practice.

Artificial intelligence, often seen as a disruptive force, should be embraced as a vital partner in this transformation. AI-powered adaptive learning platforms, predictive analytics, and decision support systems can help monitor individual progress, personalize learning, and provide continuous updates in a world where medical knowledge doubles at unprecedented speed. Rather than displacing the human role in education, AI can empower both teachers and learners—freeing faculty to focus on mentorship, professional identity formation, and the moral dimensions of practice while supporting students in navigating their own developmental pathways.

Equally important, the postgraduate curriculum must cultivate more than technical expertise. Professional identity, ethical reasoning, resilience, communication, and compassion remain at the heart of what it means to be a physician. These qualities are not acquired through textbooks alone; they emerge from safe, inclusive, and reflective learning environments where mistakes can be discussed openly and feedback is a natural part of growth.

Ultimately, the postgraduate curriculum of the future must move beyond the notion of producing "finished specialists." It must instead nurture adaptive, reflective, and compassionate physicians who see themselves as lifelong learners and responsible leaders within their communities. Such a curriculum is not only essential for the personal and professional success of individual doctors—it is a moral imperative for the quality, resilience, and equity of health systems worldwide.

References

1. Guo H, Li H, Yao Y, Li Y, Huang Y. The application of integrating medical humanities education into emergency skill-training scenario simulation teaching. Front Med. 2025;12:1561504. https://doi.org/10.3389/fmed.2025.1561504.
2. Harden RM, Lilley P, Yıldız S. The curriculum: the heart and soul of a medical school. Med Teach. 2024;46(12):1524–8. https://doi.org/10.1080/0142159X.2024.2416307. Epub 2024 Nov 1.
3. Greiner AC, Knebel E, editors. Chapter 2: Challenges facing the health system and implications for educational reform. In: Health professions education: a bridge to quality. Washington, DC: National Academies Press (US); 2003. Available from: https://www.ncbi.nlm.nih.gov/books/NBK221522/.
4. Bajwa J, Munir U, Nori A, Williams B. Artificial intelligence in healthcare: transforming the practice of medicine. Future Healthc J. 2021;8(2):e188–94. https://doi.org/10.7861/fhj.2021-0095.
5. Abdelouahed M, Yateem D, Amzil C, Aribi I, Abdelwahed EH, Fredericks S. Integrating artificial intelligence into public health education and healthcare: insights from the COVID-19 and monkeypox crises for future pandemic readiness. Front Educ. 2025;10:1518909. https://doi.org/10.3389/feduc.2025.1518909.
6. Bhardwaj V, Zhang S, Tan YQ, Pandey V. Redefining learning: student-centered strategies for academic and personal growth. Front Educ. 2025;10:1518602. https://doi.org/10.3389/feduc.2025.1518602.
7. Shah N, Desai C, Jorwekar G, Badyal D, Singh T. Competency-based medical education: an overview and application in pharmacology. Indian J Pharmacol. 2016;48(Suppl 1):S5–9. https://doi.org/10.4103/0253-7613.193312.
8. American Board of Pediatrics. Competency-Based Medical Education (CBME) [Internet]. American Board of Pediatrics; [cited 2025 Nov 13]. Available from: https://www.abp.org/content/competency-based-medical-education-cbme.
9. Herlinawati H, Marwa M, Ismail N, Junaidi LLO, Situmorang DDB. The integration of 21st century skills in the curriculum of education. Heliyon. 2024;10(15):e35148. https://doi.org/10.1016/j.heliyon.2024.e35148.
10. Organisation for Economic Co-operation and Development. Lessons for education from COVID-19. Paris: OECD Publishing; 2020. Available from: https://www.oecd.org/content/dam/oecd/en/publications/reports/2020/12/lessons-for-education-from-covid-19_ef772b31/0a530888-en.pdf.
11. Densen P. Challenges and opportunities facing medical education. Acad Med. 2011;86(4):458–64. https://doi.org/10.1097/ACM.0b013e31820f1c88.
12. Schwab K. The fourth industrial revolution. Geneva: World Economic Forum; 2016. Available from: https://law.unimelb.edu.au/__data/assets/pdf_file/0005/3385454/Schwab-The_Fourth_Industrial_Revolution_Klaus_S.pdf.
13. Pool AO, Jaarsma ADC, Driessen EW, Govaerts MJB. Student perspectives on competency-based portfolios: does a portfolio reflect their competence development? Perspect Med Educ. 2020;9(3):166–72.

14. Çınar S, Babadoğan MC. The concept of micro-credentials in the context of curriculum. Int J Educ Stud Policy. 2025;6(1):1–15. https://doi.org/10.5281/zenodo.15049507.
15. de Graaf J, Bolk M, Dijkstra A, van der Horst M, Hoff RG, ten Cate O. The implementation of entrustable professional activities in postgraduate medical education in the Netherlands: rationale, process, and current status. Acad Med. 2021;96(7 Suppl):S29–35. https://doi.org/10.1097/ACM.0000000000004110.
16. ten Cate O. Competency-based postgraduate medical education: past, present and future. GMS. J Med Educ. 2017;34(5):Doc49. https://doi.org/10.3205/zma001146.
17. de Graaf J, Bolk M, Dijkstra A, van der Horst M, Hoff RG, ten Cate O. Development of Somaliland national harmonised medical curriculum. Med Teach. 2024;46(12):1589–92. https://doi.org/10.1080/0142159X.2023.2289841.
18. Abubakar I, Aldridge RW, Devakumar D, et al. The UCL–Lancet Commission on Migration and Health: the health of a world on the move. Lancet. 2018;392(10164):2606–54. https://doi.org/10.1016/S0140-6736(18)32114-7.

3 Developing and Maintaining the Competencies of Educators Through Continuing Professional Development

Lawrence Sherman and Gohar Wajid

Key Points

- Exponential increase in HPE institutions and recent educational advancements require that educators must be formally trained to ensure the quality of education.
- Teaching clinicians in practice requires specific training that focuses on andragogy and heutagogy, as opposed to the pedagogical training seen in undergraduate HPE.
- Active engagement with the learner community has been identified as the most powerful aspect of the career pathway, providing peer support for imagining and navigating the development of dual identities of educators in the clinician and educator communities of practice.
- Leadership, a framework, and a clearly delineated plan that is responsive to the needs and context of the setting are essential for the development, implementation, and sustainability of a CPD system for healthcare professionals in less developed countries [14].
- Digital technologies, especially social media platforms, can be used as powerful tools to provide equitably accessible educational opportunities, especially for less privileged communities of practice and institutions.

L. Sherman
Meducate Global LLC, Tierra Verde, FL, USA
e-mail: ls@meducateglobal.com

G. Wajid (✉)
Visiting Faculty, Health Professions Education, The University of Lahore, Lahore, Pakistan

J. Sandars et al. (eds.), *Modern Medical Education*,
https://doi.org/10.1007/978-3-032-27958-3_3

3.1 Introduction

The overall goal of health professions education (HPE) system is to produce adequate, competent, and high-quality health professionals that are relevant and responsive to the health needs of the population they serve. Education should be well regulated and managed at the undergraduate, graduate/postgraduate, and continuing professional development (CPD) levels to achieve the above goal. Having adequate number of competent educators to ensure high-quality education is central to any health professions education strategy. This chapter delves into the need for the professional development of educators in HPE institutions and provides guidance on the need for structured CPD systems for educators. Because educators work across a continuum, faculty development must also be tiered and role-specific, with a clear CPD educator pathway, which has historically not been addressed.

Realizing the need for educational reforms, the World Health Organization [23] provided guidelines on bringing reforms in education. Five critical domains identified related to faculty development, strengthening HPE regulations, accreditation systems, increased funding for education, and the need for effective monitoring and evaluation systems. The WHO policy brief on faculty development identified gaps in research on faculty development and suggested policy options to emphasize structured faculty development programs [24]. The Lancet Commissions on transforming HPE also identified a series of reforms aimed to develop transformative and interdependent professional education system to develop competent health professionals to provide equity in health [3].

The production of high-quality health professionals requires competent educators. Educators are expected to have adequate clinical and scientific competencies, but they may not be well equipped with pedagogical preparation required to function in todays' increasingly complex educational environment. Faculty development is, therefore, important to ensure that teachers and trainers are well prepared to assume their responsibilities as competent educators. Faculty development in this context is defined as "a planned programme of events aimed at preparing individuals for their roles as teachers, clinicians, researchers and administrators with the purpose of enabling the institution to meet its goals, vision and mission, and its social and moral responsibilities to the communities it serves" [3]. The range of activities help educators in improving their professional skills that are vital for carrying out their teaching, research, or administrative activities [11].

CPD of educators is central to maintaining and upgrading the competencies of educators in the advent of rapidly changing scenario of HPE. A review conducted on the effectiveness of faculty development concluded that faculty development programs (FDPs) have been shown to foster the pedagogical skills, assessment, research, and leadership of faculty. Although no unified faculty development framework was found, the programs can be structured and tailored to match their educational needs [1].

Faculty development however may not be a straightforward task in the rapidly transforming modern education ecosystem with several complexities. Adequacy, quality, and relevance are not the only elements that shape an HPE system in a country. This is a complex highly adaptive ecosystem, with multiple actors and layers. Tens of cadres of health professionals, mostly working in silos, the complexity of the interaction between the education and health systems, and the continuum of undergraduate, postgraduate, and CPD add layers of complexities to the system. The complexity of the system is further exacerbated by the dynamic nature and fast-paced changes occurring in health professions education. The changing demographic and epidemiological landscape, digital innovations, and advances in simulations and other educational technologies are reshaping the goals, standards, and outcomes of education [3].

3.2 Exponential Increase in Health Professions Education Institutions and the Quality of Education

Globally, most countries witness the shortage of health professionals to provide adequate health services. The WHO identifies 55 countries with critical shortage of doctors, nurses, and midwives that pose a serious threat to achieving universal health coverage and other health-related targets. Countries are responding to the shortage of health professionals through opening new institutions and increasing their admission capacities. Exponential increase in the number of HPE institutions in a short time poses threats to the quality of education. Well-developed quality improvement/performance improvement (QI/PI) systems must be in place to ensure that the institutions deliver high-quality education. QI/PI is not restricted to well-developed infrastructure and the availability of facilities, but it involves elements such as processes, well-defined outcomes, competent faculty, and the critical alignment between the structure and the processes to achieve the desired outcomes. Research indicates shortage of faculty and weak faculty development as a major factor in improving the quality of education, especially in less developed countries [13].

3.3 The Role of Educators in Health Professions Education Institutions

Exponential increase in HPE institutions requires proportionate increase in the number of educators as well. Educators must be well trained on the roles of the teacher and educational delivery process and steer the curriculum change through their own professional development. The increasing complexity of the educational system requires that educators be well trained for their teaching roles. Traditionally, specialists in basic and clinical sciences have been inducted as educators without any formal training on pedagogical and educational management skills. In the recent past, there has been increasing concerns and realization that educators need to be trained on their roles as teachers, which goes beyond their basic sciences or clinical skills [22]. Harden and Laidlaw identify the multifaceted eight essential roles of a medical teacher as information provider, role model, facilitator, assessor, planner, resource developer, student support, and scholar [5]. Based on the skills, educational scholarship, and the levels of accomplishment toward excellence, the Association of Surgical Education in the USA creates a four-level educators' "pyramid" for teachers. The levels, from the bottom to the top of the pyramid, are teacher, master teacher, educator, and master educator [18].

Pedagogical training of teachers through well-structured training programs provides opportunities to teachers to prepare themselves as competent educators to consider education as a holistic approach, which stretches far beyond their own specialties. In addition, an educator is expected to play the role of a professional, leader, and change manager, exhibit emotional intelligence to advance his profession, contribute to educational research and scholarship to provide evidence base for critical decision-making, and promote interprofessional education and collaboration in the institution.

Maintenance and upgrading of these competencies in the long run are big challenges. In addition to the competencies for educators to resolve day-to-day educational issues in an HPE institution, an educator is expected to be proficient in digital technologies (e.g., execution of learning management system, e-learning tools, artificial intelligence, digital simulations, etc.). Additionally, the need for appropriate training in interprofessional education (IPE) and interprofessional continuing education (IPCE) exists, with the goal of preparing students for interprofessional collaborative practice (IPCP).

3.4 Continuing Professional Development for Educators

Teaching clinicians in practice requires specific preparation distinct from undergraduate and postgraduate medical education. Faculty development for educators must include training in professional practice gap analysis, outcome planning, interprofessional design, independence standards, and integration with quality improvement/performance improvement (QI/PI) activities. Heutagogical approaches (highly autonomous and self-determined learners, well prepared for the complexities of today's workplace) are especially relevant for CPD [7, 15, 16].

Historically, HPE has faced challenges related to unstructured teaching practices and a lack of consistent professional standards for educators. Educators specializing in basic and clinical sciences are entrusted with teaching responsibilities, yet only a handful of them have formal training in teaching and educational methods [8]. Very few formal teaching programs or formal licensing requirements can be cited for teaching in health professions education. On the other hand, there is an increasing demand on faculty members who are required to be socially responsible and to deal with the increasing demand for the professionalization of pedagogical practices. Developing competent professional educators, researchers, and educational leaders to equip them with their progressive and increasingly complex roles requires continuing faculty development, and this is not an easy task [12]. Educators play a critical role in shaping the professional identity of students at all stages of training; hence, their own development as professional teachers is essential.

Faculty development (FD) thus becomes an absolute necessity that cannot be ignored by the national governing and regulatory bodies and the HPE institutions. Steinert [19] argues that "FD should be seen more broadly, considering that faculty members' roles have been changing significantly and FD has become an increasingly important component of medical education." Educators face a range of challenges that hamper their efforts to deliver high-quality education effectively. These challenges relate to the management of education, resources, and training of staff. The infrastructure and financial support for development has also been identified as a major challenge for health professions education institutes [17]. Sheer increase in the number of educational institutions, especially in the private sector, poses significant governance and regulatory challenges in faculty development.

Supportive institutional leadership, the availability of appropriate resources, and institutional recognition of teaching excellence are pivotal to consistent faculty development [9]. Faculty development thus becomes a norm in an academic ecosystem, rather than a burden. In the USA, ACGME emphasizes the monitoring of faculty expertise in teaching, assessment, clinical knowledge, and scholarship through a formal faculty development tracking system.

There is dearth of formal professional development opportunities for educators to keep them abreast with the evolving HPE systems. While there is emphasis on competency-based education, most HPE programs may not be framed around competencies for educators, and when they do, the differences between the competencies needed at different stages of HPE are often omitted. Most notably, very few opportunities exist to prepare HPEs and clinician educators to design, develop, deliver, and evaluate CPD activities. Teaching clinicians in practice requires specific training that focuses on andragogy and heutagogy, as opposed to the pedagogical training seen in undergraduate HPE.

The rapidly shifting educational paradigm from traditional education system to community-, competency-, and interprofessional education-based curricula and the increasing role of digital technologies in education demand that FD is well planned, regulated, and governed at the national level through well-structured conceptual and regulatory framework, strategies, plans, monitoring and evaluation, and accreditation systems. Under the broad national frameworks, educational institutions and professional bodies play their roles to create FD opportunities that are well aligned with the educational needs of the faculties. So far, efforts toward such FD strategies in most countries are sporadic.

3.5 Planning and Governance of Professional Development of Educators

There is an established need for structured and formal training of educators in HPE institutions for several reasons mentioned above. Countries need to establish structured training programs for educators. Although a lot of training happens informally, in an unstructured manner, faculty developed in this context should be seen as formal and structured training of educators in the form of licensed educators followed by regulatory support to maintain their pedagogical competencies. These competencies must be well defined in this context, for example, an educator must be able to develop curriculum, set objectives, facilitate small group discussions, give effective feedback, develop multiple choice questions, conduct assessment of students, etc. Countries/institutions may consider developing core/mandatory and optional competencies for educators.

The scoping review on CPD system development conducted by Merry et al. [14] identifies that the process of CPD system development includes leadership, a well-developed framework based on thorough needs assessment, CPD policies and processes, and a monitoring and evaluation system. Other requirements include accreditation system, a robust financial plan, and an appropriate CPD content. Conceptual and regulatory frameworks provide the basis for effective planning and governance of CPD system. The system should be supported by appropriate regulations, contextualized to the local CPD requirements [14]. Regulation and standards provide CPD legitimacy, while a conceptual approach that aligns with the local culture, and values, optimizes effectiveness of the system [21].

In this context, a conceptual framework for CPD includes concepts, assumptions, expectations, beliefs, evidence, theories, and the presumed relationships among them that provide a comprehensive understanding of the phenomenon [16]. A CPD system backed by appropriate regulations and legislation ensure the structure and quality assurance of the system, whereas both approaches ensure the feasibility and appropriateness of the CPD system [14]. Regulatory frameworks should recognize CPD educators as a distinct group, with competencies including independence standards, outcome planning, and QI/PI integration. Licensing bodies and accreditors can reinforce this by recognizing educator portfolios and micro-credentials. Training specifically for CPD planners and educators is becoming more available globally [6].

Several factors could affect the performance of faculty members, for example, lack of formal pedagogical training, variations in teaching methodologies, multiple faculty roles, and heavy workloads. Faculty development programs built on a thorough assessment of situation help in addressing these issues. Several countries have major governance and regulatory gaps in FD programs [14]. Governance systems are often fragmented with poor alignment between regulatory demands and educational needs, for instance, FD must align with broader health workforce planning, accreditation frameworks, and policy governance—but misalignment remains a major issue in several countries [10].

Monitoring and evaluation (M&E) of CPD at all levels is an essential component of the CPD system. It should be included as an essential component of CPD regulatory framework. A number of tools can be used to conduct M&E of the system, for example, clinical audits, CPD credit accumulation, learning portfolios, criterion reference methods, computer diaries, peer review, chart audits, etc. [4]. CPD must be amenable to external evaluation to become transparent, demonstrable, and accountable [4]. An accreditation system provides means to ensure the quality of the CPD system. M&E and accreditation of CPD systems is usually weak. Rapid scoping review of CPD systems conducted by Merry et al. [14] found major gaps in the CPD accreditation practices in several countries, threatening the quality of the system.

3.6 Advancements in Faculty Development

Like other fields of education, there are continual yet slow advancements in FD as well. There is increasing realization among the governance and regulatory bodies and professional associations to introduce more structured programs/approaches to FD for educators. Most FD programs are based on the principles of learner centeredness (heutagogy), contextual relevance, interprofessional collaboration, community of practice, equity and inclusivity, and longitudinality [12, 20]. FD practices are widely recognized and relatively better regulated in developed countries, for example, Essential Skills in Medical Education (ESME) certificate courses run by AMEE and tens of courses for educators conducted by a large number of universities in the USA, Canada, Australia, and other countries. Recently, AMEE launched an ESME course for CPD educators. It has a six-module hybrid design, combining self-directed learning with regularly scheduled facilitated discussions.

Unfortunately, most developing countries still have informal, unregulated, and unstructured approaches to FD. Faculty development largely revolves around clinical medicine, heavily dominated and funded by the pharmaceutical industry with the primary intent of marketing of their products. FD opportunities are inadequate, especially for professions other than medical doctors. The practice is predominantly unregulated, for example, regulatory bodies in many developing countries do not have any formal regulatory (licensing, certification, or recertification) requirements to ensure that health professionals keep themselves abreast with the advancements in their fields.

There is however rising awareness, and occasional deviations are evident, for example, the regulatory body in Pakistan (Pakistan Medical and Dental Council) has made it mandatory for educators to attend a Certification Course aimed at enhancing their educational skills. Foundation for Advancement of International Medical Education and Research (FAIMER) has played a significant role in educator's training through its fellowship programs, specifically designed for developing countries and with regional institutes in India, Brazil, sub-Saharan Africa, China, and Egypt. Still, there is a room for the expansion in this program and redesigning its organization to the needs of the developing countries. Although there is an increasing trend in diploma/master in HPE programs in developing countries, these programs aim at more specialized HPE for those who need to work full time as educationists in HPE institutions. These countries still have big gaps in specific, targeted, short courses that should be designed for sharpening the pedagogical skills of educators, for example, short courses on essential roles of an educator, teaching and learning, curriculum/module development, student assessment, educational management, the use of digital technologies in HPE, quality assurance for educators, etc. These short courses should be contextualized to the needs of the educators in the specific educational environments of different countries. Governing and regulatory bodies need to have clear regulations and national strategies for the education and training of educators in all HPE institutions, develop policies on the professional development of educators, and create enough opportunities for faculty development programs to respond to the increasing training needs of educators.

As opposed to traditional pedagogical and andragogical approaches of education followed at the undergraduate and postgraduate education levels, the adoption of heutagogical approaches for faculty development should be the mainstay of any national-level faculty development strategic plan. At the level of educators, learners should be able to identify their learning needs, create learning opportunities with the help of their institutions, and take full control of their self-determined, adaptable, and longitudinal learning, backed by evidence of learning and reflective practice (e.g., online portfolios). Supported by appropriate regulatory environment and policies, once educators get internally motivated to respond to their own learning needs, eventually, these practices are transferred to their pupils at the undergraduate and postgraduate levels.

Web-based CPD events in their synchronous and asynchronous forms are providing flexibility to the providers and users alike, expanding their reach to remote communities, thus strengthening equitable CPD system. There is an increasing use of social media networks by educators/organizations for CPD activities globally. Online tools improve research efficiency, and social media is playing an important role in enhancing professional networking [2].

The use of digital technologies, especially social media platforms, is playing a transformative role in creating equitably accessible educational opportunities, especially for less developed countries. A large number of local and broader-scale communities of practice have emerged over the years that is playing a critical role in faculty development. These online communities of practice are available across the board for the developed and developing countries and across different professions, promoting interprofessional education informally. Regulatory bodies need to map and formalize these educational platforms and bring them into mainstream to play their critical role.

3.7 Conclusion

Faculty development for educators is critically important. There is an ever-increasing demand of competent and well-trained educators at HPE institutions, especially in nursing and other nonmedical fields. Educators may be qualified and trained in their respective technical specialties in basic and clinical sciences; however, there are serious gaps in their training on pedagogy. They may be experts in their specialties and still may fail in teaching. There is an increasing awareness about the need for a well-structured training of educators on pedagogy. An increasing number of teacher training programs are addressing this issue, using the traditional and advanced approaches such as communities of practice and digital technologies. Although informal channels of education have increased over the years, governing and regulatory bodies need to introduce more formal faculty development strategies and plans to fulfil the ever-increasing need of faculty development in their countries. If faculty development is not paid attention to, the quality of education may be seriously threatened in the ever-increasing number of HPE institutions. CPD educators face unique challenges and opportunities. By focusing on identifying and closing professional practice gaps, interprofessional design, outcome measurement, independence, and integration with QI/PI, they can directly impact clinician performance and patient outcomes.

References

1. Bilal, Guraya SY, Chen S. The impact and effectiveness of faculty development program in fostering the faculty's knowledge, skills, and professional competence: a systematic review and meta-analysis. Saudi J Biol Sci. 2019;26(4):688–97. https://doi.org/10.1016/j.sjbs.2017.10.024.
2. Filipe HP, Silva ED, Stulting AA, Golnik KC. Continuing professional development: best practices. Middle East Afr J Ophthalmol. 2014;21(2):134–41.
3. Frenk J, Chen L, Bhutta ZA, Cohen J, Crisp N, Evans T. Health professionals for a new century: transforming education to strengthen health systems in an interdependent world. Lancet. 2010;376(9756):1923–58.
4. Grant J. The good CPD guide. A practical guide to managed continuing professional development in medicine. 2nd ed. London, New York: Radcliffe Publishing; 2012.
5. Harden RM, Laidlaw JM. Essential skills for a medical teacher: an introduction to teaching and learning in medicine. 2nd ed. Edinburgh: Elsevier; 2017.
6. Institute of Medicine (US) Committee on Planning a Continuing Health Professional Education Institute. Redesigning continuing education in the health professions. Washington, DC: National Academies Press; 2010.
7. Interprofessional Education Collaborative (IPEC). Core competencies for interprofessional collaborative practice. Washington, DC: Interprofessional Education Collaborative; 2016.
8. Krueger PM, Neutens J, Bienstock J, et al. To the point: reviews in medical education teaching techniques. Am J Obstet Gynecol. 2004;191(2):408–11. https://doi.org/10.1016/j.ajog.2004.02.003.
9. Kolomitro K, Hamilton J, Leslie K, Hazelton L, Veerapen K, Kelly-Turner K, & Keegan D. Viewing faculty development through an organizational lens: Sharing lessons learned. Medical Teacher. 2021;43(8):894–899. https://doi.org/10.1080/0142159X.2021.1931078
10. Kumar A, Atwa H, Shehata M, Al Ansari A, Deifalla A. Faculty development programmes in medical education in the Eastern Mediterranean Region: a systematic review. East Mediterr Health J. 2022;28(5):362–80. https://doi.org/10.26719/emhj.22.014.
11. Kwan D, Barker K, Richardson D, Wagner S, Austin Z. Effectiveness of a faculty development program in fostering interprofessional education competencies. J Res Interprof Pract Educ. 2009;1:24–41.
12. McLean M, Cilliers F, Van Wyk JM. Faculty development: yesterday, today and tomorrow. Med Teach. 2008;30(6):555–84. https://doi.org/10.1080/01421590802109834.
13. Mennin S. The global challenges in medical education: wicked issues and options for action. Med Sci Educ. 2021;31(Suppl 1):17–20. https://doi.org/10.1007/s40670-021-01404-w. PMID: 34567834; PMCID: PMC8452128.
14. Merry L, Castiglione SA, Rouleau G, et al. Continuing professional development (CPD) system development, implementation, evaluation and sustainability for healthcare professionals in low- and lower-middle-income countries: a rapid scoping review. BMC Med Educ. 2023;23:498. https://doi.org/10.1186/s12909-023-04427-6.

15. Moore DE Jr, Green JS, Gallis HA. Achieving desired results and improved outcomes: integrating planning and assessment throughout learning activities. J Contin Educ Heal Prof. 2009;29(1):1–15. https://doi.org/10.1002/chp.20001.
16. Moore DE Jr, Chappell K, Sherman L, Pavan ME. A conceptual framework for planning and assessing learning in continuing education activities designed for clinicians in one profession and/or clinical teams. Med Teach. 2018. https://doi.org/10.1080/0142159X.2018.1483578.
17. Samaneh S, Hamid R, Pouran R, Mohammadreza M. Financial challenges of teaching hospitals and providing solutions. J Educ Health Promot. 2018;7:155. https://doi.org/10.4103/jehp.jehp_95_18.
18. Sherertz EF. Criteria of the "educators' pyramid" fulfilled by medical school faculty promoted on a teaching pathway. Acad Med. 2000;75(9):954–6. https://doi.org/10.1097/00001888-200009000-00022. PMID: 10995622.
19. Steinert Y. Faculty development: the road less travelled. Acad Med. 2011;86(4):409–11. https://doi.org/10.1097/ACM.0b013e31820c6fd3.
20. Steinert Y. Faculty development in the health professions: a focus on research and practice. Springer; 2014.
21. Vakani FS, Uebel K, Balasooriya C, Demirkol A. The status quo of continuing medical education in south-east Asia and eastern Mediterranean regions: a scoping review of 33 countries. J Contin Educ Health Prof. 2022;10:1097. https://doi.org/10.1097/CEH.0000000000000471.
22. Varga Z, Pótó Z, Czopf L, et al. Do we need special pedagogy in medical schools? – attitudes of teachers and students in Hungary: a cross-sectional study. BMC Med Educ. 2020;20:472. https://doi.org/10.1186/s12909-020-02385-x.
23. WHO. Transforming and scaling up health professionals' education and training: what are the key policy issues and possible responses? 2013. Available from: https://www.ncbi.nlm.nih.gov/books/NBK298944/.
24. WHO. Transforming and scaling up health professional education and training. Policy brief on faculty development. 2013.

4 Interprofessional Education of the Future

Naveed Yousuf, Komal Atta, Anuja Bhargava, and Saleema Gulzar

Key Points

- Interprofessional education (IPE) is essential to prepare healthcare professionals for collaborative practice in increasingly complex systems.
- Embedding IPE into curricula develops core competencies such as teamwork, communication, and cultural sensitivity.
- Technological innovations, including AI, simulation, and digital platforms, will redefine future interprofessional learning and practice.
- Planetary health, professional plasticity, and patient inclusion demand broader, future-oriented interprofessional collaboration.
- Policy support, faculty development, and sustainable curricular integration are critical enablers of IPE in health professions education of the future.

N. Yousuf (✉)
Department for Educational Development, Medical College, Faculty of Health Sciences, Aga Khan University, Karachi, Pakistan
e-mail: naveed.yousuf@aku.edu

K. Atta
Medical Education, University Medical and Dental College, The University of Faisalabad, Faisalabad, Pakistan
e-mail: komal.atta@tuf.edu.pk

A. Bhargava
ENT, Eras Lucknow Medical College, Era University, Lucknow, Uttar Pradesh, India
e-mail: dranujabhargava@erauniversity.in

S. Gulzar
School of Nursing and Midwifery, Aga Khan University, Karachi, Pakistan
e-mail: saleema.gulzar@aku.edu

J. Sandars et al. (eds.), *Modern Medical Education*,
https://doi.org/10.1007/978-3-032-27958-3_4

4.1 Introduction

Maximizing patient care and ensuring safety in the current healthcare environment require a comprehensive understanding of how professionals from diverse disciplinary backgrounds come together. Health systems worldwide are increasingly complex, shaped by demographic transitions such as the aging population, the rising prevalence of chronic illnesses, and the growing burden of multimorbidity.

These realities necessitate integrated responses that no single profession can provide adequately in isolation. Effective collaboration across professions has consistently been demonstrated to improve patient safety and the overall quality of care. Interprofessional collaboration, therefore, has become indispensable in addressing chronic and complex health conditions [1].

A key enabler of such collaboration is interprofessional education (IPE), which provides aspiring health professionals with the skills, attitudes, and values necessary to practice collaboratively. Embedding interprofessional principles within curricula not only equips graduates for teamwork but also creates a cultural shift toward shared responsibility for health outcomes. A robust framework of interprofessional education is thus critical for preparing the health workforce to meet contemporary and future challenges in healthcare delivery [2].

4.2 Evolution of the Interprofessional Education Concept

The concept of interprofessional education has undergone a notable evolution over time, reflecting changing understandings of what it means for professionals to learn together. The earliest definition, offered in 1987 by the Centre for the Advancement of Interprofessional Education (CAIPE), described IPE simply as occasions when two or more professions learn together with the intention of cultivating collaborative practice. By 2002, CAIPE had refined this definition to emphasize not only learning together but also learning *with, from, and about* each other, underscoring the bidirectional and interactive nature of the process.

In 2016, CAIPE advanced its definition further by highlighting that both students and members of two or more professions may engage in such learning. This broadened the scope of IPE to encompass not only prelicensure education but also continuing professional development, with the goal of improving collaboration and the quality of both care and services.

The World Health Organization (WHO), in its Framework for Action on Interprofessional Education and Collaborative Practice, reinforced this perspective. It emphasized that students, residents, and health workers across different disciplines must learn with, about, and from each other in order to enable effective collaboration and ultimately improve health outcomes. Similarly, the Canadian Interprofessional Health Collaborative defined interprofessional collaboration as the process of developing and sustaining effective working relationships among practitioners, patients, families, and communities to achieve optimal health outcomes.

Other scholars have further expanded this concept. Interprofessional learning, for example, has been described as the learning that emerges from interactions between members or students of two or more professions. This learning may be a deliberate product of structured IPE activities, or it may occur spontaneously in workplaces and educational settings. Interprofessional practice refers to the active participation of all team members in service delivery, where mutual reliance enables the achievement of common goals and strengthens the patient's overall experience of care. The concept of *interprofessionality* was later introduced to capture the deeper process through which professionals reflect upon and reshape their ways of working, creating an integrated and cohesive response to the needs of patients, families, and populations.

Together, these evolving definitions illustrate the progression from a relatively simple idea of shared learning toward a more dynamic and integrated model of practice, education, and reflection [3].

4.3 Why Is Interprofessional Education Necessary Today?

Interprofessional education (IPE) is of paramount importance in the current health professions education (HPE) framework, as it encourages collaboration, enhances patient safety, and equips students with the necessary competencies for modern healthcare [4]. As acknowledged by the WHO, the integration of IPE into curricula enhances team-building skills, which are vital to reducing medical errors and improving patient outcomes [2].

Many experts have emphasized the importance of starting IPE at the undergraduate level, enabling future healthcare professionals to develop a deep-rooted understanding of the roles and responsibilities that come with collaborations across other fields.

4.3.1 Enhancing Collaboration and Patient Outcomes

Currently, one of the most compelling rationales for IPE is its demonstrated ability to enhance collaboration among healthcare professionals (nurses, physicians, pharmacists, radiologists, nutritionists, and others) and improve patient outcomes. IPE fosters mutual understanding of team dynamics and main roles and responsibilities. This clarity leads to the streamlining of healthcare services, as everyone has a clear, assigned task, and duplication of services is avoided. Stronger communication bonds are also formed, leading to improvement in the quality of care.

Evidence also suggests that collaborative practice not only increases the accuracy of diagnosis and treatment planning but also reduces medical errors and allows for better resource utilization.

4.3.2 Fostering Professional Identity Formation

IPE plays a crucial role in shaping the professional identity of healthcare professionals. By sharing space with colleagues from other disciplines, students develop defined roles and a clear sense of purpose while cultivating respect for others' work. This leads to a hierarchical flattening and a bridging of gaps that otherwise may exist in medical fields and impede teamwork in clinical environments. Stereotypes are also broken that attribute certain medical specialties to specific behaviors [5].

4.3.3 Implementing Competency-Based Education

Another very significant dimension of the importance of IPE is the contribution to Competency-Based Education (CBE), also known as Competency-Based Medical Education (CBME). The transition from time-based to competence-based training requires students to work through competencies spanning multiple domains, most of which are inherently interprofessional [6]. Recent literature demonstrates that IPE fosters the development of essential core competencies, such as shared professional values, teamwork, and interprofessional communication. These are the "essential" competencies that transcend disciplines and technical expertise, providing the basics of frameworks such as entrustable professional activities and milestones [3].

Global frameworks, including those of the WHO, the Interprofessional Education Collaborative (IPEC), and regional accreditation bodies, now identify interprofessional collaboration as a nonnegotiable attribute of health professionals [2, 7, 8]. By explicitly integrating IPE into CBE, institutions ensure that graduates are not only clinically competent within their own discipline but also capable of functioning as synergistic members of multiprofessional teams.

While these arguments justify IPE now, the evolving health needs of societies and emerging disruptions make its role even more vital in the decades ahead.

4.4 Why Interprofessional Education Will Be Even More Important in the Future?

The future healthcare workforce will face unprecedented challenges that require innovative approaches to professional roles and collaboration. These were demonstrated during the COVID-19 pandemic, when significant improvisation and expansion of health sciences roles occurred [9].

"Professional plasticity" refers to the ability of health professionals to assume overlapping roles and functions depending on the context, for example, in some settings, advanced practice nurses may need to take roles traditionally held by physicians in primary care settings. To prepare for professional plasticity, healthcare professionals must not just develop expertise in their own fields but also embrace IPE, which will create educational experiences fostering fluidity, flexibility, and adaptability.

The integration of artificial intelligence (AI) and advanced technologies into healthcare will fundamentally transform how interprofessional teams function. Rather than replacing healthcare professionals, AI is expected to augment human capabilities and facilitate better collaboration. Successful clinicians will need to harness AI to assist in clinical practice, understanding that the combination of human expertise and artificial intelligence will be superior to either alone.

Looking toward the future, collaborative robots with augmented intelligence may become members of interprofessional teams, particularly in high-resource settings. These "cobots" will work alongside human professionals in shared workspaces, requiring healthcare teams to develop new forms of human-machine collaboration. Students will need to learn not only to work with other professionals but also to integrate technological partners into their collaborative practice.

The growing emphasis on planetary health and the impact of climate change on health outcomes presents new challenges that are ideally suited to interprofessional collaboration. Future health professionals will need to address the environmental and societal implications of global warming, pollution, and resource scarcity. These complex challenges require coordinated responses from multiple professions working together to address both immediate health needs and long-term environmental sustainability.

The concept of high-value care, providing the best possible care efficiently using resources to achieve optimal results for each patient, will become increasingly important as healthcare costs continue to rise globally. This approach requires interprofessional teams to work together to optimize resource use, reduce waste (including environmental waste from clinical supplies), and ensure sustainable healthcare delivery.

4.5 Interprofessional Competencies

Interprofessional education aims to cultivate a set of competencies that enable effective teamwork in healthcare. Four domains are widely recognized as foundational:

First, values and ethics form the moral basis of interprofessional collaboration. Working together requires professionals to maintain a climate of mutual respect, shared values, and ethical conduct. Without these, technical knowledge and skills cannot be translated into meaningful collaboration.

Second, an understanding of roles and responsibilities is essential. Learners must develop a strong sense of their own professional contributions while also appreciating the expertise and functions of other team members. This dual awareness enables teams to align their skills effectively, meeting both individual and population health needs.

Third, communication underpins all interprofessional activity. Effective collaboration demands responsive, responsible, respectful, and compassionate communication across professional boundaries. The ability to share information clearly, listen actively, and engage in dialogue that fosters trust is critical.

Ultimately, teamwork encompasses the science and practice of working together as a collective. Learners must be able to adapt their own roles within diverse team contexts while applying principles of team dynamics, decision-making, and conflict resolution.

These competencies may be understood at three levels.

Common competencies are those shared by multiple professions, forming a baseline for collaboration.

Complementary competencies are specific to each profession but essential to team functioning, since they provide the unique contributions of each discipline.

Collaborative competencies are those that emerge through interaction among professionals, reflecting the added value of teamwork beyond the sum of individual expertise [8].

4.6 Interprofessional Learning Experiences

Interprofessional learning can be structured across three broad categories: exposure, immersion, and mastery. These stages represent a continuum along which learners move as they deepen their ability to collaborate.

At the level of exposure, learners are introduced to peers from other health professions through shared activities such as common orientation programs. These encounters aim to raise awareness of professional diversity, foster familiarity with different roles, and cultivate an appreciation for teamwork.

The immersion stage extends this interaction by engaging learners in collaborative activities that require meaningful exchange and problem-solving. Examples include case discussions, bedside rounds, or participation in team meetings, where learners directly experience the interdependence of professional roles. Simulation-based interprofessional learning has also emerged as a powerful approach at this stage, allowing learners to engage in realistic scenarios that enhance their collaborative competencies in a safe and controlled environment.

Finally, the mastery stage reflects a deeper integration of critical thinking and problem-solving in complex, real-world contexts. Here, interprofessional learning is embedded in the provision of team-based care, where learners not only collaborate but also adapt their roles and responsibilities dynamically to address the multifaceted needs of patients. This stage represents the culmination of IPE, as learners demonstrate the ability to function effectively within interprofessional teams in authentic practice settings [10].

4.7 Innovative Pedagogical Approaches and Examples in Interprofessional Education

The pedagogical basis of IPE can be derived from adult learning principles that emphasize the importance of relevant, problem-based learning experiences that are directly connected to the future roles and responsibilities of students. Social learning theory is also primarily at play in IPE, highlighting the critical role of peer interaction.

Another crucial theoretical basis is contact theory, which is relevant to breaking down professional stereotyping through meaningful interactions between members of different groups, resulting in the cultivation of positive intragroup attitudes and a reduction in bias.

4.7.1 Simulation-Based Interprofessional Learning

Simulation-based learning is highly suited for IPE, as in such simulation environments students must not only navigate clinical scenarios but also work through interpersonal challenges necessary for team-based healthcare, such as developing skills in communication, coordination, and problem-solving. High-fidelity simulations are beneficial, as they mimic real-life IPE scenarios while providing the educational advantages of iterative practice, feedback, and detailed post-scenario analysis.

4.7.2 Problem-Based and Case-Based Learning

PBL methodologies have been applied effectively in interprofessional learning environments to develop learning environments that facilitate collaboration, allowing the knowledge bases and professional perspectives of students across different health disciplines to be leveraged. The interprofessional PBL is one in which a team of students, representing multiple professions, collaborates to solve a complex patient situation or community health problem that necessitates a multidisciplinary approach. Studies have shown that such interprofessional PBL experiences lead to students developing a sense of mutual appreciation and respect for other professional roles, as well as enhancing their professional identity development and conceptualization of their distinctive part in patient care. Such experiences in interprofessional learning also promote in the students an awareness of how their specific professional expertise can be used to complement the contributions made by interprofessional peers.

4.7.3 Community-Based Participatory Learning

Service learning and authentic collaboration skills are essential aspects of community-based, participatory strategies in interprofessional education. These strategies also engage learners in addressing real health issues in the community. It is well recognized that some of the most pressing health problems in the community and in the public health domain are multidisciplinary in nature and require the joint efforts of different professionals, in collaboration with community members and relevant organizations.

4.7.4 Technology-Enhanced Collaborative Learning

Collaborative online platforms enable students from various professional programs and geographic locations to work together on interprofessional projects while still meeting in virtual team meetings and engaging in asynchronous discussions that accommodate diverse schedules and needs. Collaborating Across Borders, a program from the University of Washington, uses videoconferencing technology to connect interprofessional student teams from different nations for shared learning experiences focused on global health challenges [11]. Students from nursing, medicine, pharmacy, and public health programs in the USA undertake collaborative explorations in partnership with their counterparts in Kenya, Peru, and the Philippines to find solutions to those mutually shared challenges of maternal mortality, infectious disease prevention, and healthcare workforce development. Massive Open Online Courses (MOOCs), originally developed to provide scalable learning experiences for large numbers of students from various professions and institutions, have been fully incorporated for interprofessional education.

4.7.5 Arts-Based and Creative Pedagogies

Humanities approaches in IPE encompass the incorporation of art, literature, music, and storytelling to facilitate connections and relationships between students from diverse professions, thereby enhancing their understanding of the human dimensions of healthcare.

An example of such a program is the "Literature and Medicine" course by the University of Rochester, which enrolls students from multiple health professions to discuss literary works with themes relevant to healthcare provision and ethical issues.

4.7.6 Program Models and Approaches

Current IPE implementation includes diverse models:

1. Longitudinal Integrated Programs: Year-long experiences that integrate multiple professions
2. Intensive Workshops and Retreats: Short-term immersive experiences
3. Clinical Rotations: Shared clinical experiences with interprofessional mentorship
4. Online Modules: Digital learning platforms for interprofessional competency development
5. Community-Based Projects: Real-world collaborative initiatives addressing local health needs

4.8 Future Trends in Interprofessional Education

4.8.1 Integration of Advanced Technologies: AI-Enhanced and VR/AR-Integrated Platforms

Future IPE will leverage AI to create personalized learning paths that adapt to individual learner needs while maintaining focus on collaborative competencies. These platforms will enable students from different professions to interact with knowledge and each other in more sophisticated ways, potentially reducing the need for traditional memorization-based assessments in favor of collaborative problem-solving and clinical reasoning.

As we use more immersive technologies in medical education, more opportunities for IPE via these channels will arise. Virtual environments will allow students to practice complex team-based scenarios repeatedly, learn from mistakes safely, and develop collaborative skills across professional boundaries without the logistical challenges of coordinating multiple professional programs.

4.8.2 Expanded Professional Participation

Future IPE will expand beyond the traditional medicine-nursing-pharmacy triad to include biomedical sciences, health economists, digital and environmental health specialists, and other related fields, as medicine becomes a more inclusive field.

There is also growing recognition that patients, families, and community members should be active participants in interprofessional education rather than passive recipients of care. Future IPE models will systematically include patient perspectives in curriculum design, implementation, and evaluation.

4.8.3 Interprofessional Training Wards

The development of dedicated interprofessional training wards represents a significant advancement in IPE. These clinical learning environments allow students from multiple professions to work together in providing patient care under supervision, creating authentic collaborative learning experiences.

4.8.4 Practice-Based Learning Networks

Future IPE will increasingly occur in actual practice settings, with healthcare organizations serving as learning laboratories where students and practicing professionals engage in continuous interprofessional development together [6].

4.8.5 Global and Cultural Competency

IPE programs will increasingly focus on addressing health disparities and social determinants of health, recognizing that effective collaborative practice must address systemic inequities in healthcare access and outcomes.

4.9 Challenges and Limitations

Many IPE initiatives struggle with long-term sustainability after initial funding expires. The transition from pilot projects to permanent curricular integration remains a significant challenge for many institutions.

Another major challenge is faculty development for IPE. Most faculty members have limited experience with interprofessional practice and teaching, creating a need for extensive faculty development programs. The development of interprofessional teaching competencies remains an ongoing challenge.

Institutional issues include scheduling conflicts between different programs, different academic calendars and requirements, departmental silos, and resistance to change.

Measuring interprofessional competencies and long-term outcomes remains complex, with limited validated assessment tools and difficulties in tracking graduates' collaborative practice behaviors over time.

4.10 Towards the Future of Interprofessional Education

The next decade will be decisive for interprofessional education. As health systems face pressures from technological disruption, demographic transitions, and the realities of climate change, the boundaries of professional roles will continue to shift. Future healthcare teams will need to embrace professional plasticity, integrating artificial intelligence, robotics, and digital health into their workflows without losing the human touch. Learners must therefore be prepared not only to collaborate with other professions but also with intelligent systems, patients, and communities as active partners in health.

Interprofessional education of the future must move beyond episodic interventions and pilot projects to become a structural expectation of health professions curricula. This requires embedding interprofessional competencies holistically. In doing so, IPE can evolve from being an educational innovation to becoming a transformative paradigm that shapes how health systems deliver safe, sustainable, and equitable care.

4.11 Key Recommendations

For IPE to achieve its transformative potential, systemic and policy-level reforms are essential. Accreditation bodies and licensing authorities should explicitly mandate interprofessional competencies as part of graduate outcomes and continuing professional development. In low- and middle-income countries (LMICs), where health systems often face workforce shortages and an unequal distribution of providers, such mandates can strengthen team-based care and maximize the impact of limited human resources.

Funding models must go beyond supporting pilot projects and provide sustained investment for integrating IPE into curricula, clinical placements, simulation-based learning, and faculty development initiatives. In resource-constrained settings, leveraging existing infrastructures, such as primary healthcare facilities and community-based training sites, offers cost-effective opportunities to embed interprofessional learning.

Faculty preparation is critical. Investing in the development of interprofessional teaching competencies will ensure that educators not only model collaborative behaviors but also mentor learners effectively. In LMICs, building faculty capacity through regional training hubs, online platforms, and South-South collaborations can accelerate this progress.

At the institutional level, policies must address barriers such as misaligned academic calendars, siloed curricula, and rigid professional hierarchies that discourage collaboration. Encouraging shared courses, joint clinical rotations, and community-based projects can provide practical platforms for interprofessional interaction.

At the national and regional levels, health workforce strategies should prioritize interprofessional collaboration as a core mechanism for advancing universal health coverage (UHC), improving primary healthcare, and ensuring resilience during health emergencies such as epidemics, natural disasters, and humanitarian crises. In LMICs, where healthcare delivery heavily relies on nurses, community health workers, and mid-level providers, IPE can strengthen referral systems, improve task-sharing, and enhance patient outcomes.

Finally, international and regional networks of IPE practice can foster exchange of innovations, contextually relevant evidence, and culturally informed approaches to collaborative education. For LMICs, participation in such networks offers opportunities to adapt global best practices to local realities while also showcasing indigenous models of collaboration that can inform the global discourse.

4.12 Conclusion

Interprofessional education is no longer a peripheral innovation but a central necessity for the healthcare workforce of the future. By embedding IPE into curricula, institutions can ensure that graduates develop the competencies necessary to work across disciplines, embrace technological transformation, and respond to global health challenges in equitable and sustainable ways. As healthcare becomes more complex, future professionals will need to exercise collaborative leadership, professional plasticity, and digital fluency to navigate contexts shaped by artificial intelligence, telehealth, and rapidly evolving models of care. At the same time, the health impacts of climate change and widening disparities will demand culturally competent, team-based approaches that align with planetary health goals.

To achieve this vision, academic institutions, policymakers, and faculty must commit to long-term investment in interprofessional curricula, faculty development, and robust assessment frameworks. Only by prioritizing these efforts can health professions education prepare a workforce capable of delivering safe, sustainable, and patient-centered care. In this way, IPE becomes not just an educational strategy but a cornerstone of future medical education.

References

1. Spaulding EM, Marvel FA, Hanyok LA, et al. Interprofessional education and collaboration among healthcare students and professionals: a systematic review and call for action. J Interprof Care. 2019;35(4):612–21.
2. World Health Organization. Global competency and outcomes framework for universal health coverage. Geneva: WHO; 2022.
3. Ten Cate O, Chen HC, Hoff RG, Peters H, Bok H, van der Schaaf M. Curriculum development for the workplace using Entrustable Professional Activities (EPAs): AMEE Guide No. 99.: Med Teach. 2015;37(11):983–1002.
4. Reeves S, Fletcher S, Barr H, Birch I, Boet S, Davies N, et al. A BEME systematic review of the effects of interprofessional education: BEME Guide No. 39. Med Teach. 2016;38(7):656–68.
5. Lapkin S, Levett-Jones T, Gilligan C. A systematic review of the effectiveness of interprofessional education in health professional programs. Nurse Educ Today. 2013;33(2):90–102.
6. Paradis E, Whitehead CR. Louder than words: power and conflict in interprofessional education articles, 1954–2013. Med Educ. 2015;49(4):399–407.
7. Interprofessional Education Collaborative. Core competencies for interprofessional collaborative practice: 2016 update. Washington, DC: IPEC; 2016.
8. Interprofessional Education Collaborative. Core competencies for interprofessional collaborative practice: 2023 update. Washington, DC: IPEC; 2023.
9. Fulmer T, Gaines M. Partnering with families for better care: lessons from the COVID-19 pandemic. J Am Geriatr Soc. 2020;68(10):2167–9.
10. Mohammed CA, Anand R, Ummer VS. Interprofessional Education (IPE): a framework for introducing teamwork and collaboration in health professions curriculum. Med J Armed Forces India. 2021;77(Suppl 1):S16.
11. Rosen MA, DiMeglio A, Moreno-Walton L, Clay-Williams R, Baker DP. A comparison of training methods for developing team-based skills: results from a qualitative analysis. Med Teach. 2018;40(12):1249–56.

Learning Environment of the Future

5

Noor-i-Kiran Naeem, Saadia Shahzad, and Gohar Wajid

Key Points

- Health professions education has moved from apprenticeship to technology-driven learning
- Clinical immersion provides role-modelling but can be enhanced with virtual and augmented realities.
- Blended learning environments promote flexibility but risk social isolation and inequity.
- Environments using artificial intelligence enable personalized, feedback-rich learning.
- Future-ready learning environments must balance human touch, inclusivity, and co-creation.

5.1 Introduction: Reimagining Learning Environments

A learning environment (LE) in health professions education (HPE) is the entire environment in which students acquire learning and build professional competence, including the physical environment, institutional policies and procedures, social relationships, and cultural practices that combine to facilitate learning and the well-being of students. This environment comprises classrooms, clinical settings, simulation laboratories, and online media. The LE is regarded as the

N.i.K. Naeem
Department of Medical Education, ABWA Medical College, Faisalabad, Pakistan

S. Shahzad
Department of Community Medicine, Queens Medical College, Kasur, Pakistan

G. Wajid (✉)
Visiting Faculty, Health Professions Education, The University of Lahore, Lahore, Pakistan

J. Sandars et al. (eds.), *Modern Medical Education*,
https://doi.org/10.1007/978-3-032-27958-3_5

building block since it is in this area that learners can interact with education resources, network with other learners and educators, and gain competencies and skills that enable them to become future health practitioners. Over the years, the learning environment has undergone significant changes and continues to transform.

This chapter aims to reflect on the evolution of the learning environment and its measurement system, its dynamic nature, and the future of the learning environment in HPE. It addresses the changing scenario of the LE, the aspects that make the need for change inevitable, as well as proposing new models and strategies for the creation of a more effective, inclusive, and technologically diverse learning environment. The chapter also provides guidance for educators, policymakers, and stakeholders on developing a learning environment that not only meets the current needs of the modern healthcare education sector but also exceeds them.

5.2 The Evolution of the Learning Environment in Health Professions Education

The historical development of learning environments in HPE is an indicator of the impact of pedagogical and technological progress on contemporary educational practice. Understanding this evolution not only provides a historical background but also identifies the continuous development that keeps shaping HPE.

HPE has undergone substantial change spanning across centuries, as has the rest of society and technology. Formalized educational institutions replaced the traditional apprenticeship systems, which were common until the nineteenth century. By the middle of the twentieth century, clinical experiences started to be incorporated into medical school curricula, with an increased focus on hands-on learning as well as theoretical studies [14].

Over time, HPE has undergone a paradigm shift due to several factors: Firstly, new digital tools and platforms driven by technological advancements are transforming how educational content is created and used [4]. Secondly, there has been a shift in the population health needs, which are becoming more responsive and dynamic due to demographic and epidemiologic changes, emerging diseases, and health challenges [19]. Lastly, the increasing emphasis on learner-centered models, which prioritize the needs of individual students, personalized learning, and real-life integration, is becoming widely adopted [2]. These disruptive factors highlight the need to redesign medical education to prepare health professionals for the demands of the twenty-first century (see Fig. 5.1).

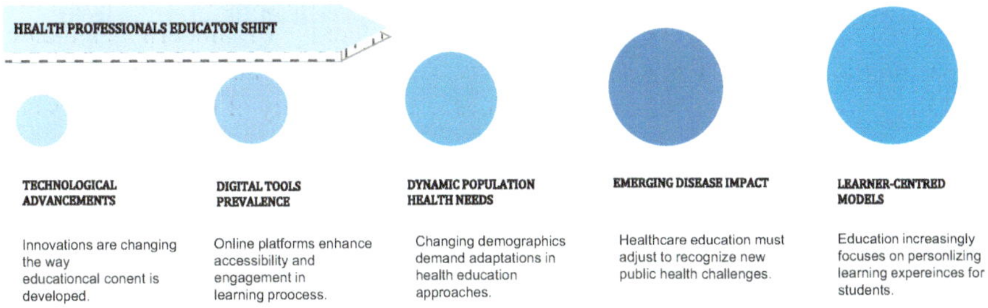

Fig. 5.1 Factors leading to transformation in health professional education

5.3 Traditional Learning Environments in Health Professions Education

Traditional medical education has been dominated by clinical immersion that allows students to train extensively with patients and health-related case scenarios at a young age. This practical exercise allows students to get acquainted with the real application of theoretical knowledge as well as acquire critical diagnostic abilities [6]. Mentorship and role modelling have also played a critical role in the development of professional identity among the students. By observing and practicing under the supervision of the mentors, learners develop clinical reasoning, ethical standards, as well as professional behavior, along with the required technical skills [10]. Apart from providing a structured experience, traditional settings encourage community feeling and peer support that are essential to emotional resilience and group learning. Direct contact with patients further provides students with invaluable practical skills that include communication skills, empathetic skills, and diagnostic skills.

On the contrary, traditional methods of teaching and learning can be rigid and unable to keep up with the current evolutions in technology and the healthcare delivery system [13]. These limitations especially become evident when the countries are trying to scale up the production of health professionals to meet the increasing health demands of the population. Bedside teaching and clinical immersion are the most resource-demanding, involving direct exposure in clinical settings. Therefore, scaling in these practices is hard to proportionate in institutions.

Such restrictions emphasize the necessity of adopting new strategies to supplement traditional learning practices to better prepare future healthcare providers. In this context, clinical immersion can be a crucial element, yet it may not prepare students to address migratory challenges by being ready to perform remote consultations or give telemedicine, which is increasingly becoming a part of the modern healthcare landscape.

5.4 Use of Digital Technologies and Learning Environment

Rapid advancements in internet-based learning approaches and advancements in virtual technologies (virtual patients, simulations, and telemedicine) provide more flexibility, accessibility, and interactivity to the learners. These technologies enable the students to access different sets of clinical situations without any limitations of time or location. Additionally, they provide an opportunity for immediate feedback and assessment, enhancing the learning process.

Virtual reality (VR) and augmented reality (AR) are valuable instruments that allow individuals to learn in an immersive world [18]. AR provides digital information over the physical world, whereas VR gives fully simulated environments capable of approximating real-world conditions. These two technologies are particularly useful in learning practical skills requiring practice that cannot be simulated in a traditional classroom. Moving forward, artificial intelligence is likely to have a deep impact on the learning environment as it provides opportunities for personalization of learning and an adaptive learning environment, development of intelligent tutoring and support systems, and more emphasis on evidence-driven educational approaches [17].

5.5 Measuring Learning Environments

The evolution of LE has a direct impact on how it is measured. Being dynamic, the nature of LE may vary across specialized clinical settings, different socio-economic settings, and cultures. The tools for measuring LE have a long history of evolution. Starting from an earlier tool developed by Stern and George in 1958, several tools were developed over the years, including the Dundee Ready Education Environment Measure (DREEM) tool and its several versions and the more recent Johns Hopkins Learning Environment Scale (JHLES) developed by Shochet and team in 2015 [22]. These tools reflect the dynamic nature of the LE and the need for continual upgrading of the tools, particularly during the current era of digital technologies.

The concept of current measurement of learning environments has now evolved into a highly complex measurement theory in that it considers a range of dimensions in a coordinated manner. The physical space must facilitate the learning process, and the social space must aid in the establishment of a spirit of working together and belonging. In addition, with the growing popularity of online education, the virtual factors like user interface design, accessibility, and technological support also matter, as shown in Fig. 5.2 representing Technology-Enhanced Learning Environment in Medical Education (TELEMED) [16]. This is a complex issue of providing a broad evaluation of these dimensions.

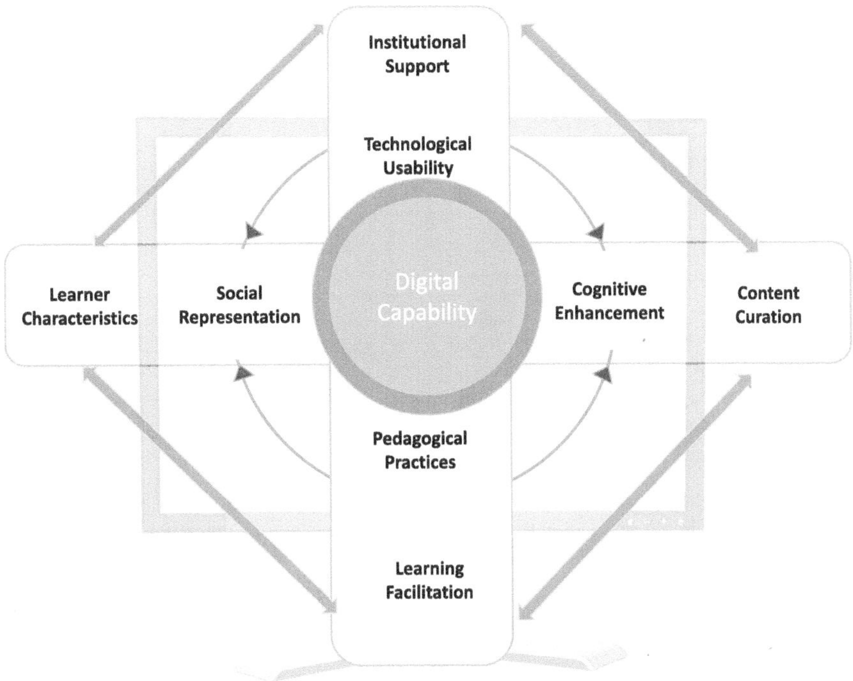

Fig. 5.2 Finalized key components of Technology-Enhanced Learning Environment in Medical Education (TELEMED) framework. (Reprinted from "Experts' consensus over key components of online learning environments in medical education: a modified e-Delphi study" By Naeem et al. [17]. Permission granted under terms of Creative Commons Attribution 4.0 International License)

5.6 Transition from In-Person to Blended Models of Education

Blended learning is the integration of classroom face-to-face learning and online learning, allowing students to receive the benefits of both the social environment of the classroom and the self-directedness of online learning. These needs for flexibility, personalization, and inclusivity are some of the drivers of this transformation, especially boosted by the COVID-19 global pandemic [23]. Digital platforms and internet use have also facilitated this revolution within the education system by utilizing the extensive collection of materials that are not present within the confines of the physical classroom. Furthermore, this transformation involves a higher degree of engagement of students in the process of their learning, which enhances self-regulated exploration and critical thinking skills. Teachers, in turn, become facilitators along with performing different roles, which also enhances the dynamic and cooperative learning process [16] (Fig. 5.3).

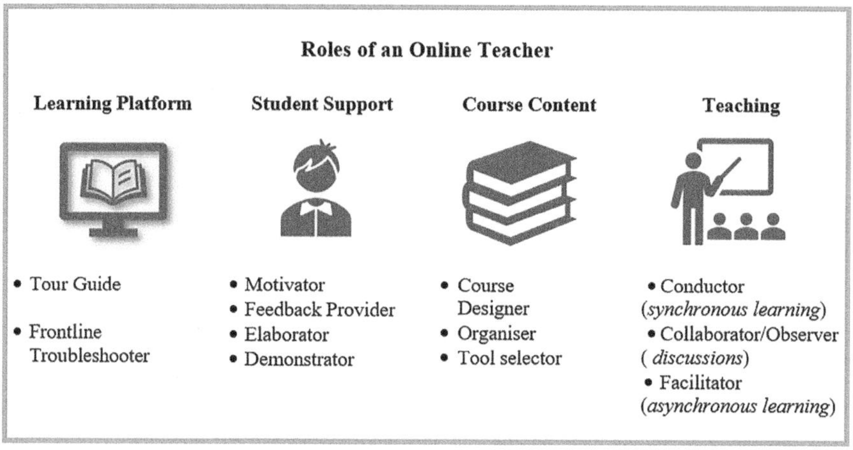

Fig. 5.3 Roles of a medical teacher in online learning environments. (Reprinted from "Understanding the scope of functional components of Technology-enhanced learning environment in medical education: A scoping review" By Understanding functional components of Technology-enhanced learning environment in medical education: A scoping review" By Naeem et al. [16]. Permission granted under terms of Creative Commons Attribution 4.0 International License)

Physical and digital spaces in education offer many benefits, such as ease of accessibility and flexibility. Nonetheless, such a combination also presents challenges, including the fair distribution of technology and digital divide issues [11]. Additionally, there is a danger of overusing digital tools at the cost of human contact, which is essential for creating strong academic communities. Teachers are key figures within the learning framework, and their professional growth should be ensured by institutions by offering extensive training and continuous support. This includes not only technical training but also the development of a mindset that is open to learning and innovation.

As online learning spaces have become more mature, there has been a change in perspective from a focus on these spaces as a short-term solution to a new way of thinking about online learning spaces as a transformative opportunity [24]. Initially regarded as a temporary solution in the times of the COVID-19 pandemic, this evolution spotlights the possibilities of the future with interconnected, dynamic learning systems to foster various educational needs.

The future of the learning environment is rapidly moving toward the integration of digital high-tech tools that enhance accessibility, interactivity, and personalization. These include learning management system (LMS), asynchronous communication, virtual simulation, and massive open online courses (MOOC) [12]. Education democratization is also a feature of MOOCs, with the courses available to a broader audience spread across the world and lacking the boundaries of geographical location and economic circumstance.

Like all other technologies, digital education is not, however, free from its downside as well. Apart from learners experiencing social isolation, digital fatigue also emerges as a problem with online learning [5]. Such a tendency of the students to have burnout due to the excessive spending of time on the screen may be a hindrance to academic performance. To reduce this effect, teachers can employ the strategies of screen breaks and promote integrated models, leading to a healthier and more efficient learning process [15]. Further, infrastructure inequality is one of the setbacks of online learning since access to a stable internet connection, computers, and software might not be equal, and this will influence the extent to which students with poor backgrounds access education. This digital gap widens the disparities present in the real world, and not all students can effectively use virtual classrooms.

5.7 Technologies Shaping the Future Learning Environment

Several digital technologies, artificial intelligence being the most recent addition, are now transforming the learning environment. By learning the strengths, weaknesses, learning speed, and preferences of individual learners, AI algorithms can build individualized lesson plans and assessment methods using large amounts of data about the learners [17]. The technology will not only boost student engagement but also assist teachers in identifying gaps in knowledge and adapting their teaching to meet the needs of the students.

Extended reality (XR), such as augmented reality (AR), virtual reality (VR), and mixed reality (MR), is transforming clinical training environments, with a simulation of a real-world environment, allowing it to be an immersive experience [7]. Unlike physical settings where medical students and professionals learn complex processes at risk, VR allows students to train in a safe, risk-free environment, while AR superimposes digital information over physical space, a step forward from limited or no practical skills and real-time assistance. As an example, a student of surgery can practice several surgeries virtually until it is mastered; thus, the probability of patient safety in surgeries is significantly increased.

With the increasing use of AI in learning environments, the presence of adaptive learning platforms and smart analytics is breaking through the education sector. The systems enable personalized learning as they allow addressing the specific needs of individual learners and working at the desired pace [8]. By means of applying adaptive algorithms, the difficulty and temporal allocation of content are optimized by dynamically reformulating based on real-time measures of content to enhance learning outcomes. In this regard, educational technology serves as an evidence-based practice, the possibility of which is ongoing improvement of curriculum by changing education standards and the needs of learners.

Though the use of technology is providing new opportunities in education, perhaps more than ever before, it is essential to keep the human touch [9]. The critical role of educators must not be substituted by technology. This entails using technology to support individualized learning, automate administrative functions, and enhance interactive learning processes. However, it is crucial to maintain the mentorship and emotional support teachers offer, which is fundamental to student success.

5.8 Considerations for Designing Future Learning Environment

Introduction of digital technologies has led to a significant shift in the way LE is perceived and will be shaped in the future. While the presence of infrastructure, face-to-face teaching and learning, and the role of the teacher remain inevitable in the learning environment, the introduction of digital technologies plays a significant role in reshaping the LE and subsequently its measurement and evaluation systems.

Learner-centeredness is an essential principle in contemporary pedagogy and puts the learner at the epicenter of the teaching course, underlining that all the elements of the educational environment should be interlocked with the interests, desires, and aspirational routes of the learners [3]. The focus of the approach has an empirical connection with the creation of individualized learning paths, responsive and time-sensitive feedback provision, and the establishment of an inclusive support group that helps to establish long-term engagement and independent studying. In order to encourage accessibility and inclusivity in education, learning environments must ensure that all learners, irrespective of their backgrounds and abilities, are afforded an equally fair chance of succeeding.

A critical balance in the digital-physical spaces preserves the coexistence between online and live communication without requiring one to substitute the other because it dictates that technology should supplement rather than take the place of the centuries-old face-to-face teaching [20]. This equilibrium reduces the distance between educators and learners, leading to actual collaboration and real, experience-based learning. An example can be seen in the utilization of virtual reality to simulate real-life environments, where classrooms that integrate breakout rooms allow students to communicate with one another.

The key to the creation of future learning environments lies in successful stakeholder engagement. It involves a close cooperation between the teachers, the students, and the technology designers so that the technologies applied in education should not only be available but also have a chance to be pedagogically viable [21]. By building a community of practice where knowledge and expertise will be shared openly, we will be capable of building resilient, inclusive, and innovative educational environments.

In the process of carrying out digital changes, the leadership of a given institution plays an imperative role [11]. There also needs to be proper governance structures for strategic planning, the allocation of resources, as well as policies that would allow technology to be integrated within all facets of education. The educational environments of the future have to be defined as flexible, inclusive, and sustainable. The pressing educational technology, pedagogical practice, and the effects of global health development emphasize the dire need to shift the paradigm in a more inclusive and fair model of HPE [1]. This revolution goes beyond the implementation of innovative apparatus such as artificial intelligence or virtual reality; it also involves developing a culture that brings about continuous education and professional development.

In order to meet these objectives, teachers, policymakers, the industry, and even the students will be required to dedicate themselves to the concept of persistent innovation and co-creation, as well as attempts to access international fairness. The latter includes the development of resilient education models that would stand a chance even in the conditions of future uncertainty. This can be ensured by nurturing the concept of lifelong learning as the means to address the new health requirements and advancing the policy frameworks that foster sustainable and inclusive approaches to HPE on a global scale.

5.9 Conclusion

The learning environment is an integral component of multidimensional and complex health professions education ecosystem. The dynamic and resilient nature of LE in HPE institutions should provide room for seamlessly integrating traditional teaching and learning approaches with advances in education due to digital technologies. The shift from apprenticeship to blended, technology-enhanced, and AI-driven environments underscores the need to balance innovation with inclusivity, equity, and human connection for professional identity formation of future health professionals. Building future-ready environments requires even more learner-centeredness, inclusivity, and co-creation among educators, learners, and policymakers. By balancing equity with sustainability, we can prepare health professionals who are not only competent but also compassionate leaders in the complex and dynamic health and education ecosystem.

References

1. Adeyele TK, Adeyele TK. Revolutionizing health education: the dynamic shift of E-learning platforms. 2024. Available at: https://doi.org/10.5772/INTECHOPEN.1004562.
2. Alamri H, et al. Using personalized learning as an instructional approach to motivate learners in online higher education: learner self-determination and intrinsic motivation. J Res Technol Educ. 2020;52(3). Available at: https://doi.org/10.1080/15391523.2020.1728449.
3. Ang WHD, et al. Resilience for undergraduate students: development and evaluation of a theory-driven, evidence-based and learner centered digital resilience skills enhancement (RISE) program. Int J Environ Res Public Health. 2022;19(19):12729. Available at: https://doi.org/10.3390/IJERPH191912729/S1.
4. Ballouk R, et al. Medical students' self-regulation of learning in a blended learning environment: a systematic scoping review. Med Educ Online. 2022;27(1). Available at: https://doi.org/10.1080/10872981.2022.2029336.
5. Büchi M. Digital well-being theory and research. New Media Soc [Preprint]. 2021. Available at: https://doi.org/10.1177/14614448211056851/ASSET/IMAGES/LARGE/10.1177_14614448211056851-FIG3.JPEG.

6. Corrao S, Argano C. Rethinking clinical decision-making to improve clinical reasoning. Front Med. 2022;9:900543. Available at: https://doi.org/10.3389/FMED.2022.900543/PDF.
7. Elendu C, et al. The impact of simulation-based training in medical education: a review. Medicine (United States). 2024;103(27):e38813. Available at: https://doi.org/10.1097/MD.0000000000038813.
8. Elmoazen R, et al. Learning analytics in virtual laboratories: a systematic literature review of empirical research. Smart Learn Environ. 2023. Available at: https://doi.org/10.1186/s40561-023-00244-y.
9. Haleem A, et al. Understanding the role of digital technologies in education: a review. Sustain Oper Comput. 2022;3:275–85. Available at: https://doi.org/10.1016/J.SUSOC.2022.05.004.
10. Hassan Khan A, et al. Role modeling in medical education and its influences on professional behaviours. Ann King Edward Med Univ. 2020;26(1):83–7. Available at: https://doi.org/10.21649/AKEMU.V26I1.3306.
11. Iqbal S, et al. Attributes of digital leaders in health professions education. J Coll Physicians Surg Pak. 2025;35(2):229–33. Available at: https://doi.org/10.29271/JCPSP.2025.02.229.
12. Littenberg-Tobias J, Reich J. Evaluating access, quality, and equity in online learning: a case study of a MOOC-based blended professional degree program. Internet High Educ. 2020;47. Available at: https://doi.org/10.1016/j.iheduc.2020.100759.
13. Maddox TM, et al. The learning healthcare system and cardiovascular care: a scientific statement from the American Heart Association. Circulation. 2017;135(14):e826–57. Available at: https://doi.org/10.1161/CIR.0000000000000480/ASSET/55716C75-E457-4526-9567-DD6FA35F930A/ASSETS/GRAPHIC/E826FIG03.JPEG.
14. Matsuo M. A revised model of cognitive apprenticeship: a qualitative study. Int J Train Dev. 2024;28(4):454–72. Available at: https://doi.org/10.1111/IJTD.12336;PAGEGROUP:STRING:PUBLICATION.
15. Naeem NK, Mushibwe CP. Navigating digital worlds: a scoping review of skills and strategies for enhancing digital resilience among higher education students on social media platforms. Discover Educ. 2025;4(1):1–15. Available at: https://doi.org/10.1007/S44217-025-00432-7/TABLES/5.
16. Naeem NK, et al. Understanding the functional components of technology-enhanced learning environment in medical education: a scoping review. Med Sci Educ. 2023;33(1):1–15. Available at: https://doi.org/10.1007/S40670-023-01747-6/TABLES/3.
17. Naeem NK, et al. Using artificial intelligence in online learning environments for positive student outcomes: a scoping review. Ann King Edward Med Univ. 2025;31(Spl2):119–29. Available at: https://doi.org/10.21649/AKEMU.V31ISPL2.5811.
18. Okwor IA, et al. Digital technologies impact on healthcare delivery: a systematic review of artificial intelligence (AI) and machine-learning (ML) adoption, challenges, and opportunities. AI (Switzerland). 2024;5(4):1918–41. Available at: https://doi.org/10.3390/AI5040095/S1.
19. Papapanou M, et al. Medical education challenges and innovations during COVID-19 pandemic. Postgrad Med J. 2022;98(1159):321–7. Available at: https://doi.org/10.1136/POSTGRADMEDJ-2021-140032.
20. Pedrero-Esteban LM, Barrios-Rubio A. Digital communication in the age of immediacy. Digital. 2024;4(2):302–15. Available at: https://doi.org/10.3390/DIGITAL4020015.
21. Peng Y, Alias BS, Mansor AN. Application of stakeholder theory in education management: a comprehensive systematic literature review (SLR). Int J Learn Teach Educ Res. 2024;23(6):1–31. Available at: https://doi.org/10.26803/IJLTER.23.6.1.
22. Shahzad S, Wajid G. Learning environment and its relationship with quality of life and burnout among undergraduate medical students in Pakistan: a cross-sectional study. BMJ Open. 2024;14(8):e080440. Available at: https://doi.org/10.1136/BMJOPEN-2023-080440.
23. So H-J, Bonk CJ. Examining the roles of blended learning approaches in computer-supported collaborative learning (CSCL) environments: a Delphi study. Educ Technol Soc. 2010;13(3):1176–3647. Available at: http://www.surveyshare.com/. Accessed 9 July 2018.
24. Younas M, et al. Unveiling digital transformation and teaching prowess in English education during COVID-19 with structural equation modelling. Eur J Educ. 2025;60(1). Available at: https://doi.org/10.1111/EJED.12818.

6 Reimagining Clinical Skills Education: Strategies for the Future Health Professionals

Jabeen Fayyaz and Gohar Wajid

Key Points

- Clinical skills education must move beyond the apprenticeship model toward structured, competency-based, and learner-centered approaches that prioritize active practice over passive observation.
- Emerging tools such as extended reality (XR), virtual patients, wearable sensors, AI-driven assessments, and adaptive platforms can enhance precision, personalization, and access in clinical training, especially when used intentionally and equitably.
- Innovations must align with competency frameworks, interprofessional collaboration, and social accountability to ensure relevance, inclusivity, and system-level impact. Curriculum redesign should reflect local health needs and global standards.
- Transformative education requires institutional commitment, strategic resource allocation, faculty development, and robust infrastructure. Long-term success depends on scalable models, meaningful assessments, and continuous stakeholder engagement.
- To prepare future-ready healthcare professionals, we must design future-ready education.

J. Fayyaz (✉)
Department of Pediatrics, Division of Emergency Medicine, The Hospital for Sick Children, University of Toronto, Toronto, ON, Canada

G. Wajid
Visiting Faculty, Health Professions Education, The University of Lahore, Lahore, Pakistan

J. Sandars et al. (eds.), *Modern Medical Education*,
https://doi.org/10.1007/978-3-032-27958-3_6

6.1 Introduction

Bedside apprenticeship has been a predominant method of teaching clinical skills for a long time. This method, however, lacks the structure, standardization, and consistent feedback [8, 16]. In addition to mastering clinical skills, today's health system demands health professionals equally competent in clinical reasoning, teamwork, leadership, technology, and data-driven decision-making. This is causing education to shift toward competency-driven and tech-enhanced models [5]. Competency-based models using simulation now enable a safe, immersive, and personalized learning [4, 6]. This chapter outlines a future where clinical training is approached as inclusive, adaptive, and aligned with the complexities of current healthcare environments.

6.2 Definition and Scope of Clinical Skills in the Changing Health Paradigm

Imagine a young medical student interacting with the patient for the first time, nervous about his interaction, trying to recall the steps given in the checklist, like smile, introduction, open-ended questions, active listening, etc., yet quickly realizing that clinical encounters are far more nuanced than a mere checklist. True clinical skill entails building trust, making decisions, and being present. In today's complex health environment, clinical competence goes beyond procedural tasks; it integrates cognitive, psychomotor, and affective domains such as communication, diagnostic reasoning, collaboration, professionalism, and other attributes, as shown in Fig. 6.1. Frameworks like Competency-Based Medical Education (CBME) and entrustable professional activities (EPAs) [9, 15] formalize this complexity. EPAs don't just assess technical ability; they evaluate whether a learner can perform independently, with sound judgment, clear communication, and patient-centered care. This approach fosters shared expectations, improves accountability, and empowers learners to take charge of their development. As Hennus et al. highlight, EPAs offer a practical way to observe and nurture complex competencies in real settings [9]. Defining clinical skills (CS) today means training clinicians who know not only what to do but also when, how, and why to do it with empathy and integrity.

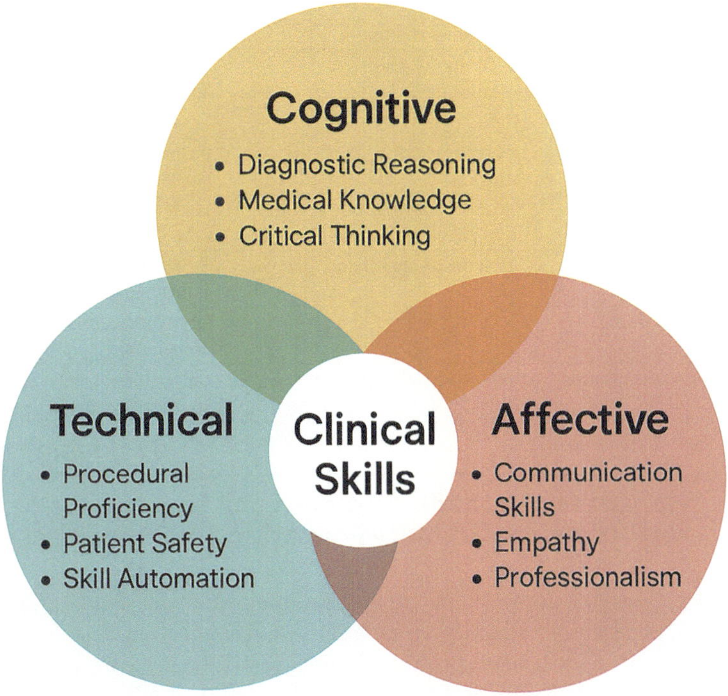

Fig. 6.1 Attributes of clinical skills

6.3 The Impact of Holistic Clinical Skills Approach on Patient Safety and Health Outcomes

In healthcare, where clinical performance directly impacts life and death, the link between CS education and patient safety is critical [17]. Evidence shows that structured training, particularly simulation-based education, enhances skill performance and care quality. A meta-analysis comparing the effects of simulation-based and traditional teaching methods on the critical thinking abilities and self-confidence of nursing students confirmed that simulation-trained learners consistently outperform those taught via traditional methods [1]. When aligned with competency frameworks, such curricula promote standardization, early error recognition, and confident decision-making, especially vital in high-stakes settings like emergency and critical care. Thus, simulation is not just an educational tool but a proven strategy to improve patient safety and team performance. Table 6.1 provides a comparison of selected outcomes metrics between traditional and simulation-based training.

Table 6.1 Comparison between traditional vs. simulation-based training

Outcome metrics	Traditional training	Simulation-based training
Procedural accuracy	Moderate (inconsistent performance)	High (reproducible, standard-aligned)
Diagnostic error rate	Higher (~15–20%)	Lower (~5–10%)
Time to intervention (e.g., sepsis)	Delayed (variable response times)	Faster (protocols practiced in simulation)
Learner confidence	Variable (self-reported low in high-stakes scenarios)	High (consistently improved post-simulation)
Team communication effectiveness	Often unstructured and reactive	Structured, anticipatory, and coordinated
Patient satisfaction	Moderate to low	High (confidence and preparedness evident)
Rate of adverse events	Higher (linked to preventable errors)	Lower (due to early recognition and management)

6.4 Holistic Clinical Skills Approach and Its Impact on Professional Identity Formation and Humanism

Clinical encounters not only are problem-solving moments but also enable the learners to experience humanity, vulnerability, and connection. Each patient interaction, listening to a difficult history or delivering bad news, shapes their professional identity, a process beyond the textbooks, enriched with lived experiences and reflections [2]. CS education supports this transformation by creating spaces where learners engage emotionally, ethically, and interprofessionally. Scenarios involving distress or ethical conflict foster empathy, cultural humility, and teamwork, but true growth comes through reflection. In a rapidly advancing healthcare system, cultivating compassion and integrity through reflective clinical education is essential. Figure 6.2 shows the pathway to professional identity formation through clinical skills training.

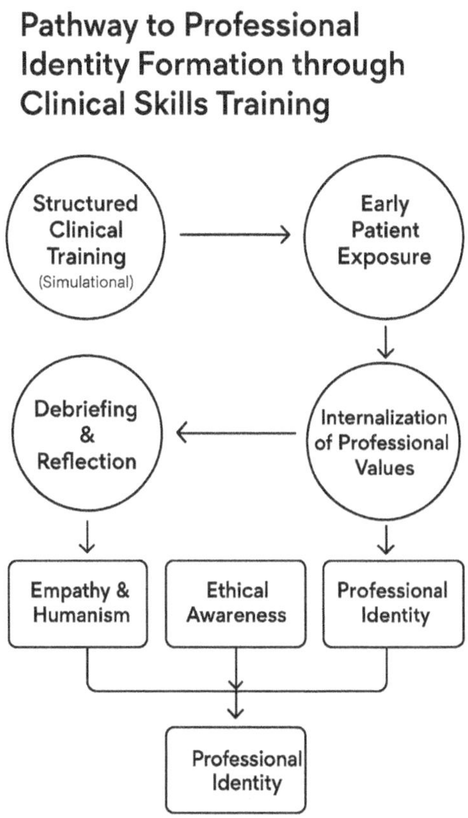

Fig. 6.2 Pathway to professional identity formation through CS training. (Created by JF using Lucidchart)

6.5 The Apprenticeship Era of Clinical Skills Teaching: Foundations and Fault Lines

CS education has long been rooted in the apprenticeship model, "see one, do one, teach one," where learners progressed from observation to supervised practice to teaching. While it emphasized experiential learning and role modelling, it was inconsistent, with wide variation based on clinical setting and supervisor engagement [11]. The interesting observation is that within a single program learner experiences could differ dramatically based on the patient exposure. This variability led to differences in skill acquisition, as illustrated by final-year students whose procedural exposure depends more on placement than curriculum. The model, though foundational, lacked standardization and failed to ensure equitable uniform readiness for clinical practice. As patient safety and care complexity increase, the need for structured, reproducible, and equitable training approaches becomes a necessity. The scope of traditional CS models gets further limited in today's education environment with an exponential increase in the number of health professions education (HPE) institutions, an increase in the number of trainees and a shortage of qualified and well-trained clinical educators. There is a sharp rise in the number of HPE institutions (medical, nursing, and other HPE institutions). In some institutions, the number of students per classroom extends even beyond 350, with equally shrinking faculty and a dearth of clinical training sites to train such a large number of students. Traditional training models cannot cope with this situation, providing room for innovative methods (such as simulations and digital technologies) to fill this crucial gap.

6.6 Rise of Structured Clinical Education

By the late twentieth century, the limitations of the apprenticeship model, variability, lack of feedback, and ethical concerns led to a shift toward structured clinical education. Innovative educators like Harden and Barrows introduced Objective Structured Clinical Examinations (OSCEs) and Standardized Patients (SPs) to bring fairness, standardization, and reproducibility to skills assessment [7, 10]. Teaching clinical skills enabled a safe, deliberate practice with immediate feedback, aligning with Ericsson's theory of expert performance through repetition and refinement. By the 2000s, OSCEs were increasingly embedded in national licensing exams globally, serving as both individual and institutional benchmarks [10]. SPs further enriched their training by simulating realistic interactions and enhancing empathy and ethical sensitivity [7]. These innovations transformed clinical education into an accountable, learner-centered model and serve as a foundation for competency-based simulation-enhanced, tech-driven approaches.

6.7 Shaping Clinical Skills Through Competency-Based Education

Competency-based education (CBE) in clinical skills (CS) moves beyond the conventional training model. The CBE emphasizes that the competencies, such as technical proficiency, communication, teamwork, clinical reasoning, and professional behaviors, are attained and standardized. CBE approach provides opportunity for deliberate practice, structured feedback, and standardized assessment that are linked to learners' clinical milestones rather than only spending a month in rotation to a specific area or on the number of patients seen. Within this model, the use of simulations plays a vital role, creating safe, realistic environments where learners can apply knowledge, refine skills, and engage in reflective practice without risk to patients [19]. By integrating simulation into competency-based education, institutions foster confident, collaborative, and practice-ready clinicians prepared for the complexities of current healthcare. Concurrently, Interprofessional Education and Collaborative Practice (IPECP) gained traction, re-establishing communication and leadership to improve patient outcomes. The IPECP competencies reinforce learning around values, roles, communication, and teamwork. Together, SBE and IPECP signify a move from fragmented, as available, individual learning, to standardized, collaborative, and goal-oriented, community-centered education, making our learners ready to face the challenges of an increasingly complex healthcare ecosystem [14].

6.8 Challenges and Opportunities in Contemporary Clinical Skills Education

CS education is impactful but also brings various systemic challenges. As institutions transition from traditional apprenticeship to competency-based, simulation-enhanced, and tech-enabled models, they face complex challenges. Overcrowded clinical settings, limited faculty, and difficulty balancing standardization with flexibility and accountability are a few to name. Technological advancements like AI and extended reality (XR) will make it more challenging for institutions in the future. Yet, these very challenges also create opportunities: simulation, virtual learning, and AI can help with scaling, while reflective practice, faculty development, and interprofessional collaboration foster safer, more compassionate care.

6.9 System-Level Constraints and Clinical Overload

Patient care and safety remain at the heart of any clinical skills development program. In reality, the rising patient loads, limited faculty time, and high-acuity demands lead to "clinical bandwidth crises," making meaningful teaching impossible. When teaching is compromised in the context of high patient load and a shortage of faculty, learners often become passive observers, especially in acute care settings. Smartly developed simulation programs with effective use of simulations provide opportunities to fill this gap, offering structured, low-risk environments for deliberate practice. When standardization in the development of clinical skills is compromised, clinical experiences and feedback remain highly variable, often determined by chance. In such situations, the creation of psychologically safe learning spaces is equally vital. Psychological safety in clinical learning is of prime importance, and simulation with structured pre-briefing and debriefing helps foster psychological and emotional safety, reflection, and resilience [3]. Faculty development is essential to embed these principles systemically, ensuring learners feel safe to question and learn. These challenges demand a shift from opportunistic to intentional, inclusive, and system-oriented CS education.

6.10 Technology and Equity in Post-COVID-19 Pandemic Clinical Education

The COVID-19 pandemic brought disruption to the education process, especially the clinical exposure and clinical skills development of students were grossly disrupted due to their confinement at home. On the other hand, the pandemic provided the opportunity to push learning into virtual spaces and accelerated the incorporation of technologies in clinical education, a paradigm shift that was never seen before. Although this paradigm shift had challenges like digital fatigue, loss of hands-on practice, and inequities in access to technology, it has resurfaced opportunities. The educators realize that the future lies in hybrid curricula that blend in-person interaction with virtual tools. In order to succeed, the integration process must be intentional, learner-centered, and inclusive [12]. Without intentional design and equitable access, technology risks deepening educational divides. The future demands not just new tools but new mindsets prioritizing accessibility, safety, and inclusion for all learners [13].

6.11 Transformative Strategies for Future Clinical Skills Education

Modern CS education is shifting from passive observation to immersive, personalized, and technology-enhanced learning. Rooted in Ericsson's theory of deliberate practice, simulation-based education (SBE) enables learners to repeat tasks, receive real-time feedback, and build mastery in a safe, standardized environment. Psychological safety during simulation encourages reflection, learning from errors, and resilience [3, 13]. Pedagogical innovations such as simulation-based learning, virtual patients, and AI-driven feedback systems are completely changing the landscape of clinical skills development approaches.

Virtual patients (VPs) offer scalable, interactive training for clinical reasoning, communication, and ethical decision-making, especially useful for remote and underserved settings. Studies confirm the effectiveness of virtual platforms to enhance diagnostic accuracy and learner confidence. In regions like the WHO Eastern Mediterranean Region, low-cost, offline VP platforms have enabled training continuity even in refugee camps. The COVID-19 pandemic further emphasized the benefits of technology-enhanced learning models and platforms [13].

Artificial intelligence (AI) is revolutionizing clinical education by enabling personalized, data-driven learning. AI systems track performance metrics like task time, error rates, hand motion, and eye movements and provide tailored feedback, even evaluating empathy and communication. However, educators need to be careful of ethical concerns such as bias, transparency, and preserving human-centered learning to maintain trust and empathy in education [18]. Table 6.2 provides a summary of the key features of the three innovative pedagogical approaches.

Other educational approaches are also playing a significant role in shaping the clinical skills development process.

Blended and flipped learning models merge digital tools (e.g., videos, quizzes) with in-person clinical teaching. The flipped classroom model is where students study content before class and apply skills during in-person sessions. Blended learning and flipped classrooms boost engagement and efficiency. In clinical settings, it

Table 6.2 Comparison of pedagogical innovations—simulation, virtual patients, and AI feedback platforms

Feature	Simulation-based learning	Virtual patient platforms	AI-driven feedback systems
Definition	Hands-on practice in controlled, realistic environments	Interactive computer-based cases mimicking real clinical scenarios	Systems that analyze learner's performance and offer feedback
Modality	In-person or virtual, high- or low-fidelity mannequins	Web-based or app-accessed digital platforms	Embedded in learning platforms or as standalone tools
Primary purpose	Procedural skills, teamwork, and crisis resource management	Diagnostic reasoning, history-taking, clinical decision-making	Personalized learning support, performance analytics
Level of interactivity	High—tactile, verbal, team-based	Moderate to high—decision trees, case branching	Variable—based on algorithms and data inputs
Feedback mechanism	Facilitator-led debriefing and peer feedback	Case-based automated responses or faculty review	Immediate, automated, data-informed feedback
Strengths	Realistic scenarios, team training, and emotional engagement	Accessibility, scalability, and cognitive skill focus	Scalability, objectivity, learner-specific insights
Challenges	Resource-intensive scheduling logistics	Limited procedural realism, variable engagement	Potential bias in algorithms, tech dependence
Ideal use cases	Emergency resuscitation, team training, procedural mastery	Remote learning, differential diagnosis, and communication practice	Continuous assessment, adaptive learning, competency tracking

improves procedural preparedness and supports equity through flexible access. However, success depends on thoughtful integration of technology and addressing the digital divide to ensure all learners benefit equally.

Interprofessional Education and Collaborative Practice (IPECP) brings together learners from multiple health disciplines to practice teamwork. It enhances mutual understanding, communication, and respect, critical for coordinated, patient-centered care [1]. Clinical scenarios can be developed to integrate learners from different disciplines, not only to demark their clinical roles in a particular situation but also to improve communication and teamwork.

Standardization in the clinical skills development process ensures reliability, fairness, and educational integrity. It involves facilitator preparation, learner assessment, and instructional delivery, aligned with competencies and entrustable professional activities (EPAs) [9]. Standardization transforms the educational delivery of clinical skills as a credible, scalable method [19]. It is especially important when a large number of students are being trained in multiple institutions across the country.

6.12 The Role of Technology-Enhanced Clinical Skills Education

In reimagining CS education for future healthcare professionals, the integration of technology-enhanced learning modalities has emerged not as a luxury but as an essential pedagogical imperative. Technology-enhanced CS education is not simply a set of tools but a strategic driver of educational transformation, bridging the gap between training and the dynamic realities of clinical practice [12].

Extended Reality (XR) Virtual, augmented, and mixed realities offer immersive, risk-free training for rare procedures and team-based scenarios. It enhances procedural accuracy, decision-making, and learner engagement. Despite cost and access challenges, XR is becoming a key pillar in scalable, future-ready curricula. Although expensive initially, the enhanced use of these modalities is likely to bring the cost down and improve their equitable access to low-resourced settings as well.

Wearable Sensors They capture real-time metrics like hand movement, gaze, and stress levels, offering objective feedback and tracking progress over time. They support self-reflective practice and competency-based education through data-driven insights.

Adaptive Learning Platforms Using AI, adaptive platforms tailor content to individual learner needs, providing just-in-time remediation or advanced challenges. They promote mastery-based progression, support self-paced learning, and align with CBME goals for personalized, efficient education [15].

6.13 Implementation: Resource Allocation, Return on Investment, and Sustainability

Integrating advanced clinical education tools such as simulation, XR, AI, and adaptive learning requires meticulous planning and strategic investment. Institutions must conduct needs-based assessments to align resources with learner needs, identify competencies for each specialty, and assess available infrastructure. High initial costs for technology, software, and faculty training demand shared resources, regional hubs and spoke models, and open-access platforms. Return on investment (ROI) should go beyond financial metrics to include educational outcomes like improved competence, reduced remediation, and enhanced patient safety. Institutional gains, such as accreditation readiness and academic reputation, also reflect ROI and leadership in health professions education. For these interventions to be sustainable, the programs required engaged faculty and robust support systems. Burnout and lack of protected time can impact the program quality, which requires faculty development and recognition. Academic networks, industry, and global organizations are important for long-term success. Ultimately, implementation is a continuous process that supports evolving technology, engaged learners, and improved clinical care.

6.14 Aligning Innovations in Clinical Education with Assessment, Interprofessionalism, and Social Accountability

As clinical education adopts digital tools, it's essential that these innovations align with competency-based assessment, interprofessional collaboration, and social accountability—mapping simulation-based assessments, digital portfolios, and AI analytics to competencies and EPAs to ensure objective, real-time evaluation. Integrating Interprofessional Education and Collaborative Practice (IPECP) into virtual and simulated environments fosters teamwork and shared decision-making across disciplines. Educational technologies should be accessible and culturally relevant, especially in low-resource settings. Ultimately, CS education and innovation are not just about following the new trends but also need educational rigor, cultural and ethical considerations, advancing both learning outcomes and their social impact.

6.15 Strategies and Framework for Curriculum Transformation

Transforming CS education requires a systemic, equity-focused redesign rooted in competency-based frameworks, as outlined in Table 6.3.

Table 6.3 Framework for curriculum transformation with focus on clinical education

Steps	Strategies	Practical actions (what to do)
1	Adopt competency-based frameworks	Define and map competencies; set measurable milestones; align skills with health-system/workforce needs
2	Integrate simulation & XR	Use a spiral curriculum: introduce core skills early; revisit with greater complexity using simulation, XR, and virtual patients
3	Sequence learning effectively	Start with foundational methods (videos, task trainers); progress to immersive, team-based, high-fidelity simulations
4	Faculty development	Train educators in simulation technology, debriefing methods, and inclusive teaching practices; provide ongoing coaching
5	Strengthen institutional capacity	Invest in infrastructure, policies, and QA systems; secure tech support and scheduling/logistics for sustainability
6	Evolve assessment strategies	Combine simulation-based exams, workplace-based assessments, and digital portfolios to capture longitudinal progress

References

1. Alamrani MH, Alammar KA, Alqahtani SS, Salem OA. Comparing the effects of simulation-based and traditional teaching methods on the critical thinking abilities and self-confidence of nursing students. J Nurs Res. 2018;26(3):152–7.
2. Aryuwat P, Holmgren J, Asp M, Radabutr M, Lövenmark A. Experiences of nursing students regarding challenges and support for resilience during clinical education: a qualitative study. Nurs Rep. 2024;14(3):1604–20.
3. Cheng A, Grant V, Eppich W. The PEARLS debriefing checklist—optimal use for faculty development. Simul Healthc. 2024;19(4):265–6.
4. Choi-Lundberg DL, Butler-Henderson K, Harman K, Crawford J. A systematic review of digital innovations in technology-enhanced learning designs in higher education. Australas J Educ Technol. 2023;39(3):133–62.
5. Dubé TV. An imperative for transforming health professions education. Med Educ. 2024;58(1):8–10.
6. Elendu C, Amaechi DC, Okatta AU, Amaechi EC, Elendu TC, Ezeh CP, Elendu ID. The impact of simulation-based training in medical education: a review. Medicine. 2024;103(27):e38813.
7. Flanagan OL, Cummings KM, Cummings K. Standardized patients in medical education: a review of the literature. Cureus. 2023;15(7):e42027.
8. Gottesman L. The history and physical, RIP. Dis Colon Rectum. 2024;67(4):487–90.
9. Hennus MP, van Dam M, Gauthier S, Taylor DR, Ten Cate O. The logic behind entrustable professional activity frameworks: a scoping review of the literature. Med Educ. 2022;56(9):881–91.
10. Kassabry MF. Evaluation of simulation using objective structured clinical examination (OSCE) among undergraduate nursing students: a systematic review. Int J Afr Nurs Sci. 2023;18:100553.
11. Lackey TG, Abaza MM. Is "see one, do one, teach one" the best way to learn procedures? Laryngoscope. 2024;134(1):1–2.
12. Lim AS, Lee SW. Is technology enhanced learning cost-effective to improve skills?: the Monash objective structured clinical examination virtual experience. Simul Healthc. 2022;17(2):131–5.
13. McDonnell JM, Ahern DP, Ross TD, Gibbons D, Synnott KA, Butler JS. The efficacy of remote virtual care in comparison to traditional clinical visits for elective orthopaedic patients: a meta-analysis of prospective randomised controlled trials. Surgeon. 2022;20(3):177–86.
14. Patel H, Perry S, Badu E, Mwangi F, Onifade O, Mazurskyy A, Walters J, Tavener M, Noble D, Chidarikire S, Lethbridge L. A scoping review of interprofessional education in healthcare: evaluating competency development, educational outcomes and challenges. BMC Med Educ. 2025;25(1):409.
15. Pirie J, Fayyaz J, Prinicipi T, Kempinska A, Gharib M, Simone L, Glanfield C, Walsh CM. Impact and effectiveness of a mandatory competency-based simulation program for pediatric emergency medicine faculty. AEM Educ Train. 2023;7(2):e10856.
16. Shahzad S, Anwar MI. Apprenticeship model in 21st century's surgical education: should it perish? Arch Surg Res. 2021;2(3):1–3.
17. Torkaman M, Sabzi A, Farokhzadian J. The effect of patient safety education on undergraduate nursing students' patient safety competencies. Community Health Equity Res Policy. 2022;42(2):219–24.
18. Vashishth TK, Sharma V, Sharma KK, Kumar B, Panwar R, Chaudhary S. AI-driven learning analytics for personalized feedback and assessment in higher education. In: Using traditional design methods to enhance AI-driven decision making. IGI Global Scientific Publishing; 2024. p. 206–30.
19. Watts PI, Rossler K, Bowler F, Miller C, Charnetski M, Decker S, Molloy MA, Persico L, McMahon E, McDermott D, Hallmark B. Onward and upward: introducing the healthcare simulation standards of best practice. Clin Simul Nurs. 2021;58:1–4.

Assessment in the Future Practice of Medical Education

7

Shahid Hassan and Gauhar Hassan

Key Points

- Assessment is moving from fixed cut-off scores toward holistic, longitudinal, workplace-based judgement.
- Competence development and entrustment now outweigh simple pass/fail thresholds.
- EPAs and milestones emphasise authentic performance, learner growth, and professional identity formation.
- Modern systems integrate WBAs, narrative feedback, reflective practice, and AI-supported analytics.
- Future assessment must be robust, fair, and valid while remaining meaningful, compassionate, and growth-oriented.

7.1 Introduction

Assessment has always played a central role in medical education, not only as a means of certification but also as a powerful driver of what and how students learn. Traditionally, assessment has been viewed primarily as summative, focusing on quantifying performance and guiding promotion or licensing decisions; however, this approach has not addressed the problem of diagnostic errors, which occur when a diagnosis is missed, delayed, or incorrect [5]. These high-stakes assessments, which are often standardized

S. Hassan (✉)
School of Medicine, American University of Barbados, Bridgetown, Barbados

G. Hassan
Department of Anatomy, School of Medicine, American University of Barbados, Bridgetown, Barbados

J. Sandars et al. (eds.), *Modern Medical Education*,
https://doi.org/10.1007/978-3-032-27958-3_7

and detached from clinical reality, have defined the boundaries of academic success in medicine for over a century [3]. Yet the practice of medicine is changing rapidly and radically. Healthcare today demands not just knowledgeable graduates but reflective practitioners, effective communicators, ethical decision-makers, and team-based problem solvers. This shift in the profile of the modern physician necessitates a corresponding transformation in how we conceptualize and implement assessment.

Educational paradigms both in pedagogy and assessment are evolving, and a move from a classroom assessment to workplace assessment has become a norm [4]. Competency-Based Medical Education (CBME), entrustable professional activities (EPAs), and professional identity formation (PIF) now shape curriculum design and learner development [1]. Assessment must adapt to support these models not as an afterthought but as an integral, dynamic part of the learning ecosystem. Technology continues to reshape education, with technological pedagogical content knowledge (TPACK) emerging as a dominant framework in response to the educational disruptions caused by COVID-19 [2]. From AI-enhanced scoring systems to virtual patients and simulation-based assessments, tools once seen as futuristic are now increasingly feasible. However, these innovations must be leveraged and thoughtfully aligned with principles of fairness, humanism, and educational value.

In current changing landscape, the traditional metrics of success (test scores, percentiles, and pass/fail thresholds) are no longer sufficient. The future of assessment in medical education must be multifaceted, contextual, and continuous. It must support growth, enable feedback, promote equity, and align with real-world clinical responsibilities. This chapter explores the future practice of assessment in medical education through three interconnected lenses:

(i) First, by defining the guiding principles that should inform any future-oriented assessment system
(ii) Second, by reviewing emerging strategies and technologies that are transforming how learners are evaluated
(iii) Finally, by proposing an original framework for future-ready assessment that integrates identity formation, authenticity, and innovation

The goal is not simply to critique existing systems but to inspire a reimagining of assessment as a powerful tool for shaping competent, compassionate, and trustworthy physicians of the future. This call for transformation is not without precedent. Over the past two decades, thought leaders have emphasized the notion of "assessment for learning," shifting attention from isolated performance snapshots to integrated feedback processes based on programmatic assessment [15]. Similarly, introduction of entrustable professional activities (EPAs) has provided a structured yet flexible framework to bridge competencies with real-world clinical responsibilities [12]. Workplace-based assessment is a central component of competency-based education, emphasizing that professional identity is not developed in classrooms but rather through supervised clinical practice [6].

These scholarly advances, combined with the growing influence of technology, have laid a solid foundation for rethinking assessment. However, despite significant progress in theory, implementation remains fragmented, and many institutions still rely on outdated paradigms that prioritize grades over growth. To move toward a future-ready model of assessment, we must revisit and realign the core principles that underlie our

Table 7.1 The difference between numeric versus narrative models of assessment

Aspect	Numeric/cutoff	Narrative/holistic model
Focus	Scores and pass/fail thresholds	Competency development over time
Measurement	Single numeric grade or cutoff	Multiple data points (scores, feedback, WBAs, portfolios)
Approach	High stakes, episodic exams	Continuous, low-stakes + high-stakes blend
Feedback	Minimal, often summative only	Rich, narrative feedback and coaching
Outcome	Gatekeeping (pass/fail decision)	Meaningful learner growth and progression

assessment philosophies and practices. These principles must embrace complexity, foster equity, promote feedback-rich learning, and respond to the needs of both learners and the health systems they serve. The next section outlines these guiding principles, cornerstones upon which a sustainable and transformative assessment culture can be built in medical education. These principles will serve as both a critique of the limitations of traditional assessment and a road map for designing assessments that are authentic, inclusive, and developmental by nature. Assessment today goes beyond numeric cutoffs; it integrates scores, feedback, and observed competencies into a holistic, programmatic model that supports meaningful learner growth and progression (see Table 7.1).

7.2 Principles Guiding Future Assessment in Medical Education

Assessment in the future practice of medical education must be guided by foundational principles that address the complexity of clinical competence, the evolving identity of the physician, and the dynamic nature of healthcare delivery [7]. These principles indicate a clear move beyond measurement toward mentorship and beyond evaluation toward evolution. Outlined below are the key principles that should shape the design, implementation, and evolution of future-ready assessment systems.

7.2.1 Competency Alignment

Future assessment should be aligned with the competency frameworks of a twenty-first-century healthcare professional, such as CanMEDS or ACGME core competencies, or locally adapted models with two important aspects addressed:

(i) Assessments should move beyond factual recall to encompass communication, collaboration, professionalism, and systems-based practice.
(ii) Integration with entrustable professional activities (EPAs) and milestones supports meaningful judgment on readiness for practice [1].

7.2.2 Continuity and Programmatic Design

Instead of fragmented and episodic exams, assessment should be longitudinal and consistent [15] and should include the following:

(i) Frequent, low-stakes formative assessments with just-in-time feedback should support high-stakes decisions.
(ii) Faculty as assessment coaches, not just judges in an assigned role of assessors.

7.2.3 Authenticity and Contextual Relevance

Assessments must reflect the real-world problem of day-to-day medical practice as under:

(i) Analytic reasoning, ethical dilemmas, communication skills, and procedural competence should be tested as an occupational job than segmented stations.
(ii) Simulations and workplace-based and narrative assessment should be aligned with authentic tasks.

7.2.4 Learner-Centeredness and Personalization

Assessment should consider learners as active participants and not in a passive role of show-how, ensuring the following practice:

(i) Learners should engage in self-assessment and peer assessment enabling personalized assessment with reflective practice prior to external rating.
(ii) Simulation technology prior to authentic assessment allowing high-tech fidelity helps in building the confidence to examine real patients.

7.2.5 Equity, Inclusivity, and Fairness

Future assessments should address inequities and promote inclusive excellence by taking care the following:

(i) Assessment be designed to avoid cultural, linguistic, or contextual biases
(ii) Multiple formats of oral, written, and visual simulation to fit in trainees' learning styles

7.2.6 Feedback-Rich and Formative by Default

Feedback must shift from being an afterthought to a primary function of assessment, checking out for two important facts:

(i) Specific, timely, and actionable feedback to guide improvement
(ii) Emphasis on narrative feedback over numeric scoring to support deep learning

7.2.7 Technology-Enabled but Human-Driven

While digital tools and AI can enhance assessment, they must support, not replace, the human elements [9] for two obvious reasons:

(i) AI can assist with scoring, pattern recognition, and early alerts.
(ii) However, human judgment, empathy, and narrative interpretation remain irreplaceable.

7.2.8 Transparency and Trustworthiness

Future assessment systems must be transparent in purpose, criteria, and outcomes as under:

(i) Learners should understand how they are being assessed and why.
(ii) Trust is built through consistency, clarity, and collaboration between learners and educators.

These guiding principles in assessment become an engine of growth rather than a gatekeeper of progress [11].

7.3 Emerging Assessment Approaches

The future of assessment in medical education is shifting away from episodic high-stakes summative examinations to periodic longitudinal formative assessment diluting the rigid boundaries between the two in a holistic and context-rich evaluation. These emerging approaches view assessment as a means to demonstrate competence in real-world contexts, support the formation of professional identity, and provide data-informed feedback, all aimed at fostering learners' growth. The following strategies may redefine how we must assess learners in the twenty-first century.

7.3.1 Programmatic Assessment: A System of Continuous Feedback

Programmatic assessment is more of a philosophy than a method, where assessment is embedded throughout the curriculum monitoring continuous improvement [15] for the following reasons:

(i) Multiple and overtime low-stakes assessments for informed and collective high-stakes decisions.
(ii) Every data point seamlessly moved from simulation to workplace-based assessments, reflections, and peer feedback is collected in a learner's portfolio.
(iii) Narrative feedback takes precedence over the numeric grades, encouraging learner reflection and growth.

(iv) Teachers in a coaching and then assessing role allow students to pair with a faculty to help interpret feedback and guide their learning growth.

This approach documents learner progression while fostering a culture of assessment for learning, not just assessment of learning.

7.3.2 Workplace-Based Assessment (WPBA): Observing Authentic Performance

Workplace-based assessment (WPBA) captures learning opportunities at the bedside, in clinics, and during interprofessional ward rounds using a variety of learning and assessment approaches like hypothetico-deductive and think aloud and problem-based inquiry strategies as under:

(i) Mini-clinical evaluation exercise (Mini-CEX): A brief observed encounter followed by immediate feedback
(ii) Direct observation of procedural skills (DOPS): Real-time evaluation of technical tasks defined as competency
(iii) Case-based discussion (CbD): Assesses clinical reasoning through overtime patient clinical care
(iv) Multisource feedback (MSF): Multiple feedback from peers, nurses, patients, and supervisors to evaluate interprofessional and communication skills

Technology-incorporated WPBA uses mobile apps and digital logbooks, allowing assessors to document behaviors, rate performance, and tag competencies to EPAs, providing rich, longitudinal data.

7.3.3 Narrative Feedback and Reflective Practice

Numeric scores often miss subtle aspects of performance, whereas narrative feedback enables educators to provide detailed comments on qualities such as empathy, ethical reasoning, and critical thinking, which are essential for the development of professional identity as under:

(i) Narrative assessment tools support holistic judgments, moving the focus beyond pass/fail to cultivating precise areas of improvement to produce confident doctors whom the community can trust.
(ii) Reflective portfolios empower self-directed learning to enable students to monitor learning, identify gaps, and reset learning objectives.
(iii) Feedback and reflection are the core skills that support lifelong learning, clinical judgment, and professional identity

Educators trained in coaching and narrative writing become essential components of faculty development in assessment.

7.3.4 Technology-Enhanced Assessment

The future of assessment is evolving through the integration of technological pedagogical and content knowledge (TPACK). Embedding a TPACK framework in the curriculum can enhance efficiency, personalize learning, and improve authenticity.

7.3.4.1 Artificial Intelligence and Learning Analytics

(i) AI-driven adaptive testing adjusts difficulty in real time to better evaluate depth of knowledge.
(ii) Natural language processing (NLP) can score open-ended responses, track sentiment in reflections, and analyze narrative feedback for themes.
(iii) Predictive analytics identify struggling learners earlier, enabling just-in-time remediation in offering them probation and decelerated program to coup up.

7.3.4.2 Simulation-Based Assessment

(i) High-fidelity simulations with embedded sensors assess procedural accuracy, decision-making, and teamwork.
(ii) Virtual medical clinics, simulated patients, and branching scenarios challenge learners with real-world ambiguity.
(iii) Simulations are ideal for evaluating crisis management, rare conditions, and ethical dilemmas without risking patient safety.

7.3.4.3 Digital Dashboards and Portfolios

(i) Interactive dashboards visualize performance across time, competency domains, and feedback trends.
(ii) Learners' portfolios while contributing artifacts like videos, reflections, annotated case logs, and feedback receiving and responding evidence.

7.3.5 Self-Assessment, Peer Assessment, and Group Assessment: Building Metacognition and Collegiality

Future-ready assessment engages learners as partners, not passive recipients; encouraging self-assessment and peer assessment fosters the following:

(i) Metacognitive skills: Learners become aware of their own factual and procedural knowledge and how they think and reason to act upon conditional knowledge demands.
(ii) Accountability: Peer feedback reinforces professional standards and shared responsibility.
(iii) Collaborative professionalism**:** In team-based learning such as group readiness assurance test (GRAT), learners assess team dynamics and shared clinical reasoning.

These approaches cultivate lifelong habits essential for team-based healthcare delivery and assessment.

7.3.6 Entrustment-Based Decisions and EPA-Aligned Assessment

Traditional numeric scores often fail to abide by real-world decisions on trainees' performance. EPAs offer a way to make judgment more meaningful in rating the trainees' performance. It acts as a road map for both trainees and supervisor, who typically uses five levels of entrustment toward independence. An assessor determines the level of supervision required to execute a task:

Level 1: Observation, not execution—A trainee observes a supervisor perform but does not execute even under supervision.

Level 2: Direct proactive supervision—A trainee performs a basic task assigned in EPA, and a supervisor observes and actively guides each step.

Level 3: Indirect reactive supervision—The trainee performs the task independently, but a supervisor is readily available nearby to call upon.

Level 4: Independent practice—The trainee is trusted to perform the task independently without a supervision; however, the trainee reports to a supervisor in the premises.

Level 5: Supervising others—A senior trainee trusted to supervise a junior trainee has achieved the level of mastery.

7.4 Assessment for Lifelong Learning and Professional Identity Formation

The ultimate aim of medical education is not only to produce graduates but also to develop professionals who are capable of continuing learning, ethical decision-making, and adaptive expertise. Assessment must therefore move beyond evaluating static competencies to more dynamic lifelong learning behavior and the development of a professional identity [10].

7.4.1 Lifelong Learning: Assessment as a Developmental Process

As medicine is evolving rapidly, technologies, therapies, disease patterns, and systems of management demand physicians to be updated with current knowledge and skills. Future assessment must prepare learners to do the following:

(i) Self-assess to identify knowledge or skill gaps.
(ii) Seek feedback purposefully and act upon it.
(iii) Engage in a reflective practice and response.
(iv) Adapt to uncertainty and unpredictable changes ahead.

Traditional high-stakes examinations therefore require a shift toward formative, low-stakes, feedback-rich assessments prominently with self-regulatory skills needed for lifelong learning as:

(i) Reflective writing and debriefing integrated into clinical education for action
(ii) Goal-setting and learning plans as part of mentorship or coaching programs
(iii) Use of digital portfolios to track growth and learning evidence overtime
(iv) Opportunities for learners to revise, retry, and resubmit in real-world learning cycles

7.4.2 Professional Identity Formation: Beyond Competency Checklists

Professional identity formation (PIF) refers to the internalization of an affective process by which learners value new knowledge. While competency frameworks describe what learners must do, PIF focuses on who learners are becoming [10]. Assessment that supports PIF must be:

(i) Narrative than numeric based on assessment
(ii) Longitudinal and developmental in growth
(iii) Mentoring and coaching in supervising role
(iv) Reflective in real-life clinical experiences

7.4.3 Feedback as a Mirror and Motivator

In above examples of lifelong learning and PIF, feedback is the linchpin; however, not every feedback is useful. Assessment in the future must ensure the following:

(i) Feedback is timely, specific, actionable, and emotionally engaging.
(ii) Learners are trained how to receive and respond to feedback constructively.
(iii) Feedback processes are part of curriculum and not treated as informal or anecdotal.

Feedback, to be functional, depends on how well it is given and received. Reflecting on feedback serves as both a mirror and a motivator. Technology and AI-assisted reports on learner's progress may not establish the relationship as human aspect of feedback will always do.

7.4.4 The Role of Coaching and Mentorship

Learner and supervisor relationships are imperative to sustainable growth that provides continuity, accountability, and support. Assessment data must be embedded within a coaching framework [8] where faculty:

(i) Help learners make sense of data.
(ii) Co-create learning plans.
(iii) Scaffold the integration of competence.

Assessment therefore becomes not an endpoint but a partner in supporting the lifelong learning physician. By aligning assessment with lifelong learning and professional identity formation, medical education can produce physicians who are fit to practice today and committed to evolving for tomorrow.

7.5 Challenges and Ethical Considerations

A range of practical, systemic, and ethical challenges in assessment in medical education evolves as it embraces technology, narrative feedback, and identity formation [14]. To keep assessment equitable, sustainable, and trustworthy, these challenges must be addressed with care to ensure that future assessment systems work well.

7.5.1 Balancing Data and Humanity

Incorporating technology into pedagogy has also enhanced assessments. AI-driven feedback and learning analytics are the examples. The most significant advantages are scalability and personalization. However, they also risk reducing learners to data points or reinforcing bias through flawed algorithms [16]:

(i) How can educators ensure that data informs but does not replace human judgment?
(ii) How do we balance efficiency with empathy and precision with mentorship?

Future assessment must remain human-driven, using technology as a support rather than a substitute.

7.5.2 Subjectivity and Bias in Narrative Assessment

Narrative assessment and workplace-based observation are more valid and contextualized; they remain subjective:

(i) Biases related to race, gender, accent, and personality can unintentionally shape faculty judgments.
(ii) Learners from underrepresented backgrounds may be disproportionately affected by implicit biases in narrative comments or entrustment decisions.

Institution's investment in faculty development, standard-setting, item analysis, and reflective practices may reduce inconsistency and promote fairness.

7.5.3 Faculty Burden and Burnout

Innovative assessment system demands time and effort from faculty, close observations, comprehensive feedback, mentoring, and coaching. No doubt valuable, these can put more pressure on clinicians and educators to question the following:

(i) How can institutions support the faculty involvement in meaningful assessment?
(ii) Can technology reduce the load without compromising the quality of interaction?

7.5.4 Learner Anxiety and Assessment Fatigue

An increased number of assessment even if low stakes can create a sense of increasing workload:

(i) Learners may feel overwhelmed, particularly if feedback is poorly framed.
(ii) High-performing students may experience static or nonlinear progress.

To overcome this, learners must be well oriented with the purpose and philosophy of programmatic assessment and the supportive role of feedback in building resilience.

7.5.5 Ethical Use of Assessment Data

Vast amounts of assessment data especially using digital platforms though raise concerns about data ownership and privacy should be used for indigenous research. Institution must decide the following:

(i) Who controls the learner's performance data?
(ii) How is it used in decisions (progression, remediation)?
(iii) Are learner's consent obtained over the use of data?

Ethical policies must address consent, transparency, and data governance to protect learners and build trust.

7.5.6 Institutional Inertia and Resistance to Change

One of the most significant barriers is the cultural resistance to historical practice of assessment reforms:

(i) Institutions with traditional grading systems may resist to adopt narrative, formative, or entrustment-based competency models.
(ii) Integrated learners and faculty provided with assessment blueprint reduces resistance to adopt to newer approaches.
(iii) The recommendations for good assessment must consider some essential key elements to ethical practice (see Fig. 7.1).

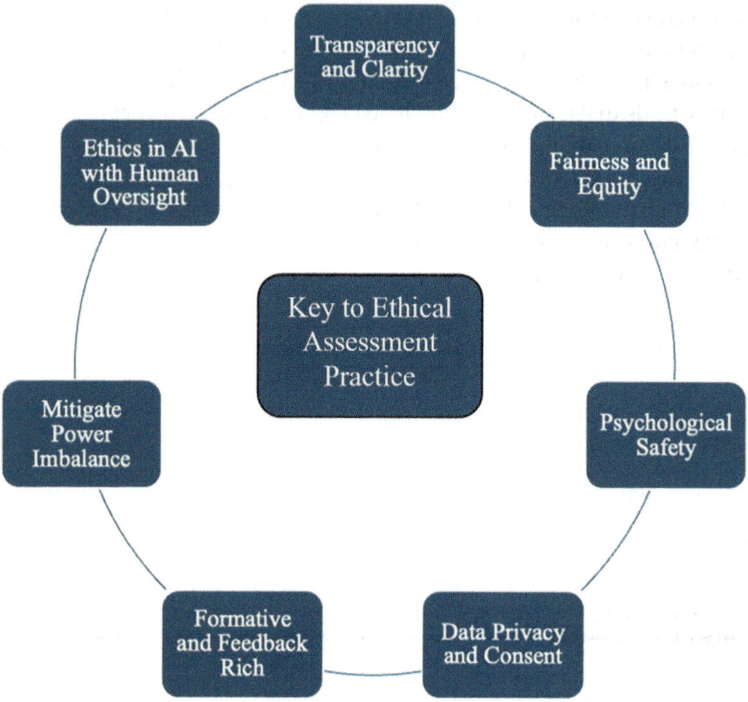

Fig. 7.1 The key recommendations for ethical assessment practice

7.6 A Proposed Framework for Future-Oriented Assessment in Medical Education

For meeting the evolving healthcare landscape needs assessment, medical education must evolve from a system of numeric measures to a system of narrative meaning with humanistic and technological support toward lifelong professionals. A learner-centered and technology-enhanced competency-driven assessment model must be reimagined beyond a measure of performance to a continuous process of growth, reflection, and professional formation. Having discussed the trends and the precedented challenges, we propose a conceptual model of FIRST assessment framework grounded in educational philosophy of reflection, competency context, trust, and growth keeping with ethical and technological imperatives of modern practice (see Fig. 7.2).

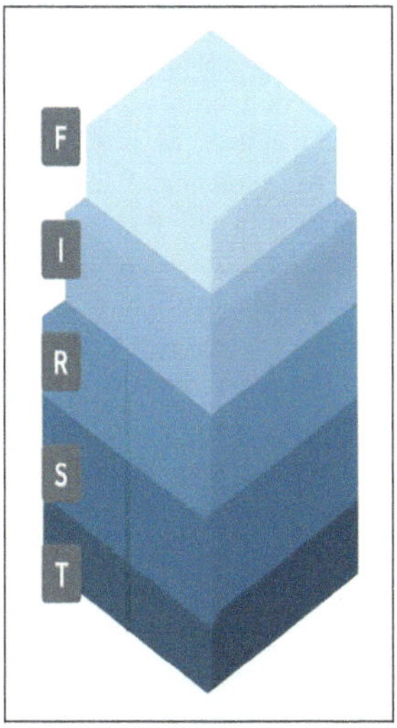

Formative Feedback Culture:
Assessment as ongoing learning provided with just-in-time narrative feedback that prompts reflection for corrective measure and improvement.

Integrated Professional Identity:
Assessment that promotes professional identity through tracking and documenting behaviour, attitude and values and not just the task accomplished by numeric ratting.

Real-world Learning Experience:
Real world experiential and authentic learning that incorporates context, test of prior knowledge, experience, reflection, feedback that leads to new learning

Smart Technology Support:
Incorporate AI, digital portfolio, simulations and data analytics that provides scalable, personalized learning and assessment preserved with human supervision.

Trust-based Entrustment of Competence:
Moving from number-based passing score to proactive rating and entrustment of EPAs observed through milestones for attainment of competency towards independent practice.

Fig. 7.2 The FIRST (formative, integrated identity, real-world, smart-tech trust-based entrustment) assessment framework

7.6.1 Positioning the FIRST Model in Theory

This framework is rooted in the following:

(i) Constructivist philosophy: Meaningful and experiential construct of competence through reflection and mentorship.
(ii) Humanistic Constructivism: Learners are guided by meaningful feedback and reflection in a personal, developmental journey and not an endpoint.
(iii) Developmental Epistemology: Competence is not a binary option but a dynamic change evolving through stages of capability provided with structured coaching and real-world practice.
(iv) Narrative Ethics: Learners' growth best captured in narrative rooted in context, storyboarding, and reflection, not just numeric scores.

7.6.2 Implementation Considerations

To personalize the FIRST framework, institutions must:

(i) Develop faculty in feedback, narrative assessment, and coaching to identify areas of improvement.
(ii) Invest in digital platforms that support e-portfolio data visualization and workplace observations.
(iii) Respect learner autonomy through self-assessment, goal-setting, and reflective practice.
(iv) Build trust with entrustment of transparency, equity, and clearly aligned learning outcomes.

Table 7.2 A comparative study of current versus the future assessment in medical education

Dimension	Current assessment practices	Future-oriented assessment
Primary purpose	Grading, ranking, gatekeeping, and certification	Growth, reflection, professional identity, and readiness for practice
Nature	High-stakes, episodic, and predominantly summative	Continuous, developmental, feedback-rich, and predominantly formative
Focus	Knowledge recall and discrete competencies	EPAs-based competencies integrated with professional identity formation
Format	Classroom exams (MCQs, SEQs) and standardized OSCEs	Programmatic assessment, portfolios, workplace-based assessments, EPAs
Feedback	Limited, delayed, often numeric	Timely, narrative, dialogic, actionable
Technology use	Test delivery platforms with or without automated scoring	Data analytics, AI adaptive testing, simulations, digital portfolios
Evaluator's role	Judge or examiner	Coach, mentor, co-learner
Learner's role	Passive recipient, numeric score no specific area of improvement	Active role, self-assessor, reflective practitioner, area of improvement
Ethical concerns	Stress, inequities, and limited transparency	Data privacy, fairness, balancing tech with human judgment
Outcome orientation	Passing exams, meeting minimal standards on onetime assessment	Lifelong learning, trust-based entrustment, adaptability in practice

The FIRST model is a holistic, future-oriented approach to assessment that honors both the science and art of competence physician. It centers learners, leverages technology, and prioritizes human oversight. Reimagine medical education for the decades ahead; it seems essential to assess not just what students know but also who they are becoming. A comparative study of current assessment practice versus future-oriented assessment practice is summarized below (see Table 7.2).

7.7 Conclusion and Call to Action

There has been a paradigm shift in medical education assessment from a fixed, summative, and numerical approach to one that is developmental, meaningful, and future-oriented. As the current chapter has outlined, the future of assessment is meeting the complexity of clinical practice, the expectations of community, and the educational needs assessment of tomorrow's healthcare professionals. Assessment in future practice will not be a measure of competence at a single point in time but a continuous evolution of learner from novice to a competent, compassionate, and professional physician. Assessment must be anchored in values, defined for purpose, and powered by technology indeed with human supervision.

The FIRST assessment framework offers a pathway to fostering (F) formative feedback culture, (I) integrated with professional identity formation, (R) real-world authenticity being assured, (S) smart technologies support leveraging, and (T)

trust-based entrustment decision. This framework aims to bridge the gap between educational ideals and practical realities that institution must vision to materialize.

The transformation of assessment should not be optional but essential. Faced with challenges of complexity, diversity, and unpredictability in global health systems, our assessment systems must evolve accordingly. Let this chapter be a starting point for a deeper insight with local innovation and global collaboration. However, time has come to move beyond traditional numeric rating and static checklists to an era of assessment that is dynamic and human-centered, aiming to produce fit-to-practice physicians.

References

1. Bremer AE, van de Pol MHJ, Laan RFJM, et al. How an EPA-based curriculum supports professional identity formation. BMC Med Educ. 2022;22:48. https://doi.org/10.1186/s12909-022-03116-0.
2. Dhurumraj T, Ramaila SM, Raban F. Transforming Assessment in Response to COVID-19. In: Mawela A, van Wyk M, Lebeloane L, Mudau A, editors. Investigating the roles of school management teams in curriculum delivery. IGI Global Scientific Publishing; 2021. p. 246–65. https://doi.org/10.4018/978-1-7998-7168-2.ch016.
3. Gliatto P, Leitman IM, Muller D. Scylla and Charybdis: The MCAT, USMLE, and degrees of freedom in undergraduate medical education. Acad Med. 2016;91(11):1498–500. https://doi.org/10.1097/ACM.0000000000001247.
4. Hodges B. Assessment in the post-psychometric era: learning to love the subjective and collective. Med Teach. 2013;35(7):564–8. https://doi.org/10.3109/0142159X.2013.789134.
5. Holmboe ES, Durning SJ. Assessing clinical reasoning: moving from in vitro to in vivo. Diagnosis. 2014;1(1):111–7. https://doi.org/10.1515/dx-2013-0029.
6. Holmboe ES, Sherbino J, Long DM, Swing SR, Frank JR. The role of assessment in competency-based medical education. Med Teach. 2010;32(8):676–82. https://doi.org/10.3109/0142159X.2010.500704.
7. Holmboe ES, Osman NY, Murphy CM, Kogan JR. The urgency of now: rethinking and improving assessment practices in medical education programs. Acad Med. 2023;98(8S):S37–49. https://doi.org/10.1097/ACM.0000000000005251.
8. Lee A, Jere A, Du Plessis L, Van Gerven PWM, Heeneman S, Ross S. Continuity of supervision: balancing continuous and episodic relationships for assessment and learning. Med Educ. 2025;59(6):596–605. https://doi.org/10.1111/medu.15595.
9. Perla L, Vinci V. Enhancing authentic assessment in higher education: leveraging digital transformation and Artificial Intelligence (short paper). Published in AIxEDU@AI*IA, Computer Science Education; 2014. https://api.semanticscholar.org/CorpusID:266965409
10. Sawatsky AP, Huffman BM, Hafferty FW. Coaching versus competency to facilitate professional identity formation. Acad Med. 2020;95(10):1511–4. https://doi.org/10.1097/ACM.0000000000003144.
11. Stables K. Assessment: feedback from our pasts, feedforward for our futures. In: Williams P, Jones A, Buntting C, editors. The future of technology education. Contemporary issues in technology education. Singapore: Springer; 2015. https://doi.org/10.1007/978-981-287-170-1_7.
12. ten Cate O. Entrustability of professional activities and competency-based training. Med Educ. 2005;39:1176–7. https://doi.org/10.1111/j.1365-2929.2005.02341.x.
13. ten Cate O. Competency-based medical education. In: Cockerham WC, Dingwall R, Quah S, editors. The Wiley-Blackwell encyclopaedia of health, illness, behavior, and society. Hoboken: Wiley; 2014. p. 1329–35.

14. Turner L, Hashimoto DA, Vasisht S, Schaye V. Demystifying AI: current state and future role in medical education assessment. Acad Med. 2024;99(4S):S42–7. https://doi.org/10.1097/ACM.0000000005598.
15. Van der Vleuten CPM, Schuwirth LWT. Assessing professional competence: from methods to programmes. Med Educ. 2005;39:309–17. https://doi.org/10.1111/j.1365-2929.2005.02094.x.
16. Zhang X. Fairness and effectiveness in AI-driven educational assessments: challenges and mitigation strategies. J Innov Dev. 2025;11(1):7–10. https://doi.org/10.54097/adcxze3.

8 Non-Technical Skills in Health Professions Education: Foundations, Pedagogy, and Evaluation

Muhammad Zafar Iqbal, Jabeen Fayyaz, and Gohar Wajid

Key Points

- Non-technical skills are inseparable from technical expertise and directly influence patient safety and outcomes.
- Experiential and simulation-based methods are highly effective for teaching non-technical skills.
- Multiple complementary assessment tools (such as OSCEs, portfolios, workplace-based methods, programmatic assessment, and digital innovations) can help in capturing the complexity of non-technical skills assessment.
- Contextualizing global frameworks within local, cultural, and institutional contexts strengthens teaching, assessment, and curricular integration of non-technical skills.
- Common challenges (such as limited faculty capacity, cultural barriers, and misalignment of assessment) can be addressed through institutional commitment, faculty development, and structured integration of non-technical skills into curricula and accreditation standards.

M. Z. Iqbal (✉)
Research Department, Acuity Insights, Toronto, ON, Canada

Department of Medical Education, University College of Medicine and Dentistry, The University of Lahore, Lahore, Pakistan

J. Fayyaz
Department of Pediatrics, Division of Emergency Medicine, The Hospital for Sick Children, University of Toronto, Toronto, ON, Canada

G. Wajid
Visiting Faculty, Health Professions Education, The University of Lahore, Lahore, Pakistan

J. Sandars et al. (eds.), *Modern Medical Education*,
https://doi.org/10.1007/978-3-032-27958-3_8

8.1 Introduction

In contemporary healthcare, non-technical skills (most commonly labeled skills include communication, teamwork, leadership, situational awareness, decision-making, self-regulation, empathy, ethics, and professionalism) are not merely adjunctive but foundational to safe, effective, and compassionate care. Increasingly complex healthcare systems, shaped by accelerating technological advances, expanding knowledge bases, and societal demands, further underscore the need for health professionals who embody these skills [1]. What distinguishes exceptional health professionals today is their capacity to communicate clearly, act with integrity, collaborate ethically, and navigate uncertainty with empathy and sound judgment. Far from being "soft skills," these competencies ensure care is ethically grounded, contextually adaptive, and deeply human.

A growing body of literature underscores the critical impact of non-technical skills on patient safety and team performance. For instance, non-technical skills training in intensive care units has been shown to significantly improve teamwork, situational awareness, leadership, and communication while also reducing response times in emergencies, as well as adjusting mortality and complication rates [2]. Similarly, a systematic review highlights how simulation-based experiences in interprofessional healthcare teams enhance both technical and non-technical skills, fostering better collaborative practice [3]. Beyond isolated interventions, broader reviews reveal that non-technical skills are often intertwined with technical performance. A recent scoping review found a positive correlation between technical and non-technical skills across multiple studies, suggesting that separating them in training design may not reflect their interdependence in practice [4].

Framing these skills within the discourse of health professions education (HPE), scholars argue that non-technical skills represent one of the greatest challenges facing contemporary HPE. They note that the complexity of modern healthcare, expanding knowledge demands, and the rise of technology and automation mean that the distinctive value clinicians bring lies in their mastery of human factors and non-technical capacities [1].

Together, these insights position non-technical skills not as peripheral extras but as vital pillars of competent practice. This chapter seeks to reposition non-technical skills at the core of HPE by examining their conceptual foundations and historical evolution, outlining practical strategies for their sustained integration into HPE curricula, and reviewing current approaches to teaching and assessment.

8.1.1 Conceptual Foundations of Non-technical Skills in Health Professions Education

Non-technical skills are commonly defined as "the cognitive, social, and personal resource skills that complement technical skills and contribute to safe and efficient task performance" [5]. Insights from psychology, human factors, and safety sciences have played a pivotal role in shaping the recognition of non-technical skills in

HPE. While technical expertise enables practitioners to perform clinical procedures, non-technical skills determine whether these procedures are carried out effectively, safely, professionally, and in ways that align with patient needs. In many ways, the conceptual foundation of non-technical skills rests on the understanding that healthcare is delivered in complex, dynamic systems where errors are rarely the result of a single technical lapse but rather stem from breakdowns in coordination, awareness, and interpersonal processes [1].

Early models in HPE have drawn heavily from the aviation industry, where structured training in crew resource management demonstrated that errors could be significantly reduced when pilots were explicitly trained in interpersonal and cognitive skills. This transfer of knowledge into healthcare led to the development of specialized frameworks for non-technical skills, such as the Anesthetists' Non-technical Skills (ANTS) system, the Non-technical Skills for Surgeons (NOTSS) taxonomy, and the Scrub Practitioners' List of Intraoperative Non-technical Skills (SPLINTS). Collectively, these frameworks provided structured taxonomies of observable behaviors for health professionals, offering educators a way to conceptualize skills that had previously been regarded as "implicit" or "soft" and lending legitimacy to their inclusion in curricula and assessment systems [6].

More recent approaches have sought to capture the dynamic and context-sensitive nature of non-technical skills. As an example, the SCOPE (Social and Cognitive Skills in Medical Education) model organizes non-technical skills into two broad domains (social and cognitive) and emphasizes their interplay during clinical tasks and learning encounters. By highlighting how the relative weight of non-technical skills shifts depending on the situation, SCOPE provides educators with a flexible yet structured conceptual tool for teaching and evaluation [7].

The theoretical underpinnings of non-technical skills also align closely with sociocultural learning theories. Vygotskian perspectives emphasize that learning occurs in interaction with others, mediated through language, collaboration, and shared problem-solving. In clinical education, this means that the way learners communicate, negotiate roles, and reflect on experiences is as critical to their development as the technical knowledge they acquire. Similarly, theories of experiential learning highlight that non-technical skills are best developed in authentic or simulated practice environments, where learners can engage in deliberate practice, receive feedback, and reflect on their performance.

Empirical research supports the value of deliberately teaching non-technical skills within HPE. A meta-analysis of educational interventions found significant improvements in communication, leadership, teamwork, situational awareness, and decision-making among healthcare professionals following structured training programs [8]. These findings suggest that non-technical skills are not fixed innate traits and can be developed through intentional pedagogical strategies. Furthermore, evidence indicates that improvements in non-technical skills positively influence technical performance, reinforcing the notion that clinical competence cannot be separated into purely technical and non-technical domains [4].

Conceptually, non-technical skills in HPE can be understood as essential enablers of safe, adaptive, and patient-centered practice. They derive legitimacy from cross-disciplinary evidence, are grounded in human factors theory, and are supported by emerging educational models that translate abstract competencies into observable behaviors. The conceptual foundations establish not only why non-technical skills matter but also how they can be systematically approached in the design of curricula and assessments. By embedding these concepts into the fabric of professional training, HPE can move beyond treating non-technical skills as peripheral attributes and instead recognize them as core dimensions of professional identity and practice.

8.2 Historical Evolution of Non-technical Skills

Throughout most of the last century, traditional apprenticeship-based model curricula had informal, implicit approaches to teaching non-technical skills with almost nonexistent formal methods of instruction or assessment. During the latter half of the century, pressures for reform in HPE began to highlight the need for more systematic attention to the behavioral and social sciences. By the 1980s, several reports in the United Kingdom and the United States had called for a broader definition of competence, signaling a shift from implicit apprenticeship learning toward a more structured educational design.

Although Competency-Based Medical Education (CBME) began taking root in the late 1970s, the 1990s marked a decisive turning point with the emergence of competency frameworks that explicitly defined non-technical skills as integral to professional practice. In 1996, the Royal College of Physicians and Surgeons of Canada launched the *CanMEDS framework* that identified roles such as communicator, collaborator, and professional as essential to medical competence. This framework was subsequently integrated into accreditation standards, training objectives, examination blueprints, and maintenance of certification programs. CanMEDS thus institutionalized non-technical skills as foundational components of professional identity and practice. In the United States, the Accreditation Council for Graduate Medical Education established its six core competencies, including interpersonal and communication skills, professionalism, and practice-based learning, in the late 1990s. These competencies formed the backbone of graduate medical education and remain central to accreditation and evaluation frameworks. The United Kingdom followed suit with frameworks such as *Tomorrow's Doctors* and the *Outcomes for Graduates* guidelines issued by the General Medical Council. These documents embedded professionalism, communication, ethics, and teamwork as expected graduate outcomes across the continuum of medical education.

Parallel developments unfolded across multiple global jurisdictions. The World Federation for Medical Education's global standards included ethics, professionalism, and cultural competence as key areas. Frameworks such as *Good Medical Practice* in the United Kingdom, *SaudiMEDS* in Saudi Arabia, and the *Seven Star Doctor* framework in Pakistan have further integrated non-technical skills into national competency models. Similarly, the World Health Organization's global competency and outcome framework for universal health coverage emphasized attributes such as ethics, cultural competence, and collaboration. Collectively, these frameworks reflect a global consensus: non-technical skills are essential to health-care delivery and must be systematically integrated into training curricula, explicitly taught, and assessed.

8.3 Integrating Non-technical Skills into Health Professions Curricula

The integration of non-technical skills into curricula represents one of the most significant shifts in HPE over the past three decades. Skills such as communication, teamwork, professionalism, cultural competence, and ethical reasoning are increasingly recognized as central to professional identity formation and patient safety, requiring deliberate curricular design, alignment with assessment strategies, and reinforcement throughout the educational continuum.

Historically, non-technical skills have often been introduced as isolated courses in ethics or communication, treated as add-ons rather than integral components of the curriculum. Effective embedding of non-technical skills requires both horizontal and vertical integration. Horizontally, these skills should be addressed across multiple subject areas, for instance, linking communication to clinical skills teaching, teamwork to simulation-based practice, ethics to case-based learning, and professionalism to bedside teaching. Vertically, these skills must be reinforced and integrated across preclinical, clinical, and postgraduate stages, with learners encountering increasingly complex challenges that mirror their expanding responsibilities, for instance, early training may focus on basic doctor-patient communication, while clinical clerkships require navigating interprofessional dynamics, and postgraduate training emphasizes leadership and conflict resolution.

Interprofessional education (IPE) has been especially influential in embedding non-technical skills. The World Health Organization identified IPE as a foundation for collaborative practice, and many medical, nursing, and allied health programs now provide shared learning opportunities. At a curricular level, IPE ensures that learners engage with peers from other disciplines throughout training, fostering mutual respect and preparing them for team-based care.

Finally, the competency frameworks (discussed earlier in this chapter) provide a blueprint for embedding non-technical skills in curricula. By aligning local curricula with competency frameworks, institutions ensure that graduates meet both national and international standards of professional practice.

Despite progress, integrating non-technical skills into curricula is not without challenges. The hidden curriculum (informal lessons conveyed through institutional culture, role modelling, and workplace behaviors) can undermine formal teaching if learners observe inconsistency between what is taught and what is practiced. Faculty development is another critical issue: educators must be equipped not only to teach these skills but also to model them consistently. In addition, cultural context adds further complexity and influences how concepts such as professionalism or hierarchy are interpreted, requiring local contextualization of global frameworks.

8.4 Teaching Non-technical Skills

Teaching non-technical skills in HPE requires deliberate pedagogical strategies that move beyond traditional lectures. Because skills such as communication, teamwork, professionalism, cultural competence, and ethical decision-making are relational and context-dependent, they are best developed through active, experiential, and reflective approaches. Over the past three decades, educators have developed structured instructional designs that not only enable learners to practice these skills but also enable them to reflect critically on their professional development.

8.4.1 Experiential and Simulation-Based Learning

Experiential learning theory emphasizes that learners acquire professional capabilities most effectively by doing, reflecting, and applying knowledge in new contexts. Simulation has evolved as one of the most powerful modalities for teaching non-technical skills. High-fidelity patient simulators, standardized patients, and virtual reality environments provide safe and controlled settings in which learners can practice teamwork, leadership, communication, and error management. Structured debriefings following simulation are critical, as they allow participants to process their emotions, receive feedback, explore and understand mental frames, and integrate lessons into their future practice. Interprofessional simulation sessions further extend these benefits by enabling students from medicine, nursing, pharmacy, and allied health to rehearse collaborative practice in realistic team environments. However, high-fidelity simulation setups might be expensive for educational settings with limited resources.

8.4.2 Case-Based and Problem-Based Learning

Case-based and problem-based learning are widely used to foster ethical reasoning, professional judgment, and collaborative decision-making. Small-group discussions centered on authentic clinical dilemmas enable learners to analyze complex situations, weigh competing values, and articulate their reasoning. These methods also model collaborative learning by encouraging students to appreciate diverse perspectives and work together to negotiate solutions. Embedding professionalism, ethical reasoning, collaboration, and communication objectives into routine case discussions reinforces the message that non-technical skills are integral to clinical reasoning, not separate from it. We discuss some of the most effective teaching methods below.

8.4.3 Reflective Practice and Narrative Medicine

Reflection is a cornerstone of teaching non-technical skills because it promotes self-awareness, empathy, and moral reasoning. Reflective journals, guided writing exercises, and learning portfolios encourage learners to examine their responses to challenging situations critically. Narrative medicine approaches, such as analyzing literature, writing personal stories, or engaging in creative arts, help students cultivate attentiveness to patients' experiences and their own professional growth. When supported by skilled faculty feedback, these exercises nurture self-awareness, motivation, and resilience and contribute to professional identity formation.

8.4.4 Role Modeling

Non-technical skills are also taught and learned informally through role modelling and the hidden curriculum. Learners keenly observe how clinicians communicate with patients, manage conflict, and uphold ethical standards. For this reason, faculty development is essential to prepare faculty for role modeling. Educators must not only teach but consistently demonstrate the behaviors they expect of learners. Structured mentorship programs can make role modelling explicit, pairing students with faculty who provide guidance, feedback, and authentic examples of professionalism in practice.

8.4.5 Interprofessional and Community-Based Learning

Interprofessional learning experiences, such as shared workshops or collaborative clinical placements, offer students opportunities to practice non-technical skills across professional boundaries. Community-based placements provide authentic contexts for developing cultural competence by exposing learners to diverse populations and the social determinants of health. These authentic encounters underscore that non-technical skills are essential to effective and equitable healthcare delivery.

While these teaching methods (discussed above) can be effective, they achieve their maximum impact when sequenced and reinforced longitudinally across the curriculum.

8.5 Assessment of Non-technical Skills

Assessment of non-technical skills is not a straightforward task due to their unique nature. Unlike technical procedures, non-technical skills are context-dependent, relational, and often intangible, which complicates efforts to evaluate them reliably and validly. Nevertheless, a wide range of methods has been developed to address these challenges, evolving from structured examinations to workplace-based approaches and innovative competency-based strategies. We briefly explain some of the commonly used methods below and summarize them in Table 8.1. A detailed comparison of their psychometric and operational strengths and weaknesses is beyond the scope of this chapter.

8.5.1 Pre-admission Assessment of Non-technical Skills

The assessment of non-technical skills begins even before students enter training programs, with selection processes that evaluate attributes such as communication, empathy, teamwork, and ethical reasoning. Although these skills can be developed during training, scholars of the opposing view suggest that foundational non-technical skills (e.g., empathy, integrity, and communication) are harder to remediate once entrenched behaviors emerge, and therefore, assessing them in advance helps identify candidates aligned with professional values and reduces risks of professionalism lapses during training. With more emphasis on initial screening, tools like multiple mini-interviews (MMIs) and situational judgment tests (SJTs) are gaining momentum as they demonstrate high validity and reliability for assessing personal and professional skills at the point of entry, complementing traditional academic metrics [9]. Early assessment ensures that admitted candidates not only are academically capable but also aligned with the professional and interpersonal demands of healthcare practice [10]. Importantly, the selection of which non-technical skills to prioritize should be guided by the institution's vision and mission, curricular goals, and/or the competencies defined in the national framework. Integrating these assessments into admission policies supports a more holistic

Table 8.1 Methods for assessing non-technical skills across the continuum of education

	Undergraduate and graduate training			
Pre-admissions	Preclinical	Clinical	Licensing exams	Continuing professional development
Multiple mini-interviews (MMI) Situational judgment tests (SJTs)	Written reflections and portfolios Case-based discussions Objective structured clinical examinations (OSCEs) Situational judgment tests (SJTs)	Objective structured clinical examinations (OSCEs) Mini-CEX Case-based discussions Multisource feedback (peers, patients, supervisors) Situational judgment tests (SJTs)	Objective structured clinical examinations (OSCEs) Situational judgment tests (SJTs) Mini-CEX	Portfolios and reflective practice Peer and multisource feedback Refresher courses and recertifications

approach to student selection, ensuring that future professionals enter training with both cognitive and human skills necessary for safe, patient-centered care.

8.5.2 In-Program Assessment of Non-technical Skills

8.5.2.1 Objective Structured Clinical Examinations (OSCE)

Initially designed to test physical examination and procedural skills, the objective structured clinical examination (OSCE) has quickly expanded to include the assessment of non-technical skills, such as communication, empathy, counseling, and professionalism. The use of standardized patients simulates clinical scenarios in which learners' abilities to listen, explain, and empathize can be observed and evaluated. Research has demonstrated that OSCEs can reliably assess aspects of doctor-patient communication and professionalism when structured checklists and trained assessors are employed. Despite their widespread adoption, OSCEs have been critiqued for capturing performance in artificial, time-limited encounters that may not fully reflect learners' behavior in authentic clinical environments.

8.5.2.2 Written and Reflective Methods

Written assessments such as reflective essays and portfolios have long been used to encourage learners to articulate their professional values and self-awareness. These methods align with the recognition that professionalism and ethical practice involve both internal dispositions and outward behaviors. Portfolios, in particular, provide a longitudinal view of development and can incorporate feedback from multiple stakeholders [11]. However, concerns about subjectivity and variability in assessor judgments remain, highlighting the need for clear rubrics and trained reviewers.

8.5.2.3 Workplace-Based Assessments

A major shift over the past two decades has been the introduction of workplace-based assessments, which allow for the direct observation of learners in authentic settings. Tools such as the mini-clinical evaluation exercise (mini-CEX), case-based discussion, and global rating forms enable supervisors to evaluate non-technical skills during routine patient care [12]. Multisource feedback, which collects evaluations from peers, nurses, patients, and other colleagues, has been particularly influential in assessing professionalism and interpersonal skills [12]. These approaches strengthen ecological validity but also raise concerns about inter-rater reliability, faculty workload, and the potential influence of personal relationships on ratings.

8.5.2.4 Simulation-Based Assessment

Simulation has emerged as a powerful tool for assessing both technical and non-technical skills. High-fidelity patient simulators, task trainers, and virtual reality platforms allow teams to practice crisis scenarios in controlled settings where non-technical skills can be observed. In surgical and anesthesia education, structured rating systems such as the Non-technical Skills for Surgeons (NOTSS) and Anesthetists' Non-technical Skills (ANTS) frameworks were developed to provide structured behavioral markers for assessment [6]. While initially developed for high-risk industries, these instruments have been adapted for use in healthcare and are now employed internationally. Simulation also enables structured debriefing, providing opportunities for both formative feedback and summative evaluation.

8.5.2.5 Entrustable Professional Activities

The move toward entrustable professional activities (EPAs) and entrustment decisions in the past two decades has transformed assessment practices. Rather than relying solely on single-point examinations, entrustment requires multiple observations over time and across contexts. EPAs, introduced by ten Cate in 2005, represent a major innovation in this regard. EPAs are units of professional practice that learners are expected to perform independently once they have demonstrated sufficient competence [13]. Each EPA integrates multiple competencies, including non-technical domains. Supervisors make entrustment decisions, whether a learner can be trusted to perform a given task without supervision, based on observed behaviors in real clinical contexts [13]. EPAs thus operationalize the assessment of non-technical skills by embedding them within authentic clinical work. Common challenges with EPAs include variability in supervisors' thresholds for entrustment, limited clarity on what constitutes sufficient evidence across contexts, and the risk of subjective bias in entrustment decisions, all of which highlight the need for contextual research, robust faculty development and shared standards.

8.5.2.6 Formative Situational Judgment Tests

Situational judgment tests (SJTs) have traditionally been used to assess noncognitive skills in admissions and selection, but recent work highlights their potential as formative tools in undergraduate training programs. Unlike high-stakes selection SJTs, formative versions are designed to support learning by presenting context-rich scenarios that elicit responses reflecting non-technical skills. These responses provide rich data to generate both quantitative scores and narrative feedback across domains, thereby guiding targeted remediation and professional growth. Evidence from a systematic review indicates that formative SJTs can help medical students link performance with professionalism, with lower scores often associated with a higher risk of unprofessional behaviors [14]. While their psychometric robustness is still developing, formative SJTs appear to add educational value by fostering self-reflection and professional identity formation, making them a promising complement to more traditional assessments of non-technical skills.

8.5.2.7 Programmatic Assessment

The concept of programmatic assessment extends competency-based approaches by integrating diverse data points into a coherent system. Instead of high-stakes single assessments, learners are evaluated continuously through multiple low-stakes observations, reflections, and feedback opportunities. This enables the capture of non-technical skills more effectively, which are inherently longitudinal and developmental [15]. In simple terms, consider programmatic assessment a combination of the above-discussed assessment methods (serving as data points) that are longitudinally integrated into the curriculum. By triangulating across different sources and contexts, programmatic assessment increases validity while also supporting learning. Faculty development and institutional culture remain crucial for effective implementation, as assessors must be equipped to provide narrative feedback and synthesize data for high-stakes decisions.

8.6 Challenges and Future Directions

Despite the diversity of available tools, assessing non-technical skills remains a complex task. Reliability is challenged by variability across contexts, raters, and patient encounters. Validity requires that tools genuinely capture constructs such as empathy or professionalism rather than superficial behaviors. Faculty development is essential, as untrained assessors may default to intuitive judgments without explicit criteria. Moreover, learners often express concerns about fairness and consistency in the evaluation of attributes that are deeply tied to personal identity and professional values.

The future of non-technical skills assessment is promising and will likely involve further integration of multiple approaches, combining simulation, workplace-based observation, reflective portfolios, and emerging digital tools within programmatic systems. Such integration aligns with the shift toward competency-based education, which emphasizes holistic, longitudinal, and contextualized judgments of competence. Ultimately, effective assessment should not only certify competence but also promote ongoing growth in the human dimensions of healthcare.

8.7 Conclusion

Non-technical skills have moved from the margins of HPE to the very center of professional identity formation and patient safety. Promising approaches emphasize integration across multiple levels of the curriculum, consistent role modelling, and alignment with assessment. The ultimate goal is to cultivate a culture in which non-technical skills are not peripheral but woven into the fabric of professional identity formation. Achieving this requires sustained institutional commitment, faculty leadership, and alignment between curricular design, teaching practices, assessment strategies, and accreditation standards. Challenges remain, particularly in addressing the hidden curriculum, ensuring meaningful faculty development, building resource capacity, and adapting global frameworks to local contexts. Nevertheless, the intentional and systematic integration of non-technical skills throughout the training continuum can prepare graduates who are not only technically proficient but also compassionate, collaborative, and ethically grounded professionals, equipped to meet the complex needs of modern healthcare.

References

1. Johnson AP, Aggarwal R. Assessment of non-technical skills: why aren't we there yet? BMJ Qual Saf. 2019;28:606–8.
2. Pimenta IDSF, Mata ÁNDS, Bezerra INM, De Araújo RMP, Santana JLA, Capucho HC, De Souza-Oliveira AC, Echevarría-Pérez P, Guillén-Martínez D, Piuvezam G. Effectiveness of non-technical skills training in intensive care units: a systematic review. BMC Med Educ. 2025;25:847.
3. Pucer P, Martinović K, Karnjuš I, Renko J. Development and improvement of non-technical skills in interprofessional healthcare teams through simulation-based experiences: a systematic review. Clin Simul Nurs. 2025;102:101726.
4. Gamborg ML, Salling LB, Rölfing JD, Jensen RD. Training technical or non-technical skills: an arbitrary distinction? A scoping review. BMC Med Educ. 2024;24:1451.
5. Flin R, O'Connor P. Safety at the sharp end: a guide to non-technical skills. 1st ed. CRC Press; 2008. https://doi.org/10.1201/9781315607467.
6. Yule S, Flin R, Paterson-Brown S, Maran N. Non-technical skills for surgeons in the operating room: a review of the literature. Surgery. 2006;139:140–9.
7. Dieckmann P, Bruun B, Mundt S, Holgaard R, Østergaard D. Social and Cognitive Skills (SCOPE) – a generic model for multi-professional work and education in healthcare. Adv Simul. 2024;9:28.
8. Sanchez-Marco M, Escribano S, Rubio-Aparicio M, Julia-Sanchis R, Cabanero-Martinez M-J. Effectiveness of nontechnical skills educational interventions in the context of emergencies: a systematic review and meta-analysis. Aust Crit Care. 2023;36:1159–71.
9. Patterson F, Knight A, Dowell J, Nicholson S, Cousans F, Cleland J. How effective are selection methods in medical education? A systematic review. Med Educ. 2016;50:36–60.
10. Iqbal MZ, Ivan R, Robb C, Derby J. Evaluating factors that impact scoring an open response situational judgment test: a mixed methods approach. Front Med. 2025;11:1525156.
11. Driessen E, Van Tartwijk J, Van Der Vleuten C, Wass V. Portfolios in medical education: why do they meet with mixed success? A systematic review. Med Educ. 2007;41:1224–33.
12. Norcini J, Burch V. Workplace-based assessment as an educational tool: AMEE Guide No. 31. Med Teach. 2007;29:855–71.
13. Ten Cate O. Entrustability of professional activities and competency-based training. Med Educ. 2005;39:1176–7.
14. Sahota GS, Fisher V, Patel B, JuJ K, Taggar JS. The educational value of situational judgement tests (SJTs) when used during undergraduate medical training: a systematic review and narrative synthesis. Med Teach. 2023;45:997–1004.
15. Torre D, Schuwirth L. Programmatic assessment for learning: a programmatically designed assessment for the purpose of learning: AMEE Guide No. 174. Med Teach. 2025;47:918–33.

9 Professionalism and e-Professionalism

Shabih Zaidi and Sakina Naqvi

Key Points

- Professionalism is the third limb of the triangle of education, alongside knowledge and skills.
- Good medical practice is the cornerstone of medical professionalism, comprising many attributes to serve the patient ethically.
- Work ethics imply attributes such as mutual respect between colleagues, care, and consideration, knowing one's limits, and avoiding harassment, among others.
- Models of professionalism mean the ways of consulting a patient, in a paternalistic, informative, interpretive, or deliberative way.
- In an emerging digital world, there is a need for e-professionalism, including netiquette, telemedicine, telehealth, and technology.

9.1 Introduction

9.1.1 The Evolution of Medical Professionalism: From Ancient Healers to AI-Driven Practice

Hippocrates (c. 460–370 B.C) was among the first to recognize the importance of professionalism in medicine. His codification of medical principles into what became known as the Hippocratic Oath laid the foundation for ethical medical practice. Though it has undergone modifications over time to reflect cultural and religious diversity, its patient-centered focus remains relevant today.

Formal medical education, as we understand it, did not emerge until the seminal Flexner Report of 1910. Until then, learning followed the informal but time-honored

S. Zaidi · S. Naqvi (✉)
al-Sadiq International Virtual University, London, UK; https://sivu.imamiamedics.com

J. Sandars et al. (eds.), *Modern Medical Education*,
https://doi.org/10.1007/978-3-032-27958-3_9

model of "see one, do one, teach one," establishing a deep mentor-mentee relationship akin to that of a *guru* and a *chela*. This intimate transmission of knowledge fostered skills not only in medicine but also in professional etiquette, bedside manners, and clinical reasoning. This model thrived until the mid-twentieth century. Following World War II, the explosion of scientific knowledge and technological advances began to outpace traditional methods of training and practice. Today, with the rapid integration of artificial intelligence (AI) and machine learning (ML), the landscape of healthcare professionalism is being reshaped in real time.

9.1.2 Profession or Trade?

The word "professionalism" stems from the root word "profession," which is typically defined as a knowledge-based occupation requiring expertise and skill. In the context of healthcare, professionalism encompasses a broad range of attributes, including demeanor, attire, communication, competence, leadership, efficiency, teamwork, time management, and ethical conduct. Medical professionalism serves as the bedrock of public trust in the healthcare system. It involves a commitment to ethical practice, clinical excellence, compassionate care, and lifelong learning. Cruess and Cruess believe that professionalism underpins the values and behaviors that society expects from its physicians [1].

9.1.3 Professional Identity

According to the Oxford Dictionary (1989), identity is defined as "a set of characteristics or a description that distinguishes a person or thing from others." Medical students enter their training with preexisting identities, which gradually evolve into a professional identity through a complex process involving experience and critical reflection. This transformation is shaped by formal curricula, clinical exposure, experiential learning, role models, and the dynamic expectations of modern healthcare. At its core, however, it remains anchored in one constant: "patient care."

In a personal communication, a learned colleague from Iraq observed that professional identity formation is often constrained by the absence of "deep reflective practices" that drive "ontological transformation" [2]—a fundamental shift in one's way of being—rather than mere epistemological growth, the accumulation of knowledge and skills. Conventional approaches, with their focus on competence and performance, risk neglecting the inner development essential to an authentic professional self.

This calls for an ontological turn in medical education: recognition that professional identity rests not only on knowing and doing but also on being and becoming. This perspective aligns with "triple-loop learning [3]," which moves beyond refining actions (single-loop) or reassessing assumptions (double-loop) toward transformative self-reflection that redefines one's core values, beliefs, and identity. Such learning fosters a professional presence that is authentic, resilient, and adaptable.

Embedding these reflective, ontological practices into medical education can help learners form identities that are deeply internalized, ethically grounded, and continuously evolving. A professional with no identity is like a silhouette in a crowd at sundown.

9.1.4 Professionalism and the Physician-Patient Relationship

Historically, the physician-patient relationship was often paternalistic, grounded in the belief that "the doctor knows best." However, this dynamic has shifted with the explosion of knowledge and technology. It has moved from being physician-centered to patient-centered. Now, all practical models, such as the (a) paternalistic, (b) informative, (c) interpretive, and (d) deliberative, promote shared decision-making and mutual respect [4]. In the Middle East, the culturally sensitive "four-gate model" professionalism was proposed to align medical ethics with regional values [5].

The first gate covers self-awareness and self-management, the second gate focuses on self-awareness and self-management, and the third and fourth gates deal with communication skills and with God awareness and divine interventions [5], respectively.

Regardless of the framework, the core objective remains unchanged: "to serve the patient with dignity, competence, and compassion" [5].

9.2 The Challenges of Professionalism in Modern Practice

The archetype of the revered family doctor—once a pillar of knowledge and trust—has evolved. In today's hyper-specialized, information-saturated world, no physician can claim omniscience. Artificial intelligence (AI) and machine learning (ML) are further redefining the role of the clinician, and traditional pedagogies are giving way to emerging paradigms that fuse technology with education.

Increasingly, the profession appears to be edging toward the nature of a trade, particularly within systems like the UK's National Health Service (NHS). Legal obligations, patient autonomy, and human rights have led to exhaustive documentation and bureaucratic consultations. Physicians are now called "health workers" and patients are called "clients." A more formal contract may be required, which is drawn and signed by both parties, such as when consent is required for a procedure. Anecdotally, a senior consultant with decades of experience may be reduced to "the man" or "the woman" in the consulting room—terminology once unthinkable in a professional setting.

This shift has significant implications. Medicine, once considered a noble and honorable vocation, now faces a decline in societal reverence. One must question: If respect and honor continue to erode, what incentive remains for young aspirants to endure the rigors of medical training, especially when other trades offer quicker routes to financial stability and social recognition?

9.2.1 The Erosion of Traditional Symbols

Professionalism was once symbolized by starched white coats, crisp nurses' hats, and an authoritative yet compassionate demeanor. These were more than uniforms—they were visual cues of responsibility, discipline, and trustworthiness. Today, such symbols are vanishing in places like the NHS, although they remain prevalent in the USA and other healthcare systems.

9.3 The Essential Attributes of Medical Professionalism

9.3.1 Integrity

One of the fundamental principles of medical professionalism is integrity. Physicians are expected to uphold high ethical standards, be honest with patients and colleagues, and maintain transparency in clinical decisions. Integrity also encompasses accountability—being responsible for one's actions and their consequences, admitting mistakes, and striving to rectify them. It is through this ethical conduct that trust is built with patients, which is essential for effective healthcare delivery.

9.3.2 Compassion and Respect

Medical professionals must treat all individuals with dignity, regardless of their background, beliefs, or circumstances. This includes honoring patient autonomy, providing culturally competent care, and maintaining confidentiality. Respectful communication fosters a therapeutic relationship that enhances patient satisfaction and compliance with treatment.

9.3.3 Competence

It is another pillar of professionalism. A physician must possess the necessary medical knowledge and technical skills to diagnose and treat illness effectively. However, competence also implies a commitment to lifelong learning. Medicine is an ever-evolving field, and staying updated with the latest evidence-based practices and technologies is a professional obligation. This continuous improvement ensures that patients receive the most effective and up-to-date care possible.

9.3.4 Altruism and Empathy

Putting the needs of patients before self-interest is central to a physician's professional identity. In practice, this may involve going beyond the minimum requirements of care, advocating for patients, and occasionally making personal sacrifices for the benefit of others. Feeling the pain or agony as if it were your own is a virtue called empathy. Altruism is sometimes questioned by psychologists as to whether there might be a hidden agenda, such as personal gain, self-interest, self-promotion, or publicity. Therefore, altruism should be practiced with caution.

Maintaining personal well-being is also crucial, as the ability to care for others is diminished when the caregiver is unwell or overburdened.

9.3.5 Collaboration and Teamwork

Multidisciplinary teams often deliver modern healthcare, and effective collaboration enhances patient outcomes and safety. Professionals must respect the roles of their colleagues, communicate clearly, and contribute to a cooperative work environment. Interprofessional education and healthcare are vital for gaining excellence.

9.3.6 Social Responsibility

Physicians must contribute to the improvement of public health and advocate for changes that promote social justice in healthcare. This includes addressing health disparities, participating in health policy discussions, and engaging in community outreach.

9.4 Theories of Professionalism

9.4.1 Behaviorism Theory of Watson, Pavlov, and Skinner [6]

It is based upon a concept that bad behaviors are often rooted in intrinsic bad habits, which may have developed during the early stages of life. They may be due to improper parenting, misfortunes, or acquiring bad traits from seniors or peers. It becomes a challenging task for a medical educator to bring about a radical change in such a medical student, requiring a mutually acceptable teacher-taught behavioristic course or plan, or strategy, eventually aiming to instill a proper professional attitude in the young mind. Initial steps outline the theoretical aspects of professionalism, thereby reaching a consensus through mutual discussion and deliberation in several meetings, demonstrating the practical application of these principles. The subsequent step is more of a reflective process, involving feedback or reinforcement from the teacher on the pupil's actions. It could be positive or negative feedback, requiring a forward movement or a revisit. Such activities become part of the student's portfolio, whether as a file or an e-portfolio. The to-and-fro process should ultimately inculcate a professional attitude in a student by conditioning, which should become part of his DNA over time.

9.4.2 The Cognitivist Theory of Piaget

This famous Swiss psychologist believed that the best way to teach or instill professionalism in medical school is through role modeling, inviting students to observe, learn, critically analyze, take notes, ask questions, and incorporate the traits into their daily life.

Through repeated practice and application of the theoretical principles, a student will learn the tips and tricks, the art and science of professionalism [7]. Modern simulation labs and structured patients as role players in educational workshops could be an alternative way, where patient contact may be limited or unavailable.

9.4.3 Good Medical Practice

The General Medical Council of Great Britain is the licensing authority that provides guidelines for best clinical care as well as medical education from time to time. The GMC's Good Medical Practice (GMP) guidance outlines the principles, values, and standards of professional behavior expected of all healthcare professionals.

In a recent publication, the GMC identified the following 4 domains: [8]

- Knowledge, skills, and performance
- Safety and quality
- Communication, partnership, and teamwork
- Maintaining trust

9.5 Work Ethics and Professionalism

Every profession follows a code of conduct, called a work ethic.

Some of the factors are covered in this subsection of medical professionalism.

9.5.1 Competence Is Based on Knowledge, Skills, and Attitude

The term attitude should be replaced with professionalism. It has wider connotations and a deeper meaning. So, every health professional and educator must keep their knowledge and skills compatible with the evolution of both in daily life. That is easily accomplished by attending courses and workshops run by different agencies, particularly the licensing bodies such as the GMC in the UK. Each country has its own licensing body that guides it from time to time.

9.5.2 Complaints and Whistleblowing

Any professional can make mistakes. It is only human. But early recognition and immediate redemption are necessary. An incident report may be recorded, and the immediate superior must be informed. Ordinary mistakes are usually managed at this level. If it happens to be a repeated mistake made by a colleague, then it should be tactfully handled. Initially, a one-to-one talk followed by a discussion with the manager should suffice. Sometimes, however, retraining may be advised, which is neither demeaning nor damaging. Everyone needs to go back to a training center periodically to reflect upon one's weakness and redemption through training, as is commonly seen in Teacher Training Programs or Faculty Enhancement Programs, which form part and parcel of a department of medical education.

Whistleblowing may be a double-edged sword as it may lead to personal animosity and ill feelings at the workplace. If it is done for sound reasons, it may benefit the institution or the organization, which is the moral reason for doing so.

9.5.3 Harassment

It is a serious offence and must be avoided. It is defined as repeated unwanted improper behavior toward a colleague. It may be verbal or digital, such as texts or emails. It may be practiced in various forms. Common examples are bullying; racial, color, and gender bias; sexual orientation; culture; and faith. Any form of harassment in a medical education environment or healthcare services must be strictly avoided. If noticed and reported to the authorities, serious consequences like expulsion or job loss may ensue. In today's environment, such notices are displayed in public transport as well as offices in many countries. There is a subtle difference between harassment and discrimination. Discrimination is evident when a colleague is unfairly treated because of his/her protected characteristics, such as gender, racial features, faith, or sexual orientation.

9.5.4 Professionalism in Education

Edmund Pellegrino (d 2013) is the only modern medical educator and clinician who promoted the concept of reintroducing humanities, social sciences, and basic philosophy in medical curricula. Humanizing medicine is a timely slogan.

It is indeed a major challenge, as many educators vehemently oppose it as if a part of their territory would be lost. Such challenges have been recognized. Efforts have been successful in some American, many British, and some Indian institutions to incorporate medical ethics into their curricula.

9.6 Teaching Professionalism

Traditional apprenticeship in the health profession did not require any special modules for teaching professionalism. It is no longer possible, especially as digital professionalism takes hold. Many educators have recommended incorporating the formal teaching of medical ethics into a curriculum to promote professionalism among students [9, 10].

The best way of teaching it is lifelike role modeling as advocated by Hafferty in the form of a hidden curriculum. It is also promoted by other educators, advocating demonstrations of professed signal behavior in either clinical setups or simulation labs, workshops, reflective practice, case-based discussion, and video libraries and developing clinical scenarios for students. Arabshahi [11] recommends Tyler's model of curriculum development, in which professionalism courses could be designed accordingly.

It could be a good model to follow in the following four steps:

1. Setting up the objectives elaborated from the definition, needs of the society, students, and updated knowledge of behavioral and ethical values
2. Selecting the learning objectives in the curriculum
3. Organizing the instructional strategies
4. Assessing and evaluating, which are both vital

9.7 Digital/e-Professionalism

e-Professionalism has encroached upon conventional professionalism in the last decade or so. It gained a huge significance from the COVID-19 pandemic when the world was deprived of face-to-face contact and virtual medical care and education took over the age-old practices. New methods had to be defined and applied in healthcare [12].

e-Professionalism or digital professionalism refers to the conduct and behavior expected of individuals in online environments, particularly in their professional interactions and communications. As the digital landscape continues to evolve, maintaining a professional online presence has become increasingly vital for students, physicians, patients, employees, and professionals alike. This concept encompasses various aspects, including how individuals present themselves on social media, the tone and style of their online communications, and their overall digital footprint.

One of the key components of e-professionalism is the understanding that online actions can have lasting consequences. In a world where information is easily accessible and often permanent, individuals must be mindful of what they post, share, and comment on. This includes being cautious with images, videos, and messages that could be perceived as unprofessional or inappropriate. This is particularly important for students, as potential employers often review candidates' social media profiles during the hiring process. A single inappropriate post can lead to missed job opportunities, medical negligence, litigation, or worse, emphasizing the need for individuals to curate their online personas carefully.

In fact, e-professionalism extends beyond social media. It includes email communications, online discussions, and participation in virtual meetings. Professionalism in emails entails using a respectful tone, proper grammar, and a clear structure. This not only reflects an individual's competence but also shows respect for the recipient. In virtual meetings, e-professionalism involves being punctual, prepared, and engaged. Participants should dress appropriately, minimize distractions, and actively contribute to discussions, demonstrating their seriousness and commitment to the professional setting.

Another aspect of e-professionalism is the awareness of digital etiquette, sometimes called netiquette. This includes understanding the nuances of online communication, such as the use of emojis, avoiding all capital letters, exclamation points, and abbreviations. While these elements can convey friendliness and enthusiasm, they may also be misinterpreted in professional contexts. Striking the right balance is essential; individuals should aim to be personable while maintaining a level of professionalism that aligns with their industry standards.

The rise of remote work has further highlighted the importance of e-professionalism. As more professionals work from home and rely on digital communication tools, the boundaries between personal and professional lives can blur. Individuals must establish clear boundaries to ensure that their professional demeanor remains intact, even in casual settings. This includes creating a dedicated workspace, adhering to a professional dress code during video calls, and being mindful of the background environment during virtual meetings.

Furthermore, e-professionalism encompasses the concept of online networking and personal branding. Building a professional online presence through platforms like LinkedIn allows individuals to showcase their skills, experiences, and accomplishments. Engaging with health-related content, connecting with professionals, and participating in discussions can enhance one's visibility and credibility within their field. However, it is crucial to remember that every interaction contributes to one's brand; therefore, maintaining professionalism in every aspect of online engagement is essential. Professionalism should be included as an important area of the curriculum in teaching, learning, and evaluating. Curricula should focus on the appropriate use of media in the social platform by including the core elements of professionalism in the medical arena [13].

E-professionalism is a critical element of modern professional life. With the increasing reliance on digital communication and the permanence of online actions, individuals must navigate their online presence thoughtfully. By being mindful of their digital footprint, adhering to professional etiquette, netiquette, by managing their online personas, individuals can cultivate a strong professional image that enhances their career prospects and fosters positive relationships within their industry. As the digital landscape continues to evolve, the principles of e-professionalism will remain a cornerstone of effective and respectful online communication.

9.8 Assessment and Valuation of Professionalism

Many non-tangible components of professionalism can only be assessed through observation, such as altruism, compassion, generosity, velour, courage, and practical wisdom. Others can be assessed by simple measures such as honesty, truth, equity, equality, and justice. No mathematical calculations can truly measure professionalism per se [14].

Some elements of a blueprint for assessment of professionalism are the following:

- Observed clinical encounters
- Multisource feedback
- Patients' opinions
- Paper-based tests or simulations
- Measures of research and/or teaching activities
- 360° evaluations
- Portfolios and logbooks
- Peer assessments
- Reflective diaries
- Self-assessment

Moreover, evidence-based knowledge and adherence to the ultimate principles of ethics are required. Altruism, selflessness, and prioritizing the best interests of patients are assessed using relevant questions.

9.9 Conclusion

Professionalism in healthcare and medical education is a deep moral commitment to the well-being of patients and society. It requires a delicate balance of scientific expertise, ethical judgment, and human compassion. Upholding these ideals not only improves individual patient care but also strengthens the integrity of the medical profession as a whole.

References

1. Cruess SR, Cruses RL. Teaching professionalism – why, what and how. Facts Views Vis Obgyn. 2012;4(4):259–65.
2. Dall'Alba G. Learning professional ways of being: ambiguities of becoming. Educ Philos Theory. 2009;41(3):34–45.
3. Tosey P, Visser M, Saunders MNK. The origins and conceptualizations of 'triple-loop' learning: a critical review. Manag Learn. 2012;43(3):291–307.
4. Emanuel EJ, Emanuel LL. Four models of the physician-patient relationship. JAMA. 1992;267(16):2221–6. https://doi.org/10.1001/jama.1992.03480160079038.

5. Al-Eraky MM, Donkers J, Wajid G, van Merrienboer JJG. A Delphi study of medical professionalism in Arabian countries: the four-gates model. Med Teach. 2014:S8–S16. https://doi.org/10.3109/0142159X.2014.886013.
6. Behaviorism theory of Watson, Pavlov, and Skinner. https://www.researchgate.net/profile/Farrelli-Hambulo/publication/341313372_The_Contribution_of_Behavioral_Theories_of_Learning_to_Education/links/5eba6b2f92851cd50dab67a9/The-Contribution-of-Behavioral-Theories-of-Learning-to-Education
7. Badyal DK, Singh T. Learning theories: the basics to learn in medical education. Int J Appl Basic Med Res. 2017;7(Suppl 1):S1–3. https://doi.org/10.4103/ijabmr.IJABMR_385_17.
8. https://www.gmc-uk.org/gmpinaction/gmc-guidance/good-medical-practice/index.asp
9. O'Sullivan H, van Mook W, Fewtrell R, Wass V. Integrating professionalism into the curriculum: AMEE Guide No. 61. Med Teach. 2012;34(2):e64–77. https://doi.org/10.3109/0142159x.2012.655610.
10. Zare S, Yamani N, Changiz T. How to develop an undergraduate medical professionalism curriculum: experts' perception and suggestions. J Adv Med Educ Prof. 2019;7(4):183–90.
11. Arabshahi S, Akbarilakeh M, Kenari H, Abdalla ME. Development of learning professionalism assessment battery for medical residents. Pak J Med Health Sci. 2021;15:1594–7.
12. Guraya SS, Rashid-Doubell F, Harkin DW, Guraya SY. Mission-driven e-professionalism in the medical field: shaping digital identity and virtual engagement. Front Med. 2024;11:1276839.
13. Jomon Lonappan PS, Aithal MJ. e-Professionalism as a professional identity in the digital era of medical education. Int J Health Sci Pharm (IJHSP). 2023;7(2):35–48.
14. Wilkinson TJ, Wade WB, Knock LD. A blueprint to assess professionalism: results of a systematic review. Acad Med. 2009;84(5):551–8.

Reflective Practice 10

John Sandars

Key Points

- Reflective practice is essential for the lifelong personal and professional development of all health professionals across the continuum of medical education.
- Important challenges and future trends include engagement, assessment, implementation of reflective practice, and both becoming and being a reflective educator.
- There is an increasing importance of technology, especially artificial intelligence, for the support of variousaspects of reflective practice.
- It is important to ensure that reflection is contextual and uses appropriate thinking frameworks that are
- aligned to the intended purpose, the reflection process is adapted to the preference of the learner, and guidance to support reflective practice is provided.

10.1 Introduction

Reflective practice is essential for the lifelong personal and professional development of all health professionals across the continuum of medical education, from undergraduate to postgraduate to continuing. The process of reflective practice requires an individual to engage in reflection on their professional practice, which can be clinical and/or educational. During reflection, an individual consciously thinks about a situation related to their daily practice, with the intention of gaining increased insights and learning that can develop their personal lives and/or professional practice. An illustrative example of reflective practice for personal development is thinking about a situation in which there was anxiety about meeting a senior

J. Sandars (✉)
Edge Hill University Medical School, Edge Hill University, Ormskirk, Lancashire, UK
e-mail: john.sandars@edgehill.ac.uk

J. Sandars et al. (eds.), *Modern Medical Education*,
https://doi.org/10.1007/978-3-032-27958-3_10

colleague. This could highlight general anxiety about encountering new situations and the subsequent need to develop new personal skills for managing similar situations in the future. An illustrative example of reflective practice for professional development is thinking about a situation in which there was uncertainty about the most appropriate clinical management of a patient. This could identify specific lack of knowledge and the subsequent need to learn more about available management approaches.

The process of reflective practice can be simply described as "do-think-act," with each component being of critical importance. *Do* highlights the importance of having an appropriate situation to stimulate reflection. These situations can trigger moments of surprise for the individual, for example, there may be an unexpected emotional response to a situation or that the intended plan was not effective. *Think* is an essential component of reflection, but it can be superficial and less meaningful for personal and professional development. In "single-loop" thinking, reflection functions like a thermostat: if the room gets too hot, the temperature is adjusted without questioning why it was too hot in the first place. In contrast, more deeper and meaningful personal and professional development requires "double-loop" thinking [1], questions underlying reasons, and requires exploration of the underlying beliefs and assumptions behind an individual's actions in a situation, for example, examining why there was reluctance to share uncertainty in clinical decision-making with colleagues can spark more lasting improvements in practice. Deeper reflection fosters greater self-awareness and learning that ultimately leads to personal and professional development. The final *act* component refers to the future actions taken by the individual in other situations and is based on the greater self-awareness and learning obtained during the *think* component.

There is increasing evidence that reflective practice increases learning and personal and/or professional development, especially about professional values and making sense of complex situations; there is the possibility that clinical practice is also improved [2]. However, there are several important challenges for the implementation of reflective practice. These challenges, and how they can be practically resolved, are discussed in this chapter. There will also be discussion of the increasing importance of ubiquitous technology, especially artificial intelligence, to support reflective practice. These discussions and recommendations are based on the author's awareness of the major trends in reflective practice, including the expected future trends.

10.2 The Challenges of Reflective Practice

The overall importance of reflective practice is recognized by health professionals but that there are also several major challenges [3]. There is often reluctance to engage in the typical extensive writing required to both promote and evidence reflection. Although any assessment and feedback are considered to be useful, the grading of reflection is not considered to be a valid approach or useful. There are also concerns about confidentiality and sharing reflections with a wider audience. Having guidance and support for reflective practice, including protected time, is important additional findings from studies.

In summary, the main identified interrelated challenges are engagement, assessment, implementation of reflective practice, and becoming and being a reflective educator.

10.3 Engagement

In this challenge, two important areas (concerns about public and private boundaries and choice of appropriate methods of reflection) will be discussed, including how technology can support reflective practice in the future.

10.3.1 Concerns About Public and Private Boundaries

Significant situations that promote personal and professional development are often intensely private, with a challenge to the individual's deeply held beliefs about self and others, for example, inappropriate management of a clinical case may challenge an individual's beliefs about being a competent doctor, and this can lead to increased vulnerability, with reluctance to share and discuss with others. In some countries, there is the additional challenge that full disclosure of any written reflection may be required by law. Practical guidance recommends taking notes focusing on the learning and future actions that have occurred, with avoidance of a full discussion of the case, or situation, and ensuring that no individual or situation can be identified.

The avoidance of full discussion of a case is an important challenge for the assessment of reflective practice. The patchwork test approach can be a useful assessment method since it analyzes several reflections to identify only the main learning points and subsequent actions in response to a variety of situations [4]. This process can increasingly be readily achieved by using artificial intelligence technology, such as by sentiment analysis [5].

10.3.2 Appropriate Methods of Reflective Practice

Writing reflection is often disliked by health professionals, and research has highlighted that this method is often not aligned to their preferences, which are more visual, creative, and active [8]. Aligning reflection to the preferences of users can increase engagement and deepen reflection, such as with LEGO® SERIOUS PLAY® and digital storytelling:

(a) LEGO® SERIOUS PLAY® can effectively engage and stimulate reflection about professional identity in student nurse education through the creation of brick models to represent specific situations and by describing the model's representation of these situations [6].
(b) Digital storytelling can promote increased engagement and reflection [7]. In digital storytelling, a variety of familiar and commonly used technology (both hardware and software) can create digital stories, by either an individual or a group, for example, a series of images that resonate with the emotions and

thoughts associated with a situation can be assembled into a digital story. During this process, there can be several prompts for reflection, such as the selection of the images, assembling a sequence to present a coherent story and following presentation to others. The overall approach of digital storytelling is versatile and can be readily adapted to promote effective reflection for personal and professional development.

10.4 Assessment

Both formative (assessment for learning) and summative (assessment of learning) types of assessments are often an integral aspect of reflective practice across the medical education continuum. These assessments are intended to understand how an individual is reflecting on their daily professional practice and progressing in their personal and professional development. However, there are two main challenges in the assessment of reflection, including reflection as a developmental process and the appropriate methods of assessment.

10.4.1 Reflection as a Developmental Process

An important consideration in the assessment of reflection is the reflective thinking developmental stage of the individual. Reflective thinking progressively develops over time, especially in relation to deeper "double-loop" reflection, and there is a wide variation in the rate of development over time [8]. An assessment can provide a useful snapshot of an individual's level of reflection at a specific moment in time, but identifying the essential progression of development requires comparison over time, such as by creating and assessing a portfolio. Increasingly, a variety of technology can be used to produce a portfolio of reflections, from a compilation of standard word-processed documents to bespoke commercial systems.

10.4.2 Appropriate Methods of Assessment

At an early developmental stage of reflection, assessment should focus on the extent to which a presented reflection is descriptive or reflective, but at further stages in the development of reflection, a more detailed measure of the depth of reflection is required. *Reflect* is a widely used and validated rubric which is based on the key features of several other rubrics for reflection [9]. This rubric includes the following levels, with each level having several explicit descriptors:

Level 1: Nonreflective—habitual action
Level 2: Nonreflective—thoughtful action
Level 3: Reflective
Level 4: Critically reflective
Level 5: Transformative learning

Artificial intelligence technology has an important future application for the assessment of reflection, especially when there are portfolios that collect a wide variety of text-based documents.

10.5 Implementation of Reflective Practice

In this challenge, the implementation of reflective practice is highlighted, with three main aspects that will be discussed: meaningful aspect of practice for reflection, need for different journeys for different destinations, and guided reflection.

10.5.1 Meaningful Aspect of Practice for Reflection

There has been an increasing recognition of the importance of identifying an appropriate stimulus for reflection, with the development of "noticing" related to an increased awareness in the individual of their emotional and/or mental responses to a situation. Some situations are more meaningful to begin the reflection process, such as experiencing a complaint from a patient, and these can prompt the individual to deepen their thinking to examine and make sense of their responses. These situations are more likely to stimulate cycles of reflection in which an individual can use their new insights from one situation to inform their actions and experiences in another situation. Through repeated cycles, the insights and actions can be progressively refined, with further deepening of reflection and increased personal and professional development.

10.5.2 Need for Different Journeys for Different Destinations

An essential aspect of reflective practice is to have contextual flexibility, with the use of different journeys, or frameworks, for the different destinations or intended outcomes. "Single-loop" thinking may be appropriate for reflection on relatively simple situations, but for more complex clinical situations, "double-loop" thinking is required, in which an individual questions underlying reasons behind their actions in a situation.

There has been an increasing interest in the development of practical wisdom and values in action, in which clinical practice is a synthesis of the essential scientific, technical, and moral dimensions. This consideration of the essential moral dimension that influences personal and professional action requires an extension of "double-loop" thinking to "triple-loop" thinking [10]. "Triple-loop" thinking leads to transformative self-reflection that redefines one's core values, beliefs, and identity. Such learning fosters a professional behavior that is authentic, resilient, and adaptable.

An important aspect of "double-loop" and "triple-loop" thinking is support and guidance so that the intended outcomes can be achieved. Appropriate reflection in this area of interest requires a structured framework (the journey) for developing practical wisdom and virtuous clinical action (the destination). An example of an appropriate framework for promoting reflection includes the following areas [11]:

1. Self-awareness: recognizing biases, assumptions, and emotional triggers
2. Ethical sensitivity: identifying moral dilemmas and value-laden situations
3. Purpose clarification: reaffirming or adjusting personal/professional purpose
4. Accountability: assessing alignment between actions and stated values
5. Continuous improvement: using values to guide personal and professional growth

10.5.3 Guided Reflection

Guided support for an individual's navigation of the reflection process is useful at all developmental levels of reflection. At an early level, the main support and guidance ha a focus on moving from being mainly descriptive (what happened) to becoming reflective (why did it happen), including action planning (what will happen next time). For more advanced levels, the main support and guidance has a focus on deepening reflection to "double loop," especially with a focus on practical wisdom and values in action. Providing individual support and guidance is highly resource-intensive, but there has been an increasing interest in group-guided reflection, and clear practical guidelines on effective reflective practice groups have been developed [12]. Artificial intelligence technology can increasingly offer a potentially useful low-resource approach for guided reflection through the use of conversational agents (chatbots) [13].

10.6 Becoming and Being Reflective Educator

There has been an increasing recognition that faculty can be champions and important role models for supporting reflective practice but requires educators to have a reflective approach to their own educational practice. An important challenge is supporting the development of becoming and being a reflective educator since this requires practical and relevant structured frameworks to stimulate "double-loop" and "triple-loop" thinking about educational situations [14] and appropriate opportunities to collaborate in group-guided reflection, such as in communities of practice [15]. Technology can offer a wide range of different online approaches for supporting these communities, from conferencing software to social media to virtual reality chat rooms.

10.7 Conclusions

The chapter highlights several current challenges and expected future trends in reflective practice, including the interrelated aspects of engagement, assessment, implementation of reflective practice, and both becoming and being a reflective educator. Technology, especially artificial intelligence, is rapidly becoming ubiquitous, and there are several future applications for applying technology to support reflection and reflective practice. Several key recommendations for current and future reflective practice are offered, including ensuring that reflection is contextual and uses appropriate thinking frameworks that are aligned to the intended purpose, the reflection process is adapted to the preference of the learner, and guidance to support reflective practice is provided.

References

1. Argyris C, Schon DA. Theory in practice: increasing professional effectiveness. San Francisco: Wiley; 1992.
2. Winkel AF, Yingling S, Jones AA, Nicholson J. Reflection as a learning tool in graduate medical education: a systematic review. J Grad Med Educ. 2017;9(4):430–9.
3. Heydari S, Beigzadeh A. Medical students' perspectives of reflection for their professional development. BMC Med Educ. 2024;24(1):1399.
4. Moen C, Brown J. Moving from patches to quilts: developing self-aware, reflective leaders through curriculum innovation based on a Patchwork Text approach. Reflective Pract. 2017;18(6):852–65.
5. Rechowicz KJ, Elzie CA. The use of artificial intelligence to detect students' sentiments and emotions in gross anatomy reflections. Anat Sci Educ. 2024;17(5):954–66.
6. Warburton T, Brown J, Sandars J. The use of LEGO® SERIOUS PLAY® within nurse education: a scoping review. Nurse Educ Today. 2022;118:105528.
7. Mojtahedzadeh R, Mohammadi A, Emami AH, Zarei A. How digital storytelling applied in health profession education: a systematized review. J Adv Med Educ Prof. 2021;9(2):63.
8. Developmental Fischer KW, Pruyne E. Reflective thinking in adulthood: emergence, development, and variation. In: Demick J, Andreoletti C, editors. Handbook of adult development. Boston: Springer; 2003. p. 169–98.
9. Wald HS, Borkan JM, Taylor JS, Anthony D, Reis SP. Fostering and evaluating reflective capacity in medical education: developing the REFLECT rubric for assessing reflective writing. Acad Med. 2012;87(1):41–50.
10. Tosey P, Visser M, Saunders MNK. The origins and conceptualizations of 'triple-loop' learning: a critical review. Manag Learn. 2012;43(3):291–307.
11. Kaldjian LC, Yoon J, Ark TK, Shinkunas L, Jotterand F. Practical wisdom in medicine through the eyes of medical students and physicians. Med Educ. 2023;57(12):1219–29.
12. Burla N, Ong RS, Chee RC, Wong RS, Neo SY, Abdul Hamid NA, Lim C, Ong EK, Somasundaram N, Krishna LK. A systematic scoping review on group non-written reflections in medical education. BMC Med Educ. 2024;24(1):1119.
13. Wolfbauer I, Bangerl MM, Maitz K, Pammer-Schindler V. Rebo at work: reflecting on working, learning, and learning goals with the reflection guidance Chatbot for apprentices. In: Albrecht Schmidt A, Väänänen K, Goyal T, Kristensson PO, Peters A, editors. Extended abstracts of the 2023 CHI conference on human factors in computing systems, April 23–28 2023, Hamburg. New York: Association for Computing Machinery; 2023. p. 1–7.
14. Sandars J, Allan D, Price J. Reflective practice by health professions educators to enhance learning and teaching: AMEE guide no. 166. Med Teach. 2024;46(7):864–73.
15. Cleland JA, Jamieson S, Kusurkar RA, Ramani S, Wilkinson TJ, van Schalkwyk S. Redefining scholarship for health professions education: AMEE guide no. 142. Med Teach. 2021;43(7):824–38.

[illegible]

7.5.1 Programmatic Assessment [illegible] of Competence [illegible]

[illegible]

7.5.3 Faculty Burden and [illegible]

[illegible]

7.5.4 Learner Anxiety and [illegible]

An important [illegible]

[illegible]

7.5.5 Ethical Use of Assessment Data

Mindfulness, Faith, Spirituality, and Mental Health in Medical Education

11

Sara Zaidi and Ali Tareq Abdulhasan

Key Points

- There is a link between mindfulness and spirituality that is described as a heightened state of awareness.
- The science behind mindfulness involves the understanding of three domains of human consciousness: the experiential process, the inner self, and the public persona and using mindfulness to allow the feeling of being with rather than avoiding or repressing emotions.
- Mindfulness has been shown to improve anxiety and depression and improve focus as illustrated by magnetic resonance imaging (MRI) studies.
- When mindfulness is implemented in professional settings, it allows for a more thoughtful, empathic response enabling stronger connection between the parties involved.
- The *Treatise on Rights* provides an ethical model for the integration of mindfulness and spirituality into medicine and can be used as a template to create patient-centered care.

11.1 Mental Well-Being and Future Trends

The three central tenets of mindfulness, according to the UK National Health Service (NHS), are the practice of paying attention to the present moment, being without judgment, and approaching it with a gentle curiosity [1]. The American Psychological Association has a similar description: it is a practice that promotes a psychological state of awareness and acceptance [2].

S. Zaidi (✉)
Department of Psychology, New York University, New York, NY, USA

A. T. Abdulhasan
Department of Medicine, University of Al-Ameed, Karbala, Iraq

J. Sandars et al. (eds.), *Modern Medical Education*,
https://doi.org/10.1007/978-3-032-27958-3_11

It is essential to distinguish between mindfulness and meditation as these can often be confused with one another. Mindfulness can be practiced anywhere anytime and merely requires one to be present in the moment while being open and accepting. Meditation is a much more formal and time-structured practice that requires mental training where an individual seeks an inner calm and a specific state of consciousness.

11.2 Mindfulness and Spirituality

Mindfulness is a practice often associated with eastern traditions with deep roots in various cultures and religions. For example, Buddhism teaches that what an individual wants to happen versus accepting what is happening is what causes suffering. In Sufism, mindfulness is central to achieving a closer relationship with God, often through meditation or "Zikr." Yoga is another ancient practice that incorporates mindfulness.

Mindfulness or "muraqaba" in Arabic is a virtue of Islam, derived from the root meaning to watch, observe, and carefully consider. It is deeply embedded in the teachings of the Quran and Hadith, where Muslims are encouraged to reflect deeply on their actions and thoughts. It is also incorporated through prayer and fasting, both of which are ways to self-reflect and allow for spiritual growth. Simply reading the Quran or listening to a surah can be meditative. Additionally, Islamic art, with its intricate designs and calligraphy, also reflects the principles of mindfulness; it is simple and repetitive and requires discipline.

The relationship between mindfulness and spirituality is reciprocal. Spiritual practices require a heightened state of awareness—the very essence of mindfulness. Spirituality is a state of comprehensive awareness of a Higher Being and our inner states in relation to Him. As we submit to the will of God in its complete form, we can reach the highest spiritual state attainable.

11.3 History of the Origins of Mindfulness

The biggest influence on bringing mindfulness from the East to the West was Jon Kabat-Zinn, a professor at the University of Massachusetts Medical School in the late 1970s [3]. He learned about and studied mindfulness under several Buddhist teachers, including Thich Nhat Hanh. Kabat-Zinn developed a program called mindfulness-based stress reduction (MBSR) to treat chronic pain. He discovered that patients would often try to avoid pain, but that avoidance would lead to deeper distress. As mindfulness shifted into mainstream practice, it was integrated into modalities such as mindfulness-based cognitive therapy, dialectical behavior therapy, and acceptance and commitment therapy.

11.4 The Science Behind Mindfulness

To understand how mindfulness works, we need to look at the consciousness processes that occur in the mind. Mindfulness assumes that there are three domains of human consciousness [4]. The first domain is the experiential domain and describes what we experience from the moment we wake up to when we go to sleep. The second domain of human consciousness is the inner self, which is an individual's internal narrator. It provides the narrative for what we are doing given our worldview, self-concept, and understanding of the current situation. The third domain is the public persona, which is what others see through our words and actions. In addition to these domains of consciousness, we must look at how they work with each other through what are known as "filters."

Within the first domain, the experiential domain—the "attentional filter" decides (a) what we choose to notice, (b) what we tend to focus on, and (c) what stays in the background. Our brains are negatively biased (resulting from the need for self-protection in primates) so we often tend to focus on the negative. For example, at work if someone gets a promotion another individual had been wanting, the person may focus on the unfairness of it instead of considering why they might not have been suited for it.

The second filter is known as the "Freudian filter," because it utilizes defense mechanisms identified by Freud. It connects the experiential domain and our inner self. Our inner self (the narrator) uses defense mechanisms to alter and filter experiences to make us feel better; typical defenses include avoidance, suppression, and cognitive dissonance. Continuing with the above example, the individual who did not get the promotion may avoid thinking about it or suppress it or convince themselves that they had not really wanted the promotion anyway.

The third filter is the "Rogerian filter," based on a counseling theory that we must approach people with positive regard; it connects the inner self and the public person in terms of how we choose to portray ourselves. What we try to keep from others, either directly by simply lying or being somewhat deceitful or more indirectly by shifting the conversation or actions to divert their attention. In the example above, the individual may tell their coworkers that they did not have time to manage the promotion and would have turned it down to convince them that they were not affected by the decision.

As more and more memories are avoided and split off, an individual's psychological state becomes increasingly destabilized, vulnerable, insecure, and defensive [5]. It can get to the point where virtually any event that triggers an association of a thought, feeling, or memory must be avoided. This results in chronic anxiety, defensiveness, lack of focus, and, over time, depression. Through mindfulness, an individual is aware and accepting of these emotions instead of avoiding or suppressing them, and this can help people from getting overwhelmed.

Mindfulness allows a reduction in stress, anxiety, and depression and improves focus and memory [6]. It does so by intercepting the negative pathways between the attentional filter, the defense mechanisms, and how we want others to perceive us. If, in our example above, the individual was to practice mindfulness, they would simply acknowledge that they are feeling upset about not being given the promotion and that they have the feelings of being sad, angry, resentful, and frustrated. The individual would stay present with those feelings and recognize that perhaps the decision that they did not get the promotion was not fair. Bringing awareness to those emotions and how the body reacts—perhaps chest heaviness, tightness in the jaw or shoulders, or dryness in the mouth—and allowing those emotions and feelings to pass instead of letting them simmer and build up inside would help them react in a healthier way.

The mechanism through which mindfulness works is through self-awareness, attention control, and emotion regulation. Magnetic resonance imaging (MRI) studies show how the brain changes after practicing mindfulness [7]. There is a significant difference on imaging that show the areas of our brain that are activated when our mind is wandering and after mindfulness, where the only activation we see is that of the prefrontal cortex. More specifically, MRIs have shown that the anterior cingulate cortex (ACC), which is associated with self-regulatory processes, including the ability to shift attention, has a higher gray matter density [6]. The amygdala which is central to switching on the stress (fight or flight) response shrinks in size. The prefrontal cortex, the logical part of the brain that is responsible for executive functioning such as planning and problem-solving, has increased gray matter density. In addition, the connections between the amygdala and the prefrontal cortex are strengthened, paving the way for higher-order brain functions to be less reactive. Researchers have also found that meditation-induced pain relief was associated with the deactivation of the ventromedial prefrontal cortex (vmPFC) [8]. These findings are consistent with the central idea of mindfulness, which is to experience thoughts and feelings without attaching one's ego or sense of self, alleviating emotional pain or discomfort.

The ability to "stop and reflect" with mindfulness practices enables the mind to stop wandering in search of a coping mechanism, to shift attention in a way that fits one's narrative, suppress those emotions, or create an inaccurate narrative. Instead, as seen on the MRI, it quietens the brain, increasing activity in the logical part of the brain, i.e., the prefrontal cortex, and shrinking the amygdala, which is the primary defense mechanism part of the brain. This allows the individual to experience difficult feelings without being overwhelmed.

11.5 Implementation of Mindfulness

Many schools and employers have begun to teach mindfulness practices and self-care. A team of researchers led by Dr. Berger decided to test whether a mindfulness program could improve the mental well-being of healthcare workers at the NIH Clinical Center in 2017 [8]. They ran a 5-week program in which participants attended one 90-min mindfulness training during the workday each week. After completing the program, their stress and anxiety levels were lower than the study's control group. These benefits persisted 2 months after the program ended, and participants also reported a greater inclination toward incorporating mindfulness into their day-to-day lives. The results of this pilot study indicate that a structured, six-week mindfulness program has the potential to benefit clinicians, personally by reducing emotional reactivity, and professionally by promoting deep listening and communication skills [9].

The ability to "stop and reflect" is associated with an improvement in the ability to listen and communicate [10]. Observing and describing are positively correlated with active listening and empathy allowing for more positive, compassionate communication with the patient and the family. The reduction in emotional reactivity allows for more time to reflect on responses and provided thoughtful guidance, rather than reacting to the situation. Nonreactivity also contributes to emotional resilience by allowing one's emotions to occur without getting overwhelmed. Emotional reactivity is directly correlated with burnout. Thus, moderating this with mindfulness techniques provides a direct mechanism of burnout prevention. Mindfulness can help in managing distractions and heighten focus particularly for clinicians performing complex and intricate tasks, thus reducing errors and mistakes [11].

In schools and universities, an effective learning environment can be created by teachers learning to control their emotions instead of trying to control the students or the class. Teachers usually have a lesson plan, an expectation of how they want the class to go, and they often tend to focus on what needs to be done. Being aware of how things are going in the moment would allow the teachers to manage their expectations and reduce their anxiety. Similarly, while wanting to get through the lesson plan, a teacher might begin to rush. Slowing down for a moment can give them time to ask themselves how they are feeling, what's happening in the classroom, and what their students need. It allows them to adapt to the situation as required. Being mindful of the classroom layout and the teachers' position within the room can help create a more positive learning environment. For example, a U-shaped orientation of desks is more conducive to discussion, rather than rows of seats in a lecture hall. Smaller classes, windows, and messaging on walls are all ways to be mindful of the space the students are in. In a virtual environment, being mindful of what tools are available online, such as whiteboards, videos, and chat options, would make the lesson more engaging. Finally, giving each student their full mindful attention for even a short period of class time gives them the message that they are valued as individuals. Recognizing the nonacademic attributes, such as helpfulness, friendliness, creativity, problem-solving, and conflict resolution, all contribute to a successful outcome.

11.6 Mindfulness and Medical Education: The *Treatise on Rights* as a Framework

Clinical overload and ethical dilemmas put a strain on medical professionals resulting in high burnout rates [12]. Conventional curricula have been known to fail to address affective dimensions of healing, including mindfulness, faith, and spirituality, that are important to psychological resilience. This gap requires embedding the *Treatise on*

Rights by Imam Zayn al-Abidin (seventh century CE), which enumerates 51 ḥuqūq (rights/duties) in self, others, and the Divine [13]. In this chapter, we recontextualize *Treatise on Rights* as an Islamic spirituality-evidence-based practice (such as mindfulness-based stress reduction [MBSR] and reflective learning) toolbox [14].

11.6.1 Mindfulness and Sufi Tradition

The focus on tawajjuh (conscious presence) and muraqaba (mindful awareness) within Islamic Sufism dates before the present interest in mindfulness. In its main exertion, tazkiyat al-nafs (self-purification), it consists of: [15]

- Dhikr (sacred remembrance)
- Muhasaba (self-examination)
- Khalwa (solitude)

They develop clinical intuition, in Arabic, we say firasah that improves the nonverbal communication with patients. Neuroscience comes to support the fact that meditation minimizes reactivity of the amygdala to negative stimulus, which helps regulate emotions in high-stress scenarios, and hence improve the intuitive function of the clinicians [16].

Imam Zayn al-Abidin as a trustee between the spirituality and practice, the work of the fourth Shiite Imam, at least that of the Al-Sahifa al-Sajjadiyya (Psalms of Islam) even when he was not a Sufi, had an enormous impact on Sufism. Such was his life:

- Spiritual asceticism (nighttime prayers which reflect Sufi dhikr (meditation)
- Moral rigor through conformance to tazkiyat al-nafs (enhance the growth and development of self)
- Literary influence (influencing themes of closeness to the divine according to Rumi) [15].

This treatise appeared in Umayyad proto-Sufi asceticism, and combined Shiite walaya (divine authority) with individual religious devotion, this became the bridge between early Islamic piety and subsequent mysticism [13].

11.7 The *Treatise on Rights*: A Paradigm of a Mindful Practice

The treatise groups the rights into three interrelated spheres: [13]

1. Self-Rights:
   - Right of the tongue: Use it to what is good, do not interfere (Treatise 3).
   - Right of the stomach/stomach: Do not eat too much or drink and/or eat what is not permitted (Treatise $8).

- Right of the sight: Protect against unethical watches (Treatise SS5).
- Implementation: The trainees are shown how to speak mindfully (e.g., not to gossip) and to take good care of themselves (e.g., balanced diet), reducing the risk of burnout (Treatise §18).

2. Other People Rights:
   - Patient right (similar to the subject through authority, (Treatise SS18): "Do justice, and mercy."
   - Rights of coworkers (Treatise): Be not a punishment, be a favor.
   - Practice: Role-playing during PBL sessions will result in a more empathetic way of settling conflict.
3. God Rights:
   - Right to ritual prayer (Treatise 10): Prayer is standing before God.

     Application: Ordered reflection is a way of matching clinical work with transcendent goals.

     B. Resilience and the Spiritual Intelligence

     The treatise makes a connection between self-awareness and ethical action:
     - Self-regulation: The right of the hand is not to grasp the unlawful (Treatise SS6) compared to methods of mindfulness concerning impulse control.
     - Compassion: Ethical obligations to others have such aspects as the right of the mother (Treatise SS22) that fosters gratitude and extends to vulnerable patients' empathy [13].

11.8 Incorporation of the *Treatise on Rights* in Medical Education

11.8.1 Problem-Based Learning (PBL)

The *Treatise on Rights* shows how Imam Zayn al-Abidin furthers the training in medical ethics using problem-based learning (PBL). A scenario that portrays the severity of a patient nearing his end of life by insisting on being told all the truth and the family refusing since it bestows protective care on that family member qualifies as a case study. The major principles are the adequate respect of the rights of patients, recognition of the family emotions, and balancing the ethical obligations. After discussing, students think about the ways of making judgments with the help of *Treatise on Rights*. The given mode aggravates the moral judgment maximizing the students to face the practical challenges of these problems with focus on rights, empathy, and responsibility toward the patients [17]. Here is a practical plan to medical educators:

11.8.1.1 Introducing a PBL Learning Session through the *Treatise on Rights*

Step 1: Clinical-Ethical Dilemma: The Presentation of Clinical-Ethical Dilemma

Owing to which I suggest that the case example on the problem of conflict of rights, for example:

The case in question is an Ahmed, a 68-year-old male patient and terminally ill, whose mental state is pretty good, as he requested his doctor to tell him about his prognosis as frequently as possible. He appreciates integrity and independence and informs him that he should work his way out. But his adult children who are too concerned about his interest advise the medical workers against revealing this information. It is due to the fact they believe that his presence would most likely make privy to all the truth and bring him to so much suffering and they believed it was their devotion to the culture to keep him out of such painful information.

Step 2: Support Group Analysis and Decision with Regard to the Conflict

Separate the students into small groups and discuss the case using the help of the following questions:

- What are we aware of regarding the medical issues?

In this instance (i.e., the right to know of the patient, the right to protect of the family), is there a conflict in the rights (Ḥuqūq)?

- How is this to the patient? For the family? For the healthcare team?

Step 3: Introducing the Treatise on Rights as an Ethical Framework

Give the students a couple of passages of the treatise relevant to this ethical dilemma, and ask them to exercise these rights so that they can research this dilemma. The better rights, which may be brought, are:

- The right of the one who has responsibility for you (Treatise section 18): this can be taken to refer to the obligation of the doctor to the patient and family and he must not be fair and must not be true.
- The right of the tongue (Treatise section 3) and why one is supposed to speak wisely and speak the truth. All around is its telling of truth against.
- The right of the self (connoted everywhere): the right of choice of the patient and his religious preparedness to death.

Step 4: The Reflection of Deliberation and Role Play

This case is an opportunity to practice mindfulness, that is, enact the scenario using role play, to get deep into feelings and thoughts of the doctor in charge, the patient, and family:

The role-players will also be asked to complete the part of the physician, Ahmed, and one of the family members. A doctor must speak about his/her initiative, and he/she must listen, but not to judge, bring up the question about the fear of the family (I hear your great love and care of your father), and reassure the patient he/ she has the free will of knowing the truth he/she could prepare (Ahmed, you have said it is important that you should know the truth so that you could prepare).

Brainstorm a Resolution: In this step, the groups will brainstorm, i.e., brainstorm a communication plan or plan of care in which, where possible, as many rights in the dispute as possible have been considered. This might involve:

- Request a patient to provide the consent to involve his family in the process of prognosis.
- Interrogatives to ask the patient—what does he hope at this moment; it may change to his hope of being cured or comforted, finding dignity and being reconciled.
- This family should be convinced to clarify their views and be considered with their cultural considerations but clarified satisfactorily about the ethical and legal natural outcomes of the physician to the patient.

Step 5: Debrief and Reflect
Key discussion points:

- What was your reaction to the dilemma to the treatise?
- Were chances in existence where the major right of all sides would be taken into account?
- What was your attitude to role-playing and mindful listening (how either of them influenced your attitude toward what you were experiencing about the situation)?

The *Treatise on Rights* is not only a text but also does not cease being an educational toolkit simultaneously. It leaves the future generation of doctors incorporating their cultural competences into their practice providing personalized care.

11.8.2 Cinemeducation

The use of cinemeducation during medical education can offer the helpful insights concerning the ethical dilemma and the doctor-patient relationship. One of the most remarkable movies to be analyzed is The Doctor (1991) which graphically shows the right of care (Treatise 2); this is a right to give the patient compassionate and empathetic treatment [13, 18]. An interesting example with which to argue the necessity of caregivers to do so with compassion and empathy is the 1991 film "The Doctor" which illustrates the importance of the right of care (Treatise section 2).

11.8.2.1 An Educator Work Planning Model

The followings are practical steps in using The Doctor film in applying the treatise of rights:

Step 1: Preparation to See

The setting of the exercise should be placed to the students before the chosen scenes are screened. The following need to be clarified:

- We are also going to watch excerpts of The Doctor which is about Dr. Jack MacKee, brilliant, but detached surgeon until his diagnosis of his own cancer makes him the patient.
- You need to consider the effects of his experiences on the other side of the stethoscope on his perceptions of dignity of his patients, communication with his patients, and the right to provide them with compassionate care.

Step 2: Be Attentive to the Important Scene that Exemplify the Dramatic Shift in Dr. MacKee Mindset

There are 3–4 important scenes in Screen 3–4, which compare the attitude of Dr. MacKee before and after. Take a break between two screening sessions to discuss.

Scene 1: The Detached Surgeon (at the beginning of the film)

- Action: MacKee is caught being rude to his patients, making jokes on their patients or putting efficiency on priority instead of compassion. As a good example, he tells one other doctor never get involved with a patient.

Group Discussion

(1) What rights of the treatise is being abused by Dr. MacKee in his course? (e.g., the right of care (2) to be treated with compassion; the right of the tongue (3) to speak wisely and kindly).

- What is the impact of the behavior on the feelings of dignity and trust of the patient?

Scene 2: The Vulnerable Patient (his experiences in early life as a patient)

- Action: Add the by now familiar example of MacKee being disciplined in the chilly, depersonalizing, disempowering fashion that is prevalent in the hospital, even the mention of the doctor pension is bureaucrat.
- Submission Guidelines

Imagine that you are in the position of MacKee. So how is he feeling now that he is the patient?

- In what way does this experience come out to challenge his past professional identity?

Scene 3: The paradigm shift, meeting June, terminally ill patient, that trigger transformation.

- Act: MacKee is seen to make contact with another patient, who is called June. MacKee gets to know how to listen, express his vulnerability, and offer emotional support to someone.

Case Discussion

- What is the example of the right of care (§2) with his relationship with June?
- What attentive skills is he beginning to cultivate here? (e.g., deep listening, nonjudgmental presence).

Scene 4: The new professional identity (at the end of the film)

- Action: This time, MacKee is playing with another style with the patient. MacKee sits, gazes the patient in his eyes, listens, and realizes his fear.

Group Discussion

- Compare this new strategy to the initial scene that we have observed. What has happened and transformed?
- How does he now respect the right of the patient to dignity and his or her emotional needs be heard?

Step 3: Encourage Reflective Summary that Plan for Future

Once the clips are screened, have the entire class debriefed on how to put the ideas to practices by the leader.

You can follow this guide:

- The suffering Dr. MacKee experienced was what brought about the change that took place in him. You, my future doctors, will have to learn to create the same sympathy without having to experience your own health problems.
- Following the structure of the *Treatise on Rights*, develop your own "Patient Bill of Rights" to use in your practice in the future. What do you think are the three rights that would rank highest in the list, according to the trip that MacKee makes?
- Think about an occasion when you were not listened to or disregarded in a workplace or other personal situation. What can you tell me about that memory that will inform your devotion to mindful patient care?

Through organized discussion, The Doctor is no longer merely the educational programming, but the simulation that has the real authority. It provides the student with the chance to foster professional identity and see the outcome of care that is detached, the outcome of mindful care, and makes him or her wish that he or she becomes a healer who cares and not just cures.

11.8.3 Using Portfolio

Write a note of a clinical situation in which the *Treatise on Rights* by Imam Zayn al-Abidin may be used in ethical decision-making. Gratitude journals (§6, "right of hearing") in order to dispel cynicism [13, 19]. Learning portfolios really gives the students the chance to reflect on the journey and think about how the ethics presented in the *Treatise on Rights* apply to the experiences in the clinical practice, because, of course, none of it is merely theoretical, but the journey will prepare the students to be resilient to negativity, with their own professional identity that will survive the good years and the hard years of the medical profession.

11.8.3.1 A Model for Teachers

This is portfolio work, which will enable all students to apply meaningfully to the treatise.

Portfolio Part 1: The Rights-Based Clinical Reflection

This is more than your average clinical journal entry. It is an inspection of ethics in operation.

What Students Should Do

Consider one of your clinical experiences from the last rotation about which you felt uncomfortable, upset, or just really emotional—good or bad.

Part A: The Story

Simply state what occurred. Who was there? What was the medical situation? What was being said or done?

Part B: The Rights-Based Analysis (The Thoughtful Pause)

Take a step back, then, and reflect on this moment with the help of the *Treatise on Rights*. This is the opportunity you have to think deeply.

Find: What particular rights from the treatise emerged in this case?

Like: "The right of care (§2), the right to be treated kindly, was challenged when our team rushed past the patient's questions."

"The right of the tongue (§3), the right to speak out or to be silent, was difficult for me to apply one time because a superior made an insulting remark about a patient."

"I felt the right of the one who wrongs you when my sibling yelled at me, so I had to think about how to react."

To Reflect: Was the right honored or disregarded? What was your response? What was the effect on you, the client, and the rest of the world?

Imagine: What would you have done differently to honor that right? Think about one thing you could have said or done to communicate the ideas of the treatise more effectively.

Why This Helps: This activity is teaching the student how to utilize the treatise as more than just something to be memorized but also how the treatise is able to help the student think about difficult situations and develop their own response to future happenings.

Portfolio Part 2: The Gratitude Journal for Keeping Cynicism Away

Negative perceptions, the result of burnout, appear readily if one focuses on problems, complaints, and inefficiency in the system. This exercise is the opposite, utilizing the "right of hearing (§6)" to help the students focus on the positive aspects, the human side of the medical world.

What Students Should Do:

"The right of hearing" is the act of listening for the good while turning your attention away from the things that bring you down. A hospital is always noisy—alarms going off, patients complaining, bad news, negativity surrounding you on all sides. Your task: maintain a gratitude journal for the "gratitude of hearing" each week while on your rotation.

Each week, record the times you heard or saw the following:

Human Kindness: Maybe it's the nice conversation between the nurse and the patient. Maybe the laughing family in the waiting room.

Good Work: Have you ever seen a resident explain something to a puzzled patient or received good advice from a doctor?

Personal Support: It could be that you received thanks from the patient or perhaps some encouragement from a colleague.

Quiet Respect: Like the moment of quiet following the difficult diagnosis, just sitting with the patients, you know, in respect. "This week, on the cancer floor, I made an attempt to hear beyond the beeps of the alarms common to the room.

Listening, I was able to hear Dr. A spending 20 min with Mr. J and his wife, just sitting there with them, allowing them time to cry, asking the same questions repeatedly, listening instead of just seeking answers. This is definitely the right of care, the importance of which has made me realize that sometimes its greatest application is just being there, rather than having the answers."

Why This Helps: This is another way to train your mind to focus on the good stuff, instead of looking only for problems. When you focus on the good, you will grow emotionally, shield your mind from negativity, and remember why you chose to go into the field of medicine in the first place.

Combining honest ethical reflection with the diligent observation of the good, this portfolio is more than just an assignment. It is also a resource for growth, grounded in the thoughtful ideas of the *Treatise on Rights*.

11.9 Conclusion

In conclusion, mindfulness is a new way of looking at age-old practices. It's a way of accepting and being at peace with oneself that improves overall well-being. There is a deep connection to faith and spirituality, simplifying one's experience to simply being present instead of overthinking. The benefit of mindfulness lowering anxiety and stress while improving overall health is a strong argument to incorporate these methods into future curriculums in all institutions. The *Treatise on Rights* provides an ethical model of integration of mindfulness and spirituality into medicine. Practicing through problem-based learning and portfolio reflection, builds resilience, ethical reasoning, and patient-centered care, turning healthcare into a place of clinical as well as spiritual intelligence where sometimes, cure, often, treat, always comfort becomes the norm.

Acknowledgments The authors declare the use of AI tools for the paraphrasing.

Competing Interests There is no conflict of interest.

References

1. NHS. Mindfulness. National Health Service. Retrieved November 11, 2025, from https://www.nhs.uk/mental-health/self-help/tips-and-support/mindfulness/.
2. American Psychological Association. Mindfulness. APA Dictionary of Psychology. Retrieved November 11, 2025, from https://dictionary.apa.org/mindfulness
3. Joaquín J. History of mindfulness: from east to west and from religion to science. Breathwork. 2018;
4. Fagan A. What is mindfulness and how does it work. Psychol Today. 2015;
5. Tang YY, Hölzel BK, Posner MI. The neuroscience of mindfulness meditation. Nat Rev Neurosci. 2015;16(4):213–25. https://doi.org/10.1038/nrn3916.
6. Keng SL, Smoski MJ, Robins CJ. Effects of mindfulness on psychological health: a review of empirical studies. Clin Psychol Rev. 2011;31(6):1041–56. https://doi.org/10.1016/j.cpr.2011.04.006.
7. Wolkin J. How the brain changes when you meditate. Mind. 2023;
8. Marchand WR. Neural mechanisms of mindfulness and meditation: evidence from neuroimaging studies. World J Radiol. 2014;6(7):471–9. https://doi.org/10.4329/wjr.v6.i7.471.
9. Levy B. Brief mindfulness program reduces healthcare workers' stress. NIH Intramural Res Program. 2021;
10. Kotecha R. Boosting resilience and Well-being: harnessing mindfulness for healthcare professionals. Mind. 2023;
11. Watson T, Walker O, Cann R, Varghese AK. The benefits of mindfulness in mental healthcare professionals. F1000Res. 2022;10:1085. https://doi.org/10.12688/f1000research.74136.2.
12. Dyrbye LN, Shanafelt TD, Sinsky CA, Cipriano PF, Bhatt J, Ommaya A, et al. Burnout among health care professionals: a call to explore and address this underrecognized threat to safe, high-quality care. NAM Perspect. 2017;7(7):1–6. https://doi.org/10.31478/201707b.
13. Imam Zayn al-ʿĀbidīn. The Psalms of Islam (al-Ṣaḥīfa al-Sajjādiyya). Chittick WC, translator. London: Muhammadi Trust; 1988. 301 p.
14. Shapiro SL, Astin JA, Bishop SR, Cordova M. Mindfulness-based stress reduction for health care professionals: results from a randomized trial. Int J Stress Manag. 2005;12(2):164–76. https://doi.org/10.1037/1072-5245.12.2.164.
15. Ernst CW. The Shambhala guide to Sufism. Boston: Shambhala; 1997. 264 p.
16. Leung MK, Lau WKW, Chan CCH, Wong SSY, Fung ALC, Lee TMC. Meditation-induced neuroplastic changes in amygdala activity during negative affective processing. Soc Neurosci. 2018;13(3):277–88. https://doi.org/10.1080/17470919.2017.1311939.
17. Parker M. Autonomy, problem-based learning, and the teaching of medical ethics. J Med Ethics. 1995;21(5):305–10. https://doi.org/10.1136/jme.21.5.305.
18. Gorring H, Loy J, Spring H. Cinemeducation: using film as an educational tool in mental health services. Health Inf Libr J. 2014;31(1):84–8. https://doi.org/10.1111/hir.12052.
19. Puchalski CM, Vitillo R, Hull SK, Reller N. Improving the spiritual dimension of whole person care: reaching national and international consensus. J Palliat Med. 2014;17(6):642–56. https://doi.org/10.1089/jpm.2014.9427.

The Use of Workshops in Modern Clinical Education 12

Syed Yaseen Naqvi and Syed Mohammad Naqvi

Key Points

- Workshops are a pedagogical necessity in modern clinical education, resolving the tension between educational scalability and authentic practice.
- The effectiveness of workshops is grounded in andragogy, experiential learning, and their alignment with the outcomes-based framework of CBME.
- Evaluating workshop efficacy requires moving beyond learner satisfaction to a rigorous framework like the Kirkpatrick model, which assesses behavioral change and impact on results.
- Overcoming implementation barriers requires a strategic institutional commitment to dismantle cultural silos and reengineer systems to support active, interprofessional learning.
- Innovations in digital learning, virtual simulation, and augmented reality are expanding the accessibility and realism of workshops.

S. Y. Naqvi (✉)
American Board of Internal Medine, Cardiovascular Diseases and Interventional Cardiology, Faculty of Medicine, University of Warith Al-Anbiyaa, Karbala, Iraq

Health Professions Education, School of Medicine, University of Limerick, Department of Medicine, University Hospital Kerry., Tralee, Ireland

S. M. Naqvi
Health Professions Education, School of Medicine, University of Limerick, Department of Medicine, University Hospital Kerry., Tralee, Ireland

J. Sandars et al. (eds.), *Modern Medical Education*,
https://doi.org/10.1007/978-3-032-27958-3_12

12.1 Introduction

Medical education has undergone an evolution over the past few decades, transitioning from traditional, lecture-based pedagogical models to more dynamic, learner-centered and interactive approaches [1, 2]. Medical education is primarily characterized by a division between preclinical lectures and subsequent clinical clerkships. While effective at scaling the dissemination of knowledge, this model often fails to effectively prepare learners for the complexities of modern healthcare systems. A central challenge today is to adequately guide the transformation of novice learners into competent, reflective, and collaborative healthcare professionals. In this context, educational strategies that emphasize active participation, contextual learning, and real-time feedback have gained attention [2]. Traditional clerkships offer a high authenticity but are unscalable, while large-group lectures provided scalability at the cost of authentic practice. In an era marked by rapid technological advancements, evolving patient safety standards, and the shift toward competency-based medical education (CBME), workshops have emerged as an adaptable, evidence-based bridge between theory and authentic clinical application.

Workshops are broadly defined as organized, group educational events that target specific learning outcomes through participatory methods, such as simulation, discussions, role-playing, and hands-on skill development [3]. They are structured interactive and scalable learning experiences in an authentic and safe environment. By engaging learners in active problem-solving and reflective practice, it promotes deeper learning and retention. Their versatility enables them to be employed effectively from undergraduate and postgraduate training to continuing professional development initiatives. This chapter explores the theoretical foundations, instructional design principles, educational benefits, implementation challenges, and emerging innovations associated with the use of workshops in clinical education.

12.2 The Pedagogical Underpinnings of Workshop-Based Learning

A common challenge in modern education is that many curricula approach learners using pedagogical models designed for children, which may result in disengagement and reduced learning effectiveness among students and trainees [2]. Workshops are consistent with current adult learning theories and established educational frameworks that prioritize active, experiential, and socially embedded learning. These approaches highlight learner autonomy, participation, and collaborative construction of knowledge.

Chief among these is Malcolm Knowles' theory of andragogy, which highlights the unique characteristics and learning preferences of adult learners [2]. Knowles proposed that adult learners are typically self-directed, possess a strong intrinsic motivation to learn, and draw upon a wealth of prior personal and professional experience in interpreting new information. They are leaning toward learning that is problem centered and directly applicable to real-world settings. Workshops inherently support these principles by fostering environments in which learners engage with clinically relevant scenarios, solve context-specific problems, and receive immediate feedback that enhances not only their knowledge but leads to professional growth. This alignment with andragogical principles reinforces learner autonomy and accountability. They are explicitly problem centered, focusing on developing specific skills or addressing clinical challenges, which satisfies the adult's task-oriented learning preference. Furthermore, by grounding learning in authentic clinical scenarios, workshops answer the adult learner's fundamental question: "Why do I need to know this?."

While andragogy explains why workshops are effective for adult learners, David Kolb's experiential learning theory explains how they work [4]. Kolb describes learning as the process whereby knowledge is created through the transformation of experience. In this theory, meaningful learning occurs through a cyclical process that involves four stages. The cycle begins with a concrete experience (the hands-on activity), followed by reflective observation (the debriefing), then abstract conceptualization (connecting the experience to broader principles), and finally active experimentation (applying the new concepts) [4]. Workshops are ideally structured to support this model. For example, a procedural skills workshop might begin with a live or simulated demonstration of a clinical task (concrete experience), proceed with group discussion and individual reflection on the process (reflective observation), introduce underlying principles and evidence-based guidelines (abstract conceptualization), and culminate in hands-on practice or simulated patient encounters (active experimentation).

The importance of the workshop facilitator is paramount for it to be successful as they are not merely instructors but are managers of the learning cycle [3]. Kolb's theory also identifies four corresponding learning styles, noting that individuals have preferences for different parts of the cycle; "accommodators" prefer doing and feeling, while "assimilators" prefer thinking and watching [4]. A learner might naturally excel at the concrete experience but struggle with abstract conceptualization. Without guidance, they can become "stuck" in one part of the cycle, leading to incomplete learning. The facilitator's primary role is to diagnose where learners are in the cycle and guide them through all four stages, ensuring they connect doing with thinking and feeling with reflection [3]. To maximize the potential of this experience, the focus of faculty development must extend beyond content expertise to train educators in the art of managing this cognitive and emotional cycle.

Social constructivism as articulated by Lev Vygotsky supports the pedagogical value of workshops. Vygotsky emphasized the importance of the "zone of proximal development" (ZPD), the range of tasks that learners can perform with guidance but not yet independently, and the central role of social interaction in cognitive development [2]. Within workshops, learners engage in collaborative activities, guided problem-solving, and peer-to-peer learning, all of which support progression through the ZPD [2]. Facilitated discussions, role-playing, and case analyses promote the co-construction of knowledge, while feedback from instructors and colleagues helps refine clinical reasoning and judgment. The social dimension of learning, combined with scaffolded support, enhances not only knowledge acquisition but also the development of professional identity and teamwork skills, which are essential in modern clinical environments.

CBME is an outcomes-based approach where progression is defined by the demonstration of observable abilities or competencies [1]. Workshops provide a controlled, observable environment where competencies like teamwork, crisis management, and communication can be actively practiced and assessed. This aligns with Ericsson's framework of deliberate practice, where skill mastery arises from focused, purposeful practice guided by immediate feedback and coaching [5]. However, this creates a significant implementation paradox: while the philosophy here is flexible, enabling trainees to advance at their own pace, the practical delivery of workshops is often logistically rigid and complex, requiring careful coordination of learners, faculty, technicians, and dedicated space. Presenting learners with realistic, context-rich case vignettes or simulations facilitates cognitive engagement and promotes the transfer of learning from the educational setting to actual patient care. For example, a workshop focused on breaking bad news should not only present structured communication frameworks but also foster the development of empathy, emotional regulation, and clarity in dialogue.

12.3 Typology, Principles, and Benefits

Clinical workshops can take various forms enhancing their appeal. Their flexibility and scalability allow them to be tailored to a wide variety of content areas, levels of learner expertise, and institutional contexts. Short, focused sessions can be used to teach discrete skills, while longitudinal workshop series may support progressive development of complex competencies. Furthermore, the adaptability of workshops to in-person, virtual, and hybrid delivery formats allows institutions to extend learning opportunities to geographically diverse or time-constrained learners, thereby promoting equity and inclusion in medical education.

Simulation-based workshops use models, mannequins, or virtual environments to replicate clinical scenarios, providing a safe setting to develop skills without risk to patients [6]. This spectrum ranges from low-fidelity task trainers for isolated procedures to high-fidelity manikins for complex emergencies. The simulation provides "concrete experience," but deeper learning is consolidated during the subsequent reflective stages of Kolb's cycle. Debriefing is an integral part of simulations, where learners participate in structured sessions to receive feedback on their performance [6, 7]. Here, mistakes are analyzed, and mental models are corrected; however, facilitating it effectively requires specific training beyond mere clinical expertise. Therefore, a greater return on educational investment is often achieved by prioritizing faculty development in debriefing over hardware acquisition [7]. This allows learners to refine their technical skills without compromising patient safety, thereby aligning with the principles of deliberate practice and mastery learning [5].

This deliberate reflection promotes self-awareness, encourages the identification of performance gaps, and guides the development of personalized learning strategies. Over time, engaging in reflective practice has been shown to improve clinical judgment, resilience, and professional identity formation. However, this approach is not without significant hurdles. The resource intensity of simulation is a primary barrier, encompassing not only the financial cost of high-fidelity equipment but also the need for dedicated space and trained technicians. Furthermore, it creates a high demand for faculty who are skilled in facilitation, a demand that often outstrips institutional capacity.

Case-based learning (CBL) and its evolution, seminar-case learning (SCL), are workshop formats that use authentic clinical cases to bridge theory and practice [8]. In these workshops, small groups analyze a clinical scenario to hone their clinical reasoning skills. Evidence shows that the SCL model, which combines collaborative problem-solving with expert-facilitated discussion, results in improved theoretical knowledge, case analysis, and clinical skill compared to traditional lectures [8]. Real-world clinical reasoning involves navigating ambiguity and incomplete information. Therefore, an effective case must be more than a simple problem; it must be an authentic scenario that mirrors the complexity and "messiness" of a real patient encounter, designed to provoke debate rather than lead to a single answer. It is important to acknowledge that designing and planning such workshops can be both challenging, requiring significant preparation to ensure their educational value.

Active participation is the hallmark of an effective workshop and distinguishes it from more didactic formats. Learners gain the most from a workshop by preparing in advance and actively participating [3]. Studies have shown a positive correlation between practice and confidence in skills [5]. Whether applied to procedural training (e.g., vascular access, airway management) or crisis resource management scenarios, the emphasis on repetition, feedback, and incremental improvement accelerates skill acquisition and long-term retention. To further enhance realism and test clinical systems, workshops can be conducted in situ, that is, within the actual clinical environment, such as an emergency department or operating room. Techniques such as role-playing, small-group case analysis, structured debates, and high-fidelity simulations promote active learning, allowing learners to test hypotheses, refine reasoning, and internalize new information. These interactive methods foster deeper cognitive engagement, stimulate metacognitive reflection, and support the development of professional identity. Importantly, a well-balanced workshop should integrate didactic content with sufficient opportunities for learners to express their views, pose questions, and engage in collaborative problem-solving.

In addition to technical skills, workshops enhance clinical reasoning, a core competency in modern medical practice. Through structured format, learners are required to generate hypotheses, prioritize differential diagnoses, and formulate diagnostic or therapeutic plans [3]. This active engagement nurtures analytical thinking, pattern recognition, and metacognitive skills essential for diagnostic accuracy. Importantly, observing and discussing the reasoning strategies of peers and facilitators exposes learners to diverse clinical heuristics and cognitive approaches, helping to refine their diagnostic frameworks and avoid common cognitive errors.

They also improve communication and interpersonal skills, which are often under-emphasized in traditional curricula. By simulating challenging scenarios, such as delivering bad news, managing difficult patients, or engaging in interprofessional collaboration, learners can rehearse and receive feedback on both verbal and non-verbal aspects of communication. These structured encounters allow for the exploration of empathy, emotional intelligence, negotiation, and assertiveness, skills that are foundational for patient-centered care and effective team functioning. Workshops focusing on communication skills have been shown to improve not only learner confidence but also actual performance in clinical interactions [6].

12.4 Challenges, Limitations, and Evaluation

Despite the advantages associated with workshops, their implementation and sustainability are not without considerable challenges which must be thoughtfully addressed to ensure long-term effectiveness. These span logistical, instructional, learner-related, and evaluative domains.

One of the prominent barriers is the resource intensity of workshops [1, 3, 6, 7, 9]. Compared to traditional lectures, workshops typically require smaller group sizes to facilitate meaningful interaction, individualized feedback, and hands-on practice. This necessitates a high facilitator-to-learner ratio, which can strain faculty availability and institutional resources. Additionally, simulation-based workshops often depend on access to expensive equipment, task trainers, audiovisual aids, and dedicated learning spaces [6]. The logistical coordination required to schedule sessions, manage learner rotations, and maintain equipment adds further complexity. These demands are particularly burdensome in low-resource settings, where the infrastructure and financial capacity to support such educational modalities may be limited. In such contexts, the adoption of workshops may be restricted, and creative solutions, such as peer-led models, low-cost simulation alternatives, and mobile workshop units may be necessary to ensure equitable access.

Maintaining consistency and quality across multiple workshop sessions poses another significant challenge [9]. Variations in facilitator expertise, pedagogical approach, and adherence to instructional protocols can lead to discrepancies in learner experience and outcomes. Furthermore, informal teaching styles and ad hoc modifications to workshop content may dilute learning objectives or introduce unintentional biases. To address this variability, institutions should invest in the development of standardized facilitator guides, clearly articulated learning objectives, and robust orientation or faculty development programs. Establishing centralized mechanisms for quality assurance, such as standardized evaluation tools, peer observation, and periodic audits, can further promote consistency across sessions and settings. Pedagogical challenges are also significant, including a shortage of faculty trained in advanced facilitation techniques like debriefing.

Healthcare is a team-based endeavor and so interprofessional education (IPE) should be foundational in clinical education [5]. IPE has been linked to improved patient outcomes, reduced medical errors, and greater system efficiency, highlighting its clinical as well as educational value. A challenge lies however as healthcare education has traditionally been siloed, cultivating distinct professional identities that can become barriers to collaboration [10]. An effective IPE workshop must therefore first facilitate the creation of a superordinate team identity that transcends individual professional affiliations. This involves incorporating activities focused on stereotype deconstruction and mutual role clarification before engaging in complex clinical problem-solving, as addressing the social and psychological preconditions of collaboration is essential for teamwork to flourish. These cultural barriers are often compounded by formidable logistical challenges. The difficulty of aligning the academic calendars and schedules of separate professional schools may be a symptom of the traditionally siloed educational structure, making IPE one of the most difficult workshop models to implement sustainably. IPE programs have demonstrated positive outcomes by teaching and developing courses across various healthcare disciplines [10].

Learner-related factors can also complicate workshop dynamics and outcomes. Heterogeneity in learners' baseline knowledge, clinical experience, motivation, and preferred learning styles may result in differential levels of engagement and satisfaction. Some participants may dominate discussions, while others remain passive, undermining the collaborative and inclusive spirit of workshops. Effective facilitation requires sensitivity to group dynamics, the ability to scaffold learning for varying levels of expertise, and the promotion of psychological safety to encourage all learners to contribute. Facilitators must also be adept at identifying disengagement or confusion and adapting their instructional strategies accordingly.

Another significant limitation lies in the evaluation of workshop effectiveness. Post-session evaluations may show high levels of learner satisfaction and increased self-reported confidence, but these subjective metrics are limited in their ability to reflect actual learning or behavioral change [1]. To justify their significant investment of time and resources, the effectiveness of workshops must be rigorously evaluated. These may include objective structured assessments, direct observation of clinical performance, longitudinal tracking of behavior change, and, ultimately, the measurement of patient-related outcomes. Integrating workshops into broader programmatic assessment frameworks, aligned with competency-based education principles, may enhance both accountability and educational impact. While workshops hold great promise as a dynamic and learner-centered modality in clinical education, their successful implementation demands careful attention to resources, instructional design, facilitator development, learner engagement, and outcome evaluation. Addressing these challenges is essential for realizing their full educational potential.

To move beyond simple satisfaction surveys, educators should adopt a structured framework like the Kirkpatrick model, which assesses training effectiveness at four progressive levels: reaction (satisfaction), learning (knowledge and skills), behavior (transfer of learning to the workplace), and results (impact on patient outcomes) [1, 7, 11]. A study by Heydari et al. using the Kirkpatrick model demonstrated significant improvements in healthcare staff's satisfaction (Level 1), learning (Level 2), and observed behavior change (Level 3) following a structured workshop on teaching and learning methods [11]. Participants reported high satisfaction (62.5% rating the workshop as excellent), demonstrated statistically significant learning gains (notably in preparation and teaching method use, $p < 0.05$), and showed measurable behavioral improvements in key teaching competencies 2 months after training ($p \leq 0.05$ in most areas) [11]. While strong evidence supports Levels 1 and 2, and some emerging research addresses Level 3, robust data demonstrating sustained changes in clinical outcomes (Level 4) remains limited. Closing this gap represents the next major frontier for research in medical education. This "Kirkpatrick gap," the paucity of high-quality research at the upper levels of the model, marks a crucial frontier for future work in medical education.

12.5 A Framework for Designing and Facilitating High-Impact Workshops

Effective workshop design requires a strategic alignment between learning objectives, instructional methods, assessment approaches, and available resources in a strategic manner. These components must cohesively support each other to ensure that the educational intervention is both pedagogically sound and practically relevant to the clinical context. The six-step approach to curriculum development, as detailed by Schneiderhan et al., provides a practical framework for creating effective educational workshops [12].

1. *Performing a needs assessment and writing a rationale statement*

This foundational step begins by identifying the professional practice gap the workshop aims to address. This is the difference between the current state (what learners know) and the ideal state (what they should know) based on evidence, guidelines, or observed performance deficits. This analysis forms the basis of a rationale statement that justifies the need for a novel educational intervention and to define its purpose.

2. *Determining and prioritizing content*

Based on the needs assessment, the next step is to determine the specific knowledge, skills, and attitudes that must be taught. This involves curating relevant and evidence-based content. The development team must prioritize this to ensure the workshop focuses on the critical information needed to close the practice gap within the allotted time. This stage also includes selecting faculty who are not only content experts but also engaging and effective teachers.

3. *Writing goals and objectives*

With the content prioritized, the focus shifts to creating clear learning objectives. These should be written as SMART objectives (specific, measurable, achievable, relevant, and time-bound). The objectives must clearly state what the learner will be able to do as a result of participating and serve as the blueprint for the activities, content, and assessments.

4. *Selecting educational strategies*

This step involves choosing the instructional methods that best align with the learning objectives. A varied approach is most effective. This includes:

- Formats: Select the overall format (e.g., simulation, IPE, CBL, SCL).
- Activities: Use interactive methods based on learning preferences, such as small-group discussions, role-playing, brainstorming sessions, or case analyses. Match the method to the objective; for instance, teach procedural skills with hands-on trainers and teamwork with interprofessional scenarios.
- Assessment and Feedback Plan: A critical part of the strategy is planning how learning will be measured. This includes designing tools for both formative assessments (conducted *during* the learning process to guide development) and summative assessment (conducted *at the end* to evaluate if competencies have been achieved) [12]. The strategy must incorporate frequent opportunities for feedback and a structured, psychologically safe debriefing session.

5. *Implementation*

This step is the practical execution of the educational plan. It involves delivering the curated content through the planned interactive activities, facilitating learner engagement, and administering the formative assessments and feedback as designed. Effective implementation relies on careful planning, prepared faculty, and a conducive learning environment.

6. *Evaluation and application of lessons learned*

The final step is a dual process.

- First, the workshop itself is evaluated, using a framework like Kirkpatrick's model to measure learner reaction, learning, and subsequent behavioral change.
- Second, the planning committee must reconvene to analyze all evaluation data, learner feedback, and faculty reflections. This "application of lessons learned" is crucial for making iterative, evidence-based improvements to future workshops, ensuring the educational process remains a continuous cycle of quality improvement.

Following this structured cycle ensures that the programs are evidence-based, learner-centered, and continuously improved to meet evolving professional practice needs.

12.6 Innovations and Future Directions

The future of clinical education is being shaped by a coming together of technological advancements and the needs of healthcare systems. Innovations in instructional design, simulation, and assessments are transforming workshops from isolated teaching events into integral components of comprehensive, competency-driven educational frameworks. At the forefront of this transformation is the integration of immersive technologies, particularly virtual reality (VR) and augmented reality (AR). These technologies can simulate complex clinical environments and patient interactions, offering learners the opportunity to rehearse both technical procedures and cognitive tasks in realistic but risk-free settings. For procedural training in fields such as dentistry, surgery, emergency medicine, and interventional radiology/cardiology, VR and AR environments replicate anatomical complexity and enable deliberate practice with real-time feedback [13, 14]. Studies show that immersive VR in surgical training improves procedure times, accuracy, and user satisfaction and is cost-effective [13]. Similarly, for cognitive skills such as diagnostic reasoning or team-based decision-making, immersive simulations offer dynamic scenarios that evolve in response to learner input. This adaptability is particularly valuable when access to live clinical exposure is limited, whether due to patient safety concerns, time constraints, or geographical barriers.

In parallel, digital platforms are extending the reach and flexibility of workshops. Online learning management systems, mobile applications, and video-based instruction enable learners to engage with didactic material asynchronously, allowing workshops to be used primarily for active learning and skill applications. This approach aligns with the "flipped classroom" model, in which foundational content is learned independently before the in-person or synchronous workshop session [15]. By reallocating didactic time to prework and reserving workshops for interaction, feedback, and practice, educators can maximize engagement and foster deeper learning. Moreover, digital tools support longitudinal learning by enabling learners to revisit workshop materials, review their performance data, and track progress toward specific competencies.

Workshops align naturally with the CBME model when specific competencies, whether related to communication, procedural proficiency, or professionalism, are mapped to learning activities and assessment tools [1]. Well-designed workshops not only provide the structured experiences needed for skill development but also generate robust data for formative and summative assessments. This can be particularly valuable in milestone-based progression models, where learners advance based on demonstrated competence rather than time-based training. As CBME becomes more widely implemented across institutions, workshops are increasingly positioned as pivotal tools for assessing clinical readiness and supporting high-stakes decisions around advancement and licensure.

Finally, there is growing advocacy for scholarly dissemination of workshop-based innovations. Publishing detailed descriptions of workshop curricula, teaching strategies, and evaluation outcomes in peer-reviewed journals fosters sharing knowledge and advances the science of medical education. Scholarly output also allows for critical peer feedback, replication, and adaptation in diverse contexts, thereby amplifying the impact of educational interventions and contributing to a more robust evidence base.

12.7 Conclusion

Workshops represent a dynamic component of modern clinical education, offering a learner-centered alternative to didactic instruction. Grounded in robust theoretical frameworks including adult learning theory, experiential learning, and social constructivism, they foster deep engagement by aligning educational strategies with how clinicians learn best. Their capacity to integrate knowledge, skills, and attitudes through hands-on practice, real-time feedback, and interaction makes them especially suited to clinical training environments. When thoughtfully designed and aligned with clear learning objectives, they enhance procedural proficiency, clinical reasoning, communication, and interprofessional collaboration.

Despite their promise, workshops are not without limitations. Resource demands, variability in facilitation quality, and difficulties in evaluating long-term impact remain ongoing challenges. These obstacles, however, can be mitigated through faculty development, standardization of content, and the incorporation of rigorous assessment frameworks. Importantly, the field continues to evolve. Innovations in digital learning, virtual simulation, and augmented reality are expanding the accessibility and realism of workshops. Integration with competency-based medical education and interprofessional training is amplifying their relevance in preparing clinicians for the complexities of real-world healthcare. As clinical education embraces continuous improvement and innovation, workshops will remain a foundation for effective, adaptive, and meaningful training across all stages of medical practice.

References

1. Alharbi NS. Evaluating competency-based medical education: a systematized review of current practices. BMC Med Educ. 2024;24:612. https://doi.org/10.1186/s12909-024-05609-6.
2. Knowles MS, Holton EF III, Swanson RA, Robinson PA. The adult learner. 9th ed. New York: Routledge; 2020. https://doi.org/10.4324/9780429299612.
3. Belay HT, Ó Ruairc B, Guérandel A. Workshops: an important element in medical education. BJPsych Adv. 2019;25:7–13. https://doi.org/10.1192/bja.2018.41.
4. Reynolds QJ, Beck Dallaghan GL, Smith K, Walker JA, Gilliland KO. Comparison of medical student learning styles and exam performance in an integrated curriculum. Med Sci Educ. 2019;29(3):619–23. https://doi.org/10.1007/s40670-019-00766-6.
5. Wang JM, Zorek JA. Deliberate practice as a theoretical framework for interprofessional experiential education. Front Pharmacol. 2016;7:188. https://doi.org/10.3389/fphar.2016.00188.
6. Elendu C, Amaechi DC, Okatta AU, Amaechi EC, Elendu TC, Ezeh CP, Elendu ID. The impact of simulation-based training in medical education: a review. Medicine. 2024;103(27):e38813. https://doi.org/10.1097/MD.0000000000038813.
7. Duff JP, Morse KJ, Seelandt J, Gross IT, Lydston M, Sargeant J, Dieckmann P, Allen JA, Rudolph JW, Kolbe M. Debriefing methods for simulation in healthcare: a systematic review. Simul Healthc. 2024;19(1S):S112–21. https://doi.org/10.1097/SIH.0000000000000765.
8. Lou J, Guo F. Comparing the seminar-case learning and lecture-based learning models in medical education: a meta-analysis of randomized controlled trials. BMC Med Educ. 2025;25:470. https://doi.org/10.1186/s12909-025-07041-w.

9. Atkinson AR, Abbott C, Oswald A, Boucher A, Cavalcanti RB, Frank JR, Snell LS. Strategies to enable transformation in medical education: faculty and trainee development in competence by design. Perspect Med Educ. 2024; https://doi.org/10.5334/pme.960.
10. Guraya SY, Barr H. The effectiveness of interprofessional education in healthcare: a systematic review and meta-analysis. Kaohsiung J Med Sci. 2018;34(3):160–5. https://doi.org/10.1016/j.kjms.2017.12.009.
11. Heydari MR, Taghva F, Amini M, Delavari S. Using Kirkpatrick's model to measure the effect of a new teaching and learning methods workshop for health care staff. BMC Res Notes. 2019;12:388. https://doi.org/10.1186/s13104-019-4421-y.
12. Schneiderhan J, Guetterman TC, Dobson ML. Curriculum development: a how to primer. Fam Med Community Health. 2019;7:e000046. https://doi.org/10.1136/fmch-2018-000046.
13. Mao RQ, Lan L, Kay J, Lohre R, Ayeni OR, Goel DP, Sa D. Immersive virtual reality for surgical training: a systematic review. J Surg Res. 2021;268:40–58. https://doi.org/10.1016/j.jss.2021.06.045.
14. Abu Arqub S, Al-Shehri NA, Meyer S, Asefi S, Al-Moghrabi D. The effectiveness of technology-enhanced learning in prosthodontic education: a systematic review. Eur J Dent Educ. 2024;28(4):995–1015. https://doi.org/10.1111/eje.13035.
15. Hew KF, Lo CK. Flipped classroom improves student learning in health professions education: a meta-analysis. BMC Med Educ. 2018;18:38. https://doi.org/10.1186/s12909-018-1144-z.

13 Simulation Is the Future: Shaping Health Professions Education

Jabeen Fayyaz and Gohar Wajid

Key Points

- Simulation-based education (SBE) enhances clinical training by providing safe, structured, and repeatable learning environments across a range of competencies from technical to team-based and systems thinking.
- Effective SBE extends beyond equipment, relying on scenario quality, learner-centered design, structured debriefing, and strong faculty development to ensure meaningful outcomes.
- Emerging technologies such as virtual reality (VR), extended reality (XR), and artificial intelligence (AI) enable scalable, personalized, and immersive simulation experiences, supporting skill acquisition and ongoing assessment across diverse settings.
- Simulation strengthens interprofessional collaboration, nontechnical skills, and health system performance, contributing to safer, more cohesive care delivery and team dynamics.
- Sustainability and equity in SBE require thoughtful implementation strategies, contextual adaptation, and investment in faculty, infrastructure, and cross-institutional partnerships.

J. Fayyaz
Department of Pediatrics, Division of Emergency Medicine, The Hospital for Sick Children, University of Toronto, Toronto, ON, Canada
e-mail: Jabeen.fayyaz@sickkids.ca

G. Wajid (✉)
Visiting Faculty, Health Professions Education, The University of Lahore, Lahore, Pakistan

J. Sandars et al. (eds.), *Modern Medical Education*,
https://doi.org/10.1007/978-3-032-27958-3_13

13.1 Introduction: The Imperative for Simulation-Based Education

The current healthcare landscape is characterized by its complex, multidisciplinary teamwork. Constant technological innovations are reshaping pedagogical approaches. Traditional models of clinical learning, apprenticeship, patient-based experiences, and observations are deemed insufficient to meet the current population's health needs, safety demands, technological advances, and the evolving scope of ethical professional practice. SBE bridges this gap, facilitating healthcare learners to practice and master the clinical and other psychomotor skills, decision-making, and interpersonal communication in a safe and supportive learning environment. It supports both individual and team-based competencies, offering near-real clinical experiences without any risk to patients [6].

Illustrative Example

A group of final-year medical students practicing cardiac arrest management in a simulation lab reported increased confidence and knowledge retention compared to peers who only observed the code team on clinical rounds. Immediate feedback during debriefing leads to identification and correction of errors in closed-loop communication—a critical nontechnical skill.

13.2 History and Evolution of Simulation-Based Education

Simulation-based education has evolved rapidly and created a remarkable transformation in the way we train health professionals. Early on, SBE was perceived merely as a method to teach procedural skills through task trainers or simple anatomical models, such as airway management or intravenous insertion. It allowed the learners to practice in a risk-free environment, which reduces their anxiety as well as minimizes errors. During this period, clinical education remained rooted in the apprenticeship model, where variability in learner exposure and experience often resulted in inconsistent outcomes [9].

The introduction of high-fidelity simulators in the 1990s and early 2000s marked a pivotal shift. These simulators replicated physiological responses and supported complex scenario-based learning. SBE moved from isolated skill development to immersive, team-based experiences that mimic real clinical scenarios and environments. Educational institutions started building dedicated simulation spaces (simulation labs), enabling the multidisciplinary teams of learners to practice the high-acuity, low-occurrence events, such as obstetric emergencies or trauma resuscitations, within controlled conditions that supported both technical and nontechnical skill development [1]. In recent years, the use of simulations has expanded beyond clinical training to systems testing, promoting critical thinking, interprofessional team-based training, and formative and summative assessments. High-stakes evaluations such as objective structured clinical examinations (OSCEs) now incorporate simulation for assessing not only procedural skills but also communication, professionalism, and clinical decision-making. Currently, simulation is increasingly being used to test new workflows, identify latent safety threats, and assess institutional readiness for crisis response. Simulation integrated with electronic health records and clinical protocols allows organizations to identify process gaps even before they affect patient care [1].

13.3 Core Concepts and Modalities in Simulation

SBE encompasses a broad range of modalities, each designed to meet specific learning goals and accommodate different types and levels of learners. At its core, simulation creates a safe, structured environment where health professionals can practice technical and nontechnical skills without risk to real patients. The selection of simulation modalities depends on the educational objectives, the learner's level and style, and the context of training [6]. Simulations are not free from their own strengths and limitations. Educators must know how to use them effectively in specific learning situations. Table 13.1 summarizes the strengths and limitations of various simulation modalities [14].

Table 13.1 Strengths and limitations of simulation-based education modalities

Modality	Definition (as per healthcare simulation dictionary)	Use cases	Strengths	Limitations
Task trainer	A representation of a part of a human body, typically used for teaching specific procedural skills (e.g., IV insertion, airway management)	Skill acquisition, practice of isolated procedures, and competency assessment	Low cost, portable, and effective for technical skill mastery	Limited to single skills, lacks contextual complexity
Manikin	A life-sized human model that may be static or computer-controlled to provide realistic physiological responses for clinical scenarios	Emergency scenarios, resuscitation, team training, pediatric care	High realism, responsive, and facilitates team-based scenarios	Expensive, requires maintenance and trained operators
Simulated participant (SP)	An individual trained to consistently portray a patient, family member, or healthcare team member in a scripted scenario	History-taking, communication skills, breaking bad news, and cultural competence	Enhances realism, develops interpersonal skills, versatile	Variability in SP performance, intensive training required

(continued)

Table 13.1 (continued)

Modality	Definition (as per healthcare simulation dictionary)	Use cases	Strengths	Limitations
Embedded participant (EP)	A person who is part of the instructional team and is placed in the simulation to play a scripted role and influence scenario flow	System testing, clinical team behavior assessment, and latent safety threat identification	Contextual realism allows testing of workflows and communication	It may be perceived as inauthentic if poorly integrated
Confederate	An individual who appears to be part of the scenario but is placed to support scenario delivery and guide participant behavior	Enhancing realism, cueing learners, and managing flow during simulations	Controls simulation flow, ensures objectives are met	Risk of influencing outcomes if not well-scripted
Virtual reality (VR)	A computer-generated environment that fully immerses the user in a simulated clinical scenario, typically using a headset	Emergency response, procedural training, and rare events (e.g., mass casualty)	Immersive, repeatable, and allows remote and scalable access	High cost, motion sickness, and hardware dependency
Augmented reality (AR)	An environment where digital elements (e.g., images, data) are overlaid on the real world to enhance learning or decision-making	Surgical navigation, anatomy overlay, point-of-care diagnostics	Combines physical and digital elements, enhances decision-making	Technology limitations require alignment with clinical workflow
Mixed reality (MR)	An interactive environment where real-world and digital elements coexist and allow physical interaction with virtual content	Real-time teamwork with digital cues, procedural practice with haptic feedback	Combines real-world interaction with digital enhancements, promotes active learning	Complex setup, costly, requires advanced technical support

Effective scenario design is essential to the success of any simulation activity. Scenarios must be grounded in well-defined learning objectives, aligned with curriculum outcomes, and customized to the learners' level of expertise. The fidelity of the environment, the role of facilitators, and the integration of cues must all be carefully considered to create meaningful and achievable goals. Equally important is the role of debriefing, which helps in transforming experience into learning. Structured debriefing promotes reflection, reinforces key messages, and encourages the application of skills in real clinical contexts. Models such as Promoting Excellence and Reflective Learning in Simulation (PEARLS) and advocacy inquiry provide facilitators with evidence-based frameworks to guide constructive feedback while maintaining psychological safety [12].

13.4 Integrating Simulation in Health Professions Education Through Immersive Simulation-Based Programs

The use of simulation in HPE has traditionally been perceived as standalone simulation labs designed to improve isolated clinical skills. Competency- and interprofessional education-based, integrated educational approaches have broadened the scope of simulation-based education, from simulation labs/centers to simulation-based programs that are well integrated in the overall curriculum. The distinction between standalone simulation centers and simulation-based programs is crucial for understanding the full scope of simulation in health professions education. This is a misnomer that SBE can only be implemented if there is a simulation center. A simulation center typically refers to a dedicated physical space equipped with high-fidelity manikins, task trainers, audiovisual systems, and technical support. These centers offer an immersive environment to the learners for hands-on practice, interdisciplinary team training, and controlled execution of the clinical scenarios. While the simulation center provides a setting for simulation experiences, the effectiveness of simulation sessions depends on more than just a space and infrastructure [11].

In contrast, a simulation-based program extends beyond the physical space. It represents an integrated educational framework including faculty development, governance structure, and evaluation strategies. These programs are characterized by clearly defined goals and objectives, learning outcomes, longitudinally integrated simulation activities, and mechanisms for feedback and evaluation. The success of SBP lies in aligning simulation with institutional mission and vision and culture of patient safety [11]. The well-developed SBP can exist even in the absence of simulation centers, because the educational impact of simulation is ultimately driven by the potential integrated role of simulation in the curriculum, faculty expertise on the use of simulation, scenario design, and structured debriefing, not just by the space or equipment. A detailed comparison of SBP and the simulation center is provided in Table 13.2.

Table 13.2 Comparison between simulation center and simulation-based program

Aspect	Simulation center	Simulation-based program
Definition	A physical facility equipped with simulation technology (e.g., manikins, audiovisual equipment) designed to conduct simulation activities	A structured educational approach integrating simulation across curricula, regardless of location or equipment level
Focus	Infrastructure, technology, and facility management	Curricular design, faculty development, and integration into teaching and assessment
Components	High-fidelity manikins, task trainers, control rooms, standardized patient suites	Faculty-led scenarios, debriefing, learner-centered pedagogy, and outcome assessment
Staff	Typically includes simulation technicians, administrators, and support staff	Includes educators, simulation facilitators, and curriculum developers
Accessibility	Dependent on the availability of the facility, often a fixed location	Can be mobile, virtual, or integrated into existing teaching spaces
Sustainability	High operational costs, requires dedicated funding and maintenance	Focus on faculty training and scenario reusability for long-term integration
Scalability	May be limited by facility capacity	Can be scaled using blended, virtual, or decentralized models
Example	A university hospital simulation lab used for OSCEs and emergency scenarios	A medical school curriculum embedding simulation in all clinical rotations using mobile carts and faculty-run sessions

13.5 Innovations in Education and the Role of Technology-Enhanced Simulation

Over the last few decades, we have seen the advancement in educational technologies, which continue to expand the possibilities for immersive, scalable, and learner-centered SBE. Technology-enhanced simulation extends beyond manikins to include in situ simulations, virtual reality (VR), extended reality (XR), artificial intelligence (AI), and digital gaming platforms, each contributing uniquely to the learning experience [10]. In situ simulation, which is conducted within actual clinical environments, allows learners and teams to rehearse real-world workflows and responses to emergencies in their actual clinical settings. In situ simulation sessions not only reinforce clinical competence and teamwork but also expose latent safety threats that have been unnoticed before they reach actual patients, for example, running a simulated pediatric code in a hospital ward may reveal delays in accessing equipment or communication breakdowns, prompting systemic improvements, thus enhancing patient safety [2, 10].

The use of artificial intelligence (AI) further enhances the SBE by enabling personalized, data-driven learning followed by effective feedback. AI-enhanced systems can monitor learner actions such as hand movements, speech patterns, or clinical decisions and provide tailored guidance, remediation pathways, or assessments in real time. As these systems evolve, they also hold potential for benchmarking learner progress and guiding the faculty to support adaptive learning strategies [8].

Gaming simulation is another innovative educational strategy that blends elements of game design, such as competition, challenges, and rewards, with clinical learning objectives to create engaging and interactive learning experiences for twenty-first-century learners. These simulations can range from simple quiz-based games to complex, scenario-driven serious games that mimic real-life clinical situations, such as emergency response or patient triage. By fostering active participation and immediate feedback, gaming simulations support experiential learning, boost learner motivation, and promote retention [4]. With all these advancements, it becomes imperative that educators adopt and implement them to fulfil the learning outcomes and not just follow the trends. The high-tech solutions should not overshadow educational quality, nor should they outdo the inequities in access.

13.6 Simulation-Based Education Across Resource Settings: Strategies for Implementation

The implementation of SBE depends largely on institutional resources, faculty expertise, and technological infrastructure. While high-resource settings often have access to large simulation spaces with high-fidelity manikins, integrated audiovisual systems, and dedicated staff, many low- and moderate-resource settings have to thrive within these financial and logistical constraints. However, regardless of setting, the core educational principles of SBE, structured debriefing, and learner-centered facilitation remain the same [3].

In resource-intensive environments, institutions can leverage advanced simulation modalities to support interprofessional team training, systems testing, and high-stakes assessments. These programs often benefit from full-time simulation faculty, research support, and integrated curricular pathways. However, maintaining such programs requires sustained investment, ongoing faculty development, and alignment with institutional goals. In contrast, resource-limited settings have demonstrated that meaningful simulation education is possible without high-cost equipment. Programs may employ low-fidelity task trainers made from locally available materials, mobile simulation carts, or shared regional hubs. Peer-to-peer learning and virtual simulation approaches can extend access to underserved or remote areas. What matters most is not the fidelity of the equipment but the relevance of the content and the quality of the educational design [3].

13.7 Simulations for Nontechnical Skills, Team-Based Learning, and Interprofessional Collaboration

In the current healthcare era, expectations from healthcare providers are not only on technical proficiency but also on the ability of professionals to communicate, lead, collaborate, and respond to high-pressure clinical situations. SBE has proven to be a powerful modality for cultivating these skills, often referred to as "soft skills," though their impact on patient safety and outcomes is enormous. By replicating clinical scenarios that require shared decision-making, delegation, situational awareness, and conflict resolution, simulation allows learners to develop these competencies in a structured and psychologically safe setting. Scenarios such as pediatric trauma resuscitations, medication reconciliation during shift handovers, or deteriorating patient management demand teamwork and clear communication. Through these experiences, participants learn not only the "what" of clinical care but also the "how," for example, how to listen, how to assert, and how to lead with humility [15].

Interprofessional simulation brings together learners from medicine, nursing, pharmacy, allied health, and beyond, providing the realistic face of healthcare delivery. It fosters clarity of roles and responsibilities and mutual respect, helps dismantle hierarchy, and supports collaborative practice. As a result, learners' readiness improves to handle the complexity of healthcare. Simulation educators act as facilitators and help learners reflect on team dynamics, identify any breakdowns in communication or leadership, and explore how the learners can apply the lessons learned to real clinical contexts. Over time, simulations enhance psychological safety, reduce medical errors, and build a culture of accountability and trust within healthcare organizations [15].

13.8 Beyond the Individuals: The Role of Simulation for Health System Improvement

While simulation has traditionally focused on individual skill development, its role in driving systemic change across healthcare organizations is increasingly recognized. SBE extends far beyond a tool for teaching and learning to function as a diagnostic and improvement tool for complex healthcare systems. This broader application supports the transition from learner-level outcomes to measurable organizational performance, capturing Kirkpatrick's level IV outcomes. System-level simulation enables healthcare teams and institutions to test workflows, protocols, and clinical pathways, for example, simulations of sepsis response, stroke codes, or maternal emergencies can reveal latent safety threats such as missing equipment, communication delays, or procedural ambiguities that might otherwise remain undetected until a real patient is harmed. Addressing these threats in advance enhances overall system reliability [5].

Moreover, embedding simulation into quality and safety initiatives cultivates a learning health system, one that provides feedback, real-time data, and iterative testing to evolve and improve healthcare delivery. By positioning simulation as both an educational and organizational strategy, health systems can not only improve training outcomes but also ensure that care delivery processes are effective, equitable, and resilient. This integration underscores simulation's dual function as a tool for learning and a lever for transformation [5].

13.9 The Central Role of Skilled Educators in Implementing Simulation-Based Education

The effectiveness and sustainability of SBE depend heavily on skilled faculty. While technology and facilities provide the infrastructure, it is the educators who bring simulation to life through well-crafted scenarios, safe learning environments, and high-impact debriefings. Faculty development, therefore, is central to the success of simulation programs. In traditional curricula settings with teacher-centered educational approaches, educators mostly have a narrow vision toward the use of simulations in enhancing a few selected clinical skills. As the curricular approaches shift toward better integration, well-defined competencies, interprofessional education, and the use of diverse learning approaches (e.g., problem-based learning, team-based learning, game-based learning, etc.), the scope of simulations in reformed curricula gets broader and more effective. This transformation inevitably creates the need for faculty training on the effective use of simulations in a transformative educational environment. Simulation educators may require a revised set of skills that include simulation design, scenario writing, facilitation skills, debriefing techniques, and comfort with technological tools such as manikins, virtual reality platforms, and AI-enabled analytics. Structured training programs, mentorship, and certification pathways (e.g., Certified Healthcare Simulation Educator (CHSE)) have emerged to formalize these skills and support educators [13].

13.10 Strategies and Framework for Effective Implementation of Simulation-Based Education

Implementing simulation-based education (SBE) effectively requires more than purchasing manikins or launching isolated training events. It demands a coherent, learner-centered, and institutionally aligned strategy. The most successful SBE programs are those that are embedded within curricula, governed by academic leadership, and supported by clear policies, evaluation frameworks, and sustained faculty engagement. Simulation interaction should be purposeful, with scenarios mapped to learning outcomes, competency milestones, and assessment blueprints. A spiral curriculum model is particularly effective: introducing foundational skills early and returning to them with increasing complexity, realism, and interprofessional engagement across the learner's progression. Institutional readiness is also essential. This includes infrastructure (simulation spaces, IT support, AV equipment), governance (policies, regulations, committees, quality assurance), and strategic planning for sustainability. Frameworks such as the International Nursing Association for Clinical Simulation and Learning (INACSL) Healthcare Simulation Standards of Best Practice^{SM} offer guidance on simulation design, operations, facilitation, debriefing, and evaluation. Institutions can adopt these frameworks to ensure consistency, align with accreditation requirements, and benchmark their programs against global best practices [16].

Collaboration at all levels of education is another pillar of effective SBE implementation. Partnerships with national academic networks, hospital alliances, or international consortia allow for shared resources, co-development of materials, faculty exchanges, and increased scalability. These collaborations are particularly valuable for resource-constrained environments. Local context is always an important consideration; therefore, scenarios should reflect community health priorities, language, cultural norms, and ethical complexities relevant to the learner's future practice. Finally, implementation must be iterative. Pilot programs, learner feedback, and continuous program evaluation help refine content and delivery. Institutions that embrace feedback, foster innovation, and prioritize inclusion will lead the way in shaping the future of SBE [7].

13.11 Conclusion

SBE has emerged as an essential pillar in health professions education, transforming how technical, cognitive, and interpersonal skills are taught and assessed. From its early use in task training to its current applications in high-fidelity scenarios, in situ simulations, virtual and extended realities, and artificial intelligence-driven platforms, simulation has evolved to meet the demands of a complex and rapidly changing healthcare landscape. More than a method, simulation is a philosophy of education, focused on safety, reflection, deliberate practice, and system-based thinking. It empowers learners to rehearse skills, make decisions, communicate effectively, and learn from mistakes without putting patients at risk. It also supports faculty development, programmatic assessment, and organizational learning, ultimately driving improvements in patient care and safety. However, the transformative potential of SBE depends on how thoughtfully it is designed, implemented, and sustained. Faculty capacity, curriculum integration, contextual relevance, and institutional commitment are key to success. Whether in resource-rich academic hospitals or low-resource rural clinics, simulation can be tailored to serve learners and systems, provided the focus remains on educational quality, not just technology.

References

1. Bienstock J, Heuer A. A review of the evolution of simulation-based training to help build a safer future. Medicine. 2022;101(25):e29503.
2. Calhoun AW, Cook DA, Genova G, Motamedi SM, Waseem M, Carey R, Hanson A, Chan JC, Camacho C, Harwayne-Gidansky I, Walsh B. Educational and patient care impacts of in situ simulation in healthcare: a systematic review. Simul Healthc. 2024;19(1S):S23–31.

3. Davis K, Gowda RR, Stone KP, Shepherd M. Factors affecting implementation of simulation-based education after faculty training in a low-resource setting. Simul Healthc. 2022;17(1):e113–21.
4. Davis K, Gowda AS, Thompson-Newell N, Maloney C, Fayyaz J, Chang T. Gamification, serious games, and simulation in health professions education. Pediatr Ann. 2024;53(11):e401–7.
5. Deutsch ES, Perry SJ, Gurnaney HG, editors. Comprehensive healthcare simulation: improving healthcare systems. Springer; 2021.
6. Elendu C, Amaechi DC, Okatta AU, Amaechi EC, Elendu TC, Ezeh CP, Elendu ID. The impact of simulation-based training in medical education: a review. Medicine. 2024;103(27):e38813.
7. Fayyaz J, Jaeger M, Takundwa P, Iqbal AU, Khatri A, Ali S, Mukhtar S, Saleem SG, Whitfill T, Ali I, Duff JP. Exploring cultural sensitivity during distance simulations in pediatric emergency medicine. AEM Educ Train. 2023;7(6):e10908.
8. Guraya SY. Transforming simulation in healthcare to enhance interprofessional collaboration leveraging big data analytics and artificial intelligence. BMC Med Educ. 2024;24(1):941.
9. Hertel JP, Millis B. Using simulations to promote learning in higher education: an introduction. Routledge; 2023.
10. Hildreth AF, Maggio LA, Iteen A, Wojahn AL, Cook DA, Battista A. Technology-enhanced simulation in emergency medicine: updated systematic review and meta-analysis 1991–2021. AEM Educ Train. 2023;7(2):e10848.
11. Jeffries P. The NLN Jeffries simulation theory. Lippincott Williams & Wilkins; 2021.
12. Le KD. Principles of effective simulation-based teaching sessions in medical education: a narrative review. Cureus. 2023;15(11).
13. Mastoras GN, Cheung WJ, Krywenky A, Addleman S, Weitzman B, Frank JR. Faculty sim: implementation of an innovative, simulation-based continuing professional development curriculum for academic emergency physicians. AEM Educ Train. 2021;5(3):e10559.
14. Pasklinsky N, Latimer B. Simulation modalities for undergraduate nursing education. In: Comprehensive healthcare simulation: nursing. Cham: Springer; 2024. p. 27–33.
15. Salih FZ, Lamsyah R, Shimi A, Arkha Y. Impact of simulation on the development of non-technical skills. In: Advanced technologies and the university of the future. Cham: Springer; 2024. p. 439–58.
16. Watts PI, Rossler K, Bowler F, Miller C, Charnetski M, Decker S, Molloy MA, Persico L, McMahon E, McDermott D, Hallmark B. Onward and upward: introducing the healthcare simulation standards of best practiceTM. Clin Simul Nurs. 2021;58:1–4.

Medical Students at the Crossroads of Adolescence and Adulthood: Rethinking Educational Strategies

14

Süleyman Yıldız, Olga Maria Rostkowska, Paul de Roos, and Cemre Yaşöz

Key Points

- *Adolescent learners enter medical training during a period of ongoing identity formation*, making professional identity development more sensitive to educational and social influences.
- *Professional identity formation is shaped by experience, role-modeling, and belonging*, while negative role models and hidden curriculum messages heighten vulnerability to moral distress.
- *The demanding structure of medical education*, including heavy coursework and long clinical rotations, *increases the risk of burnout and psychological distress*, particularly among students navigating adolescent developmental transitions.
- *Supportive strategies such as longitudinal mentorship, flexible curricula, well-being initiatives, and programmatic assessment* promote resilience, autonomy, and healthier identity development.
- *Future-ready curricula integrating digital learning, global health, crisis preparedness, EPAs, and reflective practice* are essential to meet the developmental and professional needs of adolescent medical students.

S. Yıldız (✉)
Department of General Pediatrics and Adolescent Health, Marmara University School of Medicine, Istanbul, Turkey
e-mail: email@yildizsuleyman.com

O. M. Rostkowska
Department of Transplantation, Immunology, Nephrology and Internal Diseases, Medical University of Warsaw, Warsaw, Poland

P. de Roos
Department of Neurology, Uppsala University, Uppsala, Sweden

C. Yaşöz
Department of Child and Adolescent Psychiatry, Erenköy Mental Health and Neurological Disorders, Istanbul, Turkey

J. Sandars et al. (eds.), *Modern Medical Education*,
https://doi.org/10.1007/978-3-032-27958-3_14

14.1 Introduction

The majority of medical students begin their medical school education during adolescence and complete their training while still progressing through the transition into adulthood. During this period, biological maturation, the development of executive functions, identity formation, and the redefinition of social roles advance simultaneously [1, 2]. At the same time, students are expected to demonstrate professional behavior, be attentive to patient safety, exhibit ethical reasoning skills, and function effectively within teams. Because personal developmental tasks overlap with professional expectations, curriculum design must support students' transition into the professional identity of a physician. Adolescence and emerging adulthood represent formative stages in which individuals refine their capacity for abstract reasoning, regulate emotions more effectively, establish values, and begin to envision long-term career trajectories, yet these developmental milestones do not progress uniformly; many students entering medical programs still grapple with fluctuating confidence, heightened emotional reactivity, and strong sensitivity to social evaluation. These characteristics influence how students perceive feedback, interact with peers and supervisors, and cope with the pressures inherent in medical training. As such, the trajectory of becoming a physician unfolds within the broader context of ongoing neurobiological and psychosocial maturation [2–4].

Medical education, however, has long relied on assumptions associated with adult learning. Curricula often presuppose high levels of autonomy, resilience, and self-direction—attributes typically associated with mature adult learners. However, this group of learners—who are in a phase of "emerging adulthood"—are neither fully adolescents nor fully adults [5]. In this period, the need for autonomy coexists with the need for guidance, and tendencies toward risk-taking intersect with responsibilities related to patient safety [2, 5]. Students may experience difficulty navigating hierarchical clinical settings, balancing academic and personal demands, and managing the emotional weight of early patient encounters, all while still negotiating their own identity formation.

This tension necessitates a comprehensive reconsideration of the curriculum, assessment systems, faculty awareness, and the overall learning environment [4]. Teaching and evaluation strategies must accommodate developmental variability, foster psychological safety, normalize help-seeking, and provide structured mentorship. Likewise, faculty members must recognize that learners' emotional and cognitive capacities are still evolving, and that professional identity formation requires deliberate support rather than passive immersion alone [5, 6].

The central argument of this chapter is that medical students who are still progressing through the developmental transition out of adolescence experience a structural mismatch when placed within curricula built upon assumptions of adult learning. Bridging this gap requires aligning educational strategies with the developmental realities of learners, acknowledging the interplay between adolescence and medical professionalism, and creating learning environments that intentionally support the complex process of becoming a physician.

14.2 Developmental Context: From Adolescence to Young Adulthood

The World Health Organization defines adolescence as the 10–19 age range [1]. This period is characterized by rapid biopsychosocial changes encompassing identity development, cognitive maturation, and the redefinition of social roles. In many countries, medical students enter medical school between the ages of 17 and 19 and continue their training into their early twenties. As a result, this learner population intersects with both the WHO definition of adolescence and Arnett's conceptualization of emerging adulthood. Throughout this process, adolescents simultaneously experience a desire for independence and a need for guidance. Emotional fluctuations, increased social comparison, strengthened peer relationships, and the shaping of self-concept constitute core elements of this stage. At the same time, individuals begin to form their future academic and career trajectories, making adolescence a critical developmental threshold that influences long-term life pathways [2, 3].

Nevertheless, the specific needs of adolescents are frequently overlooked within health and education systems, resulting in substantial unmet mental health and behavioral needs. In many countries, health services draw a sharp distinction between childhood and adulthood, without adequately recognizing the unique developmental dynamics of adolescence. Similarly, education systems often disregard the fact that the cognitive capacities of this age group are still maturing, while expecting students to demonstrate adult-level self-regulation and decision-making skills. This mismatch negatively affects both academic achievement and psychosocial well-being, contributing to increased anxiety, depression, and engagement in risk behaviors [1, 7].

Professional identity formation (PIF) holds a particularly distinctive significance for students who enter medical education during adolescence. At this developmental stage, individuals are simultaneously engaged in an ongoing search for identity—seeking answers to the question "Who am I?"—while also attempting to internalize the professional values, norms, and responsibilities embodied in the statement "I am a physician" during the early years of medical school [4, 8]. The PIF process takes shape through experience, observation, role-modeling, feedback, and the gradual development of a sense of belonging to a professional community. Importantly, PIF is also shaped by cultural norms, institutional structures, and locally embedded professional hierarchies, resulting in meaningful variation across countries and educational settings. The heightened sensitivity of adolescence with regard to identity formation makes students more vulnerable to both positive and negative environmental influences during this process. Age-related power imbalances between young learners and senior clinicians further complicate the transition, influencing psychological safety, the quality of feedback, and the willingness to seek help. Particularly in clinical rotations, the pronounced hierarchy between younger students and authority figures can directly affect feedback relationships, role modeling experiences, and the overall culture of learning from mistakes [4, 8]. Consequently, role models who fail to align with developmental needs do not reflect contemporary professional standards, or convey harmful attitudes—along with distorted messages transmitted through the hidden curriculum—may contribute to more profound moral distress among adolescent medical students [9].

The inherent demands of medical education—including a heavy theoretical workload, prolonged clinical duties, shift-based schedules, and chronic sleep deprivation—significantly increase the risk of psychological distress among students [10, 11]. Large-scale studies have consistently demonstrated that medical students exhibit substantially higher rates of depression, anxiety, and burnout than age-matched peers in the general population. Rotenstein et al., in a meta-analysis of more than 129,000 medical students, reported a pooled prevalence of depressive symptoms of 27%, with suicidal ideation rates reaching 11% [11]. Similarly, Dyrbye and Shanafelt have documented burnout rates ranging between 45% and 50% among medical students, levels that are markedly higher than those observed in the general young adult population [10]. These mental health challenges are especially pronounced among students who enter their training during adolescence, a developmental period characterized by heightened emotional reactivity and limited experience with complex stressors. The coexistence of an evolving identity structure and increasing academic-professional expectations may magnify vulnerability to stress and reduce the capacity to cope adaptively. Moreover, the hidden curriculum—through messages such as "You must not make mistakes" or "Seeking help is a weakness"—further exacerbates psychological burden at a time when students are not yet developmentally equipped to manage such pressures. These converging factors help explain why medical students demonstrate elevated rates of depression, anxiety, and emotional exhaustion, underscoring the need for robust institutional mental health support systems. As a result, it is not surprising that medical students exhibit higher rates of depression, anxiety, and suicidal ideation compared with the general population. Nevertheless, the persistence of inadequate mental health support mechanisms in many medical schools further elevates the risks faced by adolescent learners, whose developmental stage already places them in a more vulnerable position [10, 11].

14.3 Rethinking Educational Models and Mentorship

It is evident that traditional educational models in medical schools must be comprehensively re-evaluated through the lens of adolescent developmental characteristics. In this sensitive period—already challenging on its own—adolescent medical students are simultaneously navigating cognitive, emotional, and identity-related maturation. The presence of educators who understand these developmental processes is indispensable. Therefore, teaching approaches and curricular expectations must be intentionally designed with adolescents in mind rather than assuming a uniform level of adult readiness. Traditional models that prioritize autonomy, high levels of responsibility, and self-directed learning may unintentionally create barriers for adolescent learners who are still developing confidence, self-regulation, and help-seeking behaviors. Consequently, educational redesign should be grounded in principles of developmental sensitivity, psychological safety, and structured support [8, 9].

Within this framework, mentorship relationships represent a fundamental element supporting both professional identity formation and emotional resilience. Effective mentorship extends far beyond academic advising; it includes role-modeling, socio-emotional support, normalization of challenges, and guided socialization into the professional community. Contemporary mentors should help adolescent learners express themselves without fear of judgment, navigate hierarchical clinical environments, and make sense of emotionally demanding early clinical encounters. Mentorship also contributes to continuity and stability, shaping long-term career goals while strengthening students' sense of professional belonging [8, 12].

Today, flexible curricula increasingly accommodate the cognitive and emotional developmental pace of adolescent learners, thereby fostering healthier developmental trajectories [7, 12]. Autonomy-supportive environments enhance intrinsic motivation, reduce anxiety associated with rigid learning structures, and enable students to explore emerging interests without compromising foundational competencies. Complementing this approach, well-being programs, resilience strategies, and supportive institutional cultures function as protective buffers against burnout, stress symptoms, and disengagement from learning [10, 13]. Institutions that integrate guidance services and support systems that are sensitive to adolescent identity are likely to demonstrate better outcomes in student satisfaction and continuity in education.

Programmatic assessment constitutes another key component of developmentally aligned educational design because it reduces overreliance on high-stakes examinations, which frequently amplify stress among adolescent learners [14]. Instead, programmatic assessment emphasizes repeated low-stakes feedback, narrative evaluations, and multisource assessment. This model not only promotes steady progression toward competence but also enables students to engage in self-reflection, identify support needs early, and interact more constructively with feedback processes.

A central element of this redesign is the implementation of Entrustable Professional Activities (EPAs). EPAs allow for the graded delegation of responsibility based on demonstrated competence [6]. In doing so, they enable adolescent learners to build confidence safely while ensuring patient safety. Through clearly defined expectations, structured supervision, and progressive entrustment, EPAs strengthen trust between students and supervisors and reinforce the foundational elements of professional identity. Alignment between developmental readiness and responsibility allocation is especially critical for learners who are still forming adult decision-making capacities.

Additionally, reflective practice represents another essential process supporting healthy identity development. Engagement in guided reflection helps students cope with uncertainty, moral dilemmas, emotional responses, and complex clinical encounters. Reflection enhances metacognition, meaning-making, and resilience—all of which are core developmental objectives for adolescents transitioning into professional roles. In parallel, normalizing uncertainty and reframing mistakes as natural components of learning can reduce the perfectionism and fear of failure often reinforced by the hidden curriculum. Ensuring coherence between the formal and hidden curricula is similarly vital for building trust, authenticity, and a sustainable professional identity [8].

Taken together, these strategies aim to create learning environments in which adolescent medical students—whose identity formation is still ongoing—can complete the PIF process in a healthy, safe, and developmentally coherent manner. Aligning educational models with developmental science will enable medical schools to support students' professional growth while also protecting their well-being and long-term commitment to the medical profession.

14.4 Global Shifts and AI Transformation

Future directions in medical education also necessitate a transformation that aligns with the developmental needs of adolescent learners. Although digitalization and AI-supported adaptive learning systems have the potential to enhance student motivation and engagement, they also introduce risks of distraction and social isolation. Therefore, it is essential that digital education models be designed in ways that preserve social connectedness and promote meaningful interaction among students [15]. Although digitalization and AI-supported adaptive learning environments hold strong potential to enhance engagement and personalize instruction, they also introduce developmental vulnerabilities that are particularly relevant for adolescent and emerging adult learners. During this period—when executive functions such as attention regulation, impulse control, and sustained focus are still maturing—constant digital stimulation may exacerbate distractibility and impair deep learning processes [2]. AI-driven platforms that streamline cognitive effort may unintentionally promote passive learning, reducing opportunities for critical reasoning and self-regulated learning skills that form the foundation of professional competence. Moreover, adolescents' heightened sensitivity to social feedback places them at increased risk of negative psychological effects associated with digital comparison, surveillance, and online academic competition. Excessive screen exposure and reliance on algorithmic content curation have also been linked with increased loneliness, social withdrawal, and sleep disturbances, all of which can hinder the development of a stable professional identity. In addition, early evidence suggests that intensive AI use may influence self-concept by blurring boundaries between human reasoning and machine-generated feedback, potentially undermining confidence in personal judgment among younger learners. For medical students who are simultaneously navigating identity formation and demanding academic expectations, these risks highlight the need for digital education models that balance technological efficiency with social connectedness, reflective practice, and human mentorship. Such a balanced approach ensures that digital innovation strengthens, rather than disrupts, the developmental foundations upon which professional identity is built [7, 16].

It is anticipated that future curricula will place greater emphasis on student participation, opportunities for autonomous learning, and participatory co-design approaches [13]. Moreover, components such as global health education, disaster and crisis preparedness, and the strengthening of resilience skills will play a crucial role in meeting the developmental and professional needs of adolescent learners, who are particularly vulnerable to global crises [7].

14.5 Conclusion

Medical education has traditionally been constructed upon assumptions of adult readiness, self-regulation, and emotional maturity. However, a substantial proportion of medical students begin this journey while still progressing through adolescence and emerging adulthood—developmental stages characterized by ongoing identity exploration, heightened emotional sensitivity, and incomplete maturation of executive functions. The findings synthesized throughout this chapter demonstrate that the structural expectations of medical training often misalign with the developmental realities of these learners, creating a hidden mismatch that influences academic performance, psychological well-being, and professional identity formation.

The transition from adolescence to early adulthood is a period marked by rapid cognitive, emotional, and social evolution. When these developmental processes intersect with the rigorous demands of medical education—intensive coursework, clinical responsibilities, role ambiguity, and exposure to suffering—students face a dual burden: managing their own internal maturation while simultaneously attempting to embody the values and responsibilities of the medical profession. Evidence consistently shows that medical students experience disproportionately high levels of burnout, anxiety, depression, and moral distress, challenges that are magnified among those still solidifying their sense of self. These realities underscore the urgency of integrating developmental science into the design of learning environments, assessment strategies, and institutional support systems.

A developmental approach does not lower expectations of professionalism; rather, it strengthens the foundation upon which professional identity is built. Strategies such as longitudinal mentorship, flexible curricula, reflective practice, EPAs aligned with readiness, and programmatic assessment offer pathways to support competence while preserving well-being. These practices ensure that responsibility is delegated in a manner that respects both patient safety and learner growth. At the same time, fostering psychological safety and reducing stigma surrounding help-seeking are essential to counteracting the harmful messages sometimes embedded in the hidden curriculum.

As medical education enters an era shaped by digitalization, globalization, and rapid technological innovation, the needs of adolescent and emerging adult learners must remain central. AI-supported learning, virtual platforms, and global health challenges create both opportunities and vulnerabilities that require thoughtful integration. Ultimately, recognizing the medical student as a developing individual—not merely a future physician—will enable institutions to cultivate healthier, more resilient, and more grounded professionals.

A medical curriculum that aligns with developmental transitions is not a luxury; it is a necessity for safeguarding both learner well-being and the future integrity of the medical profession.

References

1. World Health Organization. Adolescent health. WHO; 2023.
2. Casey BJ, Jones RM, Somerville LH. Braking and accelerating of the adolescent brain. J Res Adolesc. 2011;21(1):21–33. https://doi.org/10.1111/j.1532-7795.2010.00712.x.
3. Steinberg L. A social neuroscience perspective on adolescent risk-taking. Dev Rev. 2008;28:78–106. https://doi.org/10.1016/j.dr.2007.08.002.
4. Cruess RL, Cruess SR, Steinert Y. Supporting the development of a professional identity. Med Teach. 2019;41(6):641–7. https://doi.org/10.1080/0142159X.2018.1536260.
5. Arnett JJ. Emerging adulthood: the winding road from late teens through the twenties. Oxford University Press; 2015.
6. ten Cate O. Entrustability of professional activities. Acad Med. 2013;88(10):e12–6. https://doi.org/10.1097/ACM.0b013e31829a3b94.
7. Viner RM, et al. Adolescence and public health. Lancet. 2012;379:1641–52. https://doi.org/10.1016/S0140-6736(12)60191-5.
8. Jarvis-Selinger S, et al. Identity formation in medical education. Acad Med. 2012;87(9):1185–90. https://doi.org/10.1097/ACM.0b013e3182602804.
9. Talbot SG, Dean W. Moral injury in healthcare. BMJ. 2018;362:k4601. https://doi.org/10.1136/bmj.k4601.
10. Dyrbye LN, Shanafelt TD. A narrative review: burnout among medical students. Acad Med. 2016;91:354–73. https://doi.org/10.1097/ACM.0000000000001137.
11. Rotenstein LS, et al. Prevalence of depression among medical students. JAMA. 2016;316:2214–36. https://doi.org/10.1001/jama.2016.17324.
12. Sambunjak D, et al. Mentoring in academic medicine. JAMA. 2006;296:1103–15. https://doi.org/10.1001/jama.296.9.1103.
13. Slavin SJ, et al. Medical student well-being programs. Acad Med. 2014;89:1–6. https://doi.org/10.1097/ACM.0000000000000321.
14. van der Vleuten CPM, et al. Programmatic assessment. Med Teach. 2012;34:205–14. https://doi.org/10.3109/0142159X.2012.652240.
15. Ellaway RH, et al. Digital professionalism. Med Teach. 2015;37:759–64. https://doi.org/10.3109/0142159X.2015.1044956.
16. Rose S. Medical student education in the COVID-19 pandemic. JAMA. 2020;323:2131–2. https://doi.org/10.1001/jama.2020.5227.

Personalized and Lifelong Learning 15

Sucheta Dandekar, Nirmala Rege, and Farzana Mahdi

Key Points

- Lifelong learning and personalized learning represent distinct but complementary pillars within contemporary education.
- The integration of lifelong learning and personalized learning enables sustained professional, personal, and societal advancements in an environment characterized by rapid change and increasing complexity.
- Combining the temporal reach of lifelong learning with the individualized strategies of personalized learning is essential to prepare individuals for ongoing growth, resilience, and success in an evolving global landscape.
- Patients, community, policymakers, and regulators can be important stakeholders in the learning process.
- Creating enjoyable learning through personal choice, relevant content, and supportive teaching encourages students to develop greater independence and sustained motivation over time.

15.1 Understanding Personalized Learning

Personalized learning puts the individual learner at the center stage of education. Instead of following a fixed path for all students, it adapts teaching methods, goals, content, and assessments to match each student's unique background, pace, and learning preferences [1]. The goal is to create a learning journey that is relevant and meaningful to the student—not just efficient. This method encourages learners to take on an active role in their education by thinking critically, reflecting on their experiences, and guiding their own learning process.

S. Dandekar (✉) · N. Rege · F. Mahdi
Era's Lucknow Medical College and Hospital, Era University, Lucknow, India

J. Sandars et al. (eds.), *Modern Medical Education*,
https://doi.org/10.1007/978-3-032-27958-3_15

Personalized learning has become increasingly important in health professions education. It offers a unique educational model that supports the individual learner. With the ever-changing knowledge landscape, evolving educator/learner roles, and varying technological advances, there is a need to alter the approach to learning. The models used have to be more flexible and learner-friendly. It works by respecting each student's journey and personal goals, which in turn promotes their motivation, fosters a deeper understanding of concepts, and ultimately leads to long-term retention of knowledge.

When students are encouraged to talk about their real-life experiences, they are able to relate to the situations, and learning becomes more pertinent. This personal connect helps them to internalize what they learn because the information is not abstract but is meaningful.

15.2 Core Aspects of Personalized Learning in Health Professions Education

Personalized learning in the context of health professions education focuses on adapting learning experiences to meet students where they are—intellectually, emotionally, culturally, and professionally. Below are key dimensions that outline this approach [2]:

1. *Flexible Pathways and Pacing*
   Students' progress at a pace that suits them, often through modular, competency-based curricula that offer different ways of learning.
2. *Tailored Support and Mentorship*
   Students benefit from individualized support systems, including academic advising, mentorship, and wellness resources that reflect their personal and professional development needs.
3. *Technology-Enabled Customization*
   Tools like AI-driven platforms, adaptive learning software, and learning analytics are used to monitor progress and adjust content or difficulty levels in real time.
4. *Culturally Inclusive Learning Design*
   Effective approach appreciates the diverse identities and experiences students bring. It involves creating inclusive learning environments.
5. *Ongoing Feedback and Adaptive Learning*
   Feedback is continuous. Students receive regular, constructive input and opportunities to reflect and adjust their learning strategies.
6. *Learner Profiles and Strength Mapping*
   Educators use tools to develop detailed learner profiles, helping them understand each student's learning style, prior knowledge, and goals. The information obtained can be used for developing personalized ways to teach.

15.3 Strategies for Implementing Personalized Learning in Health Professions Education

Personalized learning places the learner at the center, where the focus is on individual preferences, abilities, and goals. While terms like adaptive, individualized, and customized learning are often used interchangeably, each represents a distinct approach. Educators can understand these fine differences and work out more thoughtful and effective educational strategies.

Adaptive learning refers to the use of technology to monitor student performance in real time and adjust instructional content accordingly. It keeps learners engaged by providing challenges that are neither too easy nor too difficult. In contrast, individualized learning modifies the pacing and order of instruction based on the learner's performance but may not always reflect their personal interests or goals [3]. Customized learning takes a more all-inclusive view—shaping the educational experience around what the learner wants to achieve. It combines elements of the other two methods and may or may not involve technology but always revolves around the learner's needs and goals.

By understanding these subtle differences, educators can make sensible choices about which model best fits a given learning context. The main idea is that different learners and settings may require different approaches—and understanding the "why" and "how" behind each model enables educators to make conscious decisions. Tools like the VARK (visual, auditory, read/write, and kinesthetics) inventory, baseline assessments, and reflective exercises can be used to collect this information.

Technology can significantly support this process. Learning management systems (LMS), multimedia content, interactive e-modules, and immersive technologies such as augmented or virtual reality offer varied ways of presenting material, making learning more engaging and accessible. Large language models (LLMs) can serve as virtual teaching assistants—simulating clinical cases, generating questions, and even supporting student reflection or reasoning exercises. They also offer support to faculty in tasks such as creating lesson plans, drafting assessments, or developing learning materials, allowing for more personalized mentoring moments.

The use of AI in education must be approached with care. Both students and educators should be trained in its responsible and ethical use, keeping in mind issues like algorithmic bias and misinformation. Institutions should establish transparent policies that govern AI usage in learning environments. This evolution also calls for a shift in how assessments are designed. With AI capable of producing well-structured answers in seconds, traditional knowledge-recall exams may need to give way to evaluations that assess higher-order thinking—such as clinical judgment, communication skills, and applied competencies [4]. When used thoughtfully, digital tools and AI can help create more learner-centered, flexible, and effective educational environments in health professions training.

Active learning methods and continuous feedback also play a crucial role in supporting personalized learning. Techniques such as problem-based, team-based, and case-based learning promote deeper understanding by encouraging students to engage with real-world scenarios. Frequent formative assessments along with prompt feedback, whether from peers, teachers, or self-assessment, enable students to consider their development and modify their study techniques accordingly. These methods aid in the development of self-sufficient, driven students who are more equipped to meet the requirements of lifelong learning [5].

15.4 Conceptualizing Personalized Learning: The Simple, Complicated, Complex, and Chaotic [6]

Implementing personalized learning is not a one-size-fits-all process—it unfolds across a range of complexities, from straightforward tasks to highly unpredictable situations. Recognizing these different layers can help educators and institutions plan more effectively [6].

15.4.1 The Simple (Known Knowns)

Some aspects of personalized learning are relatively easy to work on and will meet with least resistance, for instance, adapting lessons to suit different learning styles, ensuring common access to diverse learners, or modifying assessments to reflect individual abilities are all problems with clear solutions.

15.4.2 The Complicated (Known Unknowns)

At this level, deeper thinking and analysis are required. Educators may agree on personalization but disagree on how best to apply it. Which tools work best, whether all learners benefit equally, and how to measure progress effectively using technology could be some of the misgivings. These challenges may require thoughtful planning, collaboration, and refinement.

15.4.3 The Complex (Unknown Unknowns)

In complex situations, the path forward is not always evident. Teachers may face large class sizes, limited time, and rigid syllabi that make personalization difficult. In such situations, solutions may need experimentation, reflection, and adaptation.

15.4.4 The Chaotic (Unknowable)

This is the most unpredictable situation, where cause and effect are hard to trace. Teachers may find the process of personalizing learning overwhelming or unclear. Managing varied issues could make the educators feel disorganized—especially when too much flexibility creates confusion or inconsistency. In these situations, structure and support become crucial.

To successfully integrate personalized learning, educators and institutions must recognize that aspects that shift between the simple and the chaotic require both strategic planning and a willingness to adapt.

15.5 Understanding Lifelong Learning

Lifelong learning in healthcare is a mindset. It refers to the ongoing, self-directed, and voluntary pursuit of knowledge and growth that extends well beyond the classroom. It involves sharpening of skills, adapting attitudes, and staying curious about the constant changing world. Reflective practice, critical thinking, collaboration, and adaptability form the heart of this approach. It keeps professionals up to date with the latest in clinical care, medical technologies, and patient-centered approaches. The urgency and importance of such learning were brought into sharp focus during the COVID-19 pandemic, when the ability to think on one's feet made all the difference. By embedding lifelong learning into health professions education, health professionals can be prepared for a lifetime of evolving practice [2].

15.6 Core Aspects that Support Lifelong Learning

One of the most pressing questions in education is how can students be prepared for a career that will span decades of change.

The answer lies in cultivating the habits of lifelong learners—curiosity, self-awareness, resilience, and a commitment to growth and development. These qualities cannot be taught in a single lecture. They must be nurtured over time, within learning environments that mirror real-world healthcare.

15.6.1 Designing Curricula that Reflect Real Practice

Education becomes truly meaningful when it connects with the real-world experiences that learners will encounter. Textbook examples cannot do justice. Students benefit more when their learning includes real patient stories, up-to-date case studies, and immersive simulations. These experiences help bridge the gap between theory and practice.

15.6.2 Helping Students Take Charge of Their Own Learning

Lifelong learners seek out knowledge. Educators can help by creating spaces where students can reflect on their learning styles, engage in honest conversations with mentors, and learn from their peers [7]. Activities like reflective journaling, peer feedback, and guided discussions are powerful tools that help students to keep growing, even in the face of uncertainty [7].

15.6.3 Making Continuous Professional Development Appealing

Students feel the need to keep learning by understanding how ongoing development can directly improve their ability to care for patients and open doors in their careers.

This means designing opportunities that are engaging and meaningful: interactive workshops, hands-on sessions with emerging technologies, and conversations with experienced professionals who model what growth looks like in real life. When students can connect the dots between learning and impact, they begin to see continuous professional development not as a burden—but as a path to excellence and purpose [8].

15.7 Strategies for Implementing Lifelong Learning in Health Professions Education

In today's fast-changing healthcare environment, health professionals need to be comfortable using new technologies. Digital literacy is therefore a critical skill for supporting continuous learning throughout one's professional life. Good educational technology supports different ways of learning and encourages teamwork and critical thinking. Mobile-friendly platforms let students' study while they are on clinical rounds or traveling. Interactive tools, like simulations, allow learners to practice difficult procedures in a safe way. Virtual reality can help link textbook knowledge with real-life practice [9]. These tools also help learners connect with others across different places and time zones. Online forums, virtual group discussions, and peer mentoring remind students that they are not alone—they are part of a global learning community.

Making this kind of learning possible is not easy. Many students face challenges like heavy course loads, money problems, family duties, and the pressure of big exams. To help with this, schools can offer materials in different formats, provide scholarships or discounts for extra learning, allow flexible learning times, and create support systems among peers. The main aim is to make it easier for students to keep learning throughout their careers. Involving former students and creating learning groups can also show which methods really help students build lifelong learning habits [9]. However, this should not just add more contents to the already packed curricula. We should fundamentally reimagine how education is approached—shifting from information delivery to learning facilitation, from passive absorption to active exploration, and from individual achievement to collaborative growth.

When we succeed in cultivating these habits, we do not just prepare competent health professionals—we develop practitioners who will continue growing, adapting, and improving patient care throughout their careers. This benefits not only individual professionals but also the patients they serve and the healthcare systems they work within.

The journey toward lifelong learning could begin with a single question, a moment of curiosity, or an experience that shows students how much more there is to discover. Our role as educators is to create as many of these moments as possible while providing the support and tools students need to continue the journey long after they graduate.

Students who use learning strategies aligned with lifelong learning do not always perform better than those who rely on more surface-level approaches, as shown by van Woezik et al. in 2020. The authors emphasize that it is important to carefully design assignments and assessments to ensure that both students and teachers share a clear understanding of the goals and expectations related to developing lifelong learning skills [10].

15.8 Instruments Available for Evaluating Lifelong Learning Skills Among Healthcare Professionals [11]

Lifelong learning is a skill, and an overview of tools for evaluating this skill for professionals is needed. Verkooijen et al. [11] in their systematic review of articles published until October 2023 identified 28 unique instruments used to assess lifelong learning skills. Some of the most frequently cited ones include:

- *Jefferson Scale of Physician Lifelong Learning (JSPLL)*—One of the most widely used, especially in medical contexts.
- *Revised Jefferson Scale of Lifelong Learning for Health Professions Students (JeffSLL-HPS)*—Adapted for use with students.
- *Self-Directed Learning Readiness Scale (SDLRS)*—Evaluates readiness for self-directed learning.
- *Effective Lifelong Learning Inventory (ELLI)*—Broader, general population-focused, occasionally applied in healthcare.
- Several locally developed or adapted tools used in specific contexts or countries.

These instruments vary in scope, length, and domains covered, with a predominant reliance on self-reporting Likert-type questionnaires. The review points out both advantages and shortcomings of these instruments, and the tools can be used as per researchers' requirements.

15.9 Learning Environment and Enjoyment of Learning [12]

The idea of learning enjoyment is about how much students like the process of learning. When students enjoy learning, they get more interested, motivated, and are willing to learn even when it is difficult. Enjoyment in learning can help students feel more positive about education and can support better performance and deeper understanding.

Personalized learning and lifelong learning are both useful approaches that can increase learning enjoyment. Personalized learning gives students opportunities to study in ways that match their own needs, interests, and learning styles. It lets them make choices about what they learn and how they learn it. Thus, the students feel more in control of their own learning and more connected to the learning process. When students have a "voice and choice," they feel their opinions are respected, and they start enjoying the experience [12].

To include personalized and lifelong learning in health professions education, we need changes in how we design courses, train teachers, and shape policies. With strong leadership, teacher training, steady funding, and institutional support, flexible systems can be built that prepare students for both present and future challenges. These elements in the learning environments help to build new skills and growth throughout a health professions' career.

If people enjoy learning, they are more likely to continue learning new skills and knowledge as they grow older. Creating enjoyable learning experiences through personal choice, meaningful content, and supportive teaching can help students become more independent and motivated learners in the long term.

15.10 Recommendations for Integrating Personalized and Lifelong Learning

All over the world, concepts of personalized learning and lifelong learning are being advocated. Continuing professional development with digital platforms can use massive open online courses (MOOCs) to integrate career-long learning framework across health institutions. In order to achieve this, AI-powered personalized learning platforms, personal development plans, learning portfolios that track professional growth over time, and AI analytics to suggest learning paths based on gaps in performance are some of the innovations being tried. All this, no doubt comes with their own challenges—lack of balanced standardization in exams with individualized learning paths, inequity in access to digital tools for personalized learning, limited digital infrastructure and faculty training in rural areas, time and resource constraints for personalized mentorship, faculty resistance or lack of training in new technologies or inability to keep up with rapid technological change, and breach in data privacy [13].

The following are the suggestions to overcome the challenges, with respect to curriculum design, faculty development, and institutional policy:

1. Embed personalized learning technologies (e.g., simulations, learning analytics).
2. Integrate portfolio-based and competency-based assessments.
3. Allow modular, flexible course structure.
4. Train educators in adaptive teaching and AI tools.
5. Support them in becoming learning coaches and mentors rather than just content deliverers.
6. Establish institutional frameworks for continuing professional development as a career-long requirement.
7. Encourage innovation through pilot programs and educational research [8].

15.11 Toward a Sustainable Future in Health Professions Education

The thoughtful merging of personalized learning and lifelong learning with technologies such as LLMs has the promise to revolutionize health professions education [4].

Putting personalized learning into practice is far from simple. On one hand, it is easy to grasp the concept: "tailor education to fit each student's needs." On the other hand, educators face the unpredictable student behavior, diverse learning styles, and institutional limitations. The two ends of the spectrum—the "simple" concept and the "chaotic" implementation—highlight just how complex the educational landscape really is. And that complexity must be acknowledged if progress has to be made [6].

Ultimately, the goal of health professions education is to shape professionals who are competent, compassionate, and prepared for the ever-changing demands of healthcare. To achieve this, institutions must be intentional about how they navigate different layers of complexity, build systems that support flexible learning, and invest in leadership that values innovation and ethics.

Medical schools, hospitals, and professional organizations need to work together to make sure learning is relevant and future-ready. Patients, community, policymakers, and regulators can also be important stakeholders in the learning process. The experiences and feedback from patients can be used to identify areas for improvement and personalize learning approaches to address patient needs, thus fostering better health outcomes [14]. Community learning centers and libraries can be hubs for lifelong learning by providing social interactions. Policymakers and regulators can create policies and set standards, by establishing frameworks and vision, for lifelong and personalized learning initiatives. When these groups collaborate, they create stronger, more supportive environments where lifelong learning can thrive. This collective effort ensures that healthcare professionals continue to grow and that patients benefit from safe, high-quality care—even as the system around them continues to evolve [15].

15.11.1 Conceptual Framework

Lifelong learning and *personalized learning* represent distinct but complementary pillars within contemporary education. These frameworks address separate foundational questions central to learning and development:

- *Lifelong learning* focuses on *the temporal dimension of education*, asking the following: "When should learning occur and how can it persist throughout life?"
- *Personalized learning* addresses *the methodological dimension*, inquiring the following: "How can learning experiences be tailored to meet individual needs and preferences?"

15.11.2 Distinct Dimensions

15.11.2.1 Lifelong Learning: Temporal Emphasis

- Encompasses education across the entire human lifespan, from early childhood through senior adulthood.
- Integrates formal, informal, and nonformal educational opportunities.
- Recognizes the importance of adapting to evolving career requirements, personal aspirations, and societal changes.
- Encourages continuous, self-directed, and voluntary engagement in learning activities.

15.11.2.2 Personalized Learning: Methodological Emphasis

- Prioritizes adaptation of instructional methods, content, and pacing to suit the unique attributes of each learner.
- Employs technological tools, data analytics, and adaptive systems to refine educational delivery.
- Fosters environments responsive to individual abilities, interests, and learning preferences.
- Seeks to maximize engagement and efficacy by ensuring that educational experiences are directly relevant and accessible.

15.11.2.3 Integration and Synergy

The synthesis of lifelong and personalized learning forms a robust paradigm for twenty-first-century education:

- Lifelong learning establishes a framework that values continuous development and adaptability over the entire course of life.
- Personalized learning operationalizes this framework by delivering tailored, dynamic educational experiences that respond to the ever-changing needs of individuals.
- The integration of these dimensions enables sustained professional, personal, and societal advancement in an environment characterized by rapid change and increasing complexity.

This dual approach—combining the temporal reach of lifelong learning with the individualized strategies of personalized learning—is essential to preparing individuals for ongoing growth, resilience, and success in an evolving global landscape.

References

1. Ali M, Wahab IB, Huri HZ, Yusoff MS. Personalised learning in higher education for health sciences: a scoping review protocol. Syst Rev. 2024;13(1):99.
2. Walkington C, Bernacki ML. Appraising research on personalized learning: definitions, theoretical alignment, advancements, and future directions. J Res Technol Educ. 2020;52(3):235–52.

3. Hussain T, Yu L, Asim M, Ahmed A, Wani MA. Enhancing e-learning adaptability with automated learning style identification and sentiment analysis: a hybrid deep learning approach for smart education. Information. 2024;15(5):277.
4. Sharma S, Mittal P, Kumar M, et al. The role of large language models in personalized learning: a systematic review of educational impact. Discov Sustain. 2025;6:243. https://doi.org/10.1007/s43621-025-01094-z.
5. Pahi K, Hawlader S, Hicks E, Zaman A, Phan V. Enhancing active learning through collaboration between human teachers and generative AI. Comput Educ Open. 2024;6:100183.
6. Gunawardena M, Bishop P, Aviruppola K. Personalized learning: the simple, the complicated, the complex and the chaotic. Teach Teach Educ. 2024 Mar;1(139):104429.
7. Hardie P, O'Donovan R, Jarvis S, Redmond C. Key tips to providing a psychologically safe learning environment in the clinical setting. BMC Med Educ. 2022;22(1):816.
8. van der Burgt SM, Kusurkar RA, Wilschut JA, Tsoi SL, Croiset G, Peerdeman SM. Motivational profiles and motivation for lifelong learning of medical specialists. J Contin Educ Health Prof. 2018;38(3):171–8.
9. Hennessy S, D'Angelo S, McIntyre N, Koomar S, Kreimeia A, Cao L, Brugha M, Zubairi A. Technology use for teacher professional development in low-and middle-income countries: a systematic review. Comput Educ Open. 2022;3:100080.
10. Van Woezik T, Koksma J, Reuzel R, Jaarsma D, Jan Van Der Wilt G. How to encourage a lifelong learner? The complex relation between learning strategies and assessment in a medical curriculum. Assess Eval High Educ. 2020;45(4):513–26.
11. Verkooijen MH, van Tuijl AA, Calsbeek H, Fluit CR, van Gurp PJ. How to evaluate lifelong learning skills of healthcare professionals: a systematic review on content and quality of instruments for measuring lifelong learning. BMC Med Educ. 2024;24(1):1–4.
12. Mötteli C, Grob U, Pauli C, Reusser K, Stebler R. The influence of personalized learning on the development of learning enjoyment. Int J Educ Res Open. 2023;5:100271.
13. Pendergast D, Main K, McManus S. The effectiveness of a MOOC as a form of professional learning: an examination of an adolescent learner social and emotional well-being course. Educ Sci. 2024;14(10):1114. https://doi.org/10.3390/educsci14101114.
14. Bosveld MH, Hermans M, Verhoeven M, Smeenk F, Sehlbach C. Partners in care: training healthcare professionals in using patient feedback. Clin Teach. 2025;22(4):e70130.
15. Mitchell S, Phaneuf JC, Astefanei SM, Guttormsen S, Wolfe A, de Groot E, Sehlbach C. A changing landscape for lifelong learning in health globally. JCME. 2023;12(1):2154423.

Application of Behavioral Economics in Medical Education

16

Maryam Soleimani Movahed, Fakhrosadat Mirhosseini, and Shoaleh Bigdeli

Key Points

- Behavioral economics applies psychology and economics to explain decision-making under the influence of biases, heuristics, and emotions in learning.
- Behavioral economics employs instruments like nudges, frames, defaults, loss aversion, and feedback loops in medical education to influence good behavior.
- Behavioral economics minimizes cognitive overload and bias, with medical students being motivated to learn and become reflective clinicians.
- A nudge is a gentle direction of decisions that maintains liberty and leads learners to improved decisions in medical education.
- The future of behavioral economics is AI-based intelligent smart nudging that is personalized to learners, with an emphasis on long-term effects on competence and patient outcomes being measured.

M. S. Movahed
Education Development Center (EDC), Iran University of Medical Sciences, Tehran, Iran

F. Mirhosseini
Trauma Research Center, Kashan University of Medical Sciences, Kashan, Iran

Department of Anesthesiology, School of Allied Medical Sciences, Kashan University of Medical Sciences, Kashan, Iran

S. Bigdeli (✉)
Center for Educational Research in Medical Sciences (CERMS), Department of Medical Education, School of Medicine, Iran University of Medical Sciences, Tehran, Iran
e-mail: sbigdeli@alumni.sfu.ca

J. Sandars et al. (eds.), *Modern Medical Education*,
https://doi.org/10.1007/978-3-032-27958-3_16

16.1 Introduction

In the complex, high-stakes world of medical training, learners and educators face information overload, cognitive biases, and motivational challenges. In this world, behavioral economics (BE) combines concepts from psychology and economics to better understand decision-making and offers tools to address the current challenges. In this regard, BE interventions (called "nudges") use subtle changes in how choices are presented to guide behavior without eliminating options [1].

In their book *Nudge*, Thaler and Sunstein describe several practical examples of how the way options are organized influences the decisions people make [2]. We consider that "choice architecture" can be a critical element for designing effective medical education systems, with small adjustments by using conditional incentives (defaults, framing, and feedback) guiding learners toward beneficial behaviors while respecting their autonomy.

Generally, in education, BE concepts are increasingly recognized as promising and experts argue that nudging could be "a valuable means to influence behavior in educational contexts" [1]. Medical education is not an exception and in healthcare systems, using conditional incentives (nudges) improves clinic attendance and medication adherence in patients referring to medical clinics.

Thaler and Sunstein also highlight that people tend to stick with pre-set default options that influence their choices. Setting beneficial defaults, such as automatic enrollment in foundational skills workshops or peer mentoring programs that can significantly increase participation without coercion [2]. In medical education contexts, where time scarcity and cognitive overload (e.g., tiredness and extra workload) negatively affect decision-making, decision simplification is crucial for engagement.

However, the formal use of BE in medical education is still emerging and unrecognized. This chapter reviews how BE principles are being applied or could be applied to train better doctors around the world, drawing on examples from Asia, Africa, Europe, North America, and beyond (Table 16.1). We discuss key BE techniques, technological delivery methods, current challenges, ethical considerations, and the need to prepare educators to use these methods.

Table 16.1 The selected examples of BE mechanisms and desired outcomes according to world regions

Region	Example	BE mechanism	Outcome
Africa	WhatsApp-based nudges; BE training via Indlela Nudge Unit [3]	Timely prompts, capacity building	Greater engagement in discussions; expanded BE expertise
Asia	Rural service incentives (India); social media leaderboards (Indonesia); BE-enhanced SBME in China [4]	Loss aversion, social proof, framing	Increased rural placement commitments; improved simulation scores
Australia	CME leaderboards; performance bonds for skill checklists [5]	Social norms, loss aversion	+40% optional module completion; higher checklist compliance
Europe	Public pledge for course evaluation (Germany) [6]; social norm emails (UK) [7]	Commitment device, social proof	+50% evaluation submission; improved module completion
North America	Debt lotteries for elective completion; default study plans [8]	Loss aversion, default effect	Increased early elective completion; reduced choice overload

16.2 Behavioral Economics: Key Principles

Traditional economics assumes fully rational decision-makers, while BE recognizes that real-world decisions, including medical education, are shaped by cognitive biases, heuristics, and emotional factors which influence how learners prioritize study time, respond to feedback, or make clinical decisions under uncertainty.

16.2.1 Behavioral Economics: Concepts

Nudge as a central concept in BE indicates a subtle change in how choices influence behavior while preserving freedom of choice [1]. In their book *Nudge*, Thaler and Sunstein discuss how the structure of the decision-making environment (choice architecture) shapes outcomes even when no explicit instruction is given [2]. For example, reorganizing an online learning portal so that essential modules appear first can significantly increase completion rates without making them mandatory.

Default effect is one of the most powerful tools within choice architecture. Since individuals usually stick to pre-set options, well-designed defaults (e.g., automatic enrollment in core competency workshops) can reduce decision fatigue and increase participation [2]. This is particularly important in medical education, where learners juggle multiple responsibilities and may avoid optional but beneficial activities simply due to inertia.

BE also leverages other psychological mechanisms such as loss aversion, framing effect, and feedback loops.

(a) Humans prefer to avoid a loss (loss aversion) more than achieving a promising success (e.g., "be aware of not falling behind your classmates").
(b) The information presentation method (framing effect), such as providing statistics about survival rather than mortality rate, affects human decision-making. For example, in medical settings designing an Objective Structured Clinical Examination (OSCE) scenario at the cardiopulmonary resuscitation station with a positive frame such as "Your correct performance will save the patient's life, while each of your mistakes may lead to death" results in learner's decreased anxiety and a higher chance of success.

Specific feedback provided with appropriate timing will prevent establishment of improper habits (feedback loop). For example, using technologies such as software or simulators that provide immediate feedback on performance help correct behavior.

Thaler and Sunstein also propose the "Real Third Way" approach by designing systems where the path of least resistance leads to better outcomes, without restricting autonomy [2]. In medical education, setting up automated study reminders, peer-comparison dashboards, or structured debrief sessions can guide learners toward more effective study and clinical decision-making patterns.

16.2.2 Technological Innovations in Behavioral Interventions

Advances in educational technology have created new opportunities for applying principles of BE in scalable, cost-effective ways [3]. Learning Management Systems (LMS), mobile apps, and AI-driven tools can integrate choice architecture directly into their design to shape learner decisions while preserving autonomy.

Thaler and Sunstein duly emphasize that no choice environment is neutral and arrangement of options inevitably influences behavior and it is essential that thoughtfully set defaults are used to guide learners toward beneficial actions while preserving autonomy [2]. In addition, pre-enrolling students in specific courses or sending them automatic reminders by default reduces cognitive load and improves their engagement (default effect). The technology can enhance feedback loops [2, 11]; and, progress dashboards, instant quiz scoring, automated notifications and performance alerts by providing immediate actionable information, make feedback systems efficient and motivating [3]. Defaults in these systems, such as pre-activating reminders or auto-enrolling learners in recommended modules, leverage inertia to encourage engagement and, framing effects such as presenting progress in comparative or loss-aversion terms can further influence learner motivation in digital contexts [2].

16.3 Applications of Behavioral Economics in Medical Education

BE principles are increasingly applied in medical education across diverse cultural, institutional, and resource contexts [1]. While the specific strategies vary, the central aim is to design learning environments and experiences that align with human cognitive tendencies, making beneficial educational behaviors the easiest and most natural to adopt.

Here is a summary of selected examples from different regions, which indicates that effective nudges using various BE mechanisms can produce desired outcomes (Table 16.1).

16.3.1 Curriculum and Technology-Enabled Choice Architecture

A well-designed curriculum can embed BE principles to streamline decision-making and highlight learning priorities [1]. Defaults and structured pathways are central tools; for example, medical programs may automatically enroll students in a standard set of foundational modules (e.g., diagnostic reasoning, basic sciences) while leaving advanced topics as opt-in choices. This reduces choice overload (a form of decision fatigue) and ensures that essential competencies receive consistent attention.

Importantly, curricular nudges must adapt to cultural contexts. In hierarchical educational cultures, strongly recommended pathways may be followed more readily, whereas in more individualistic settings, overtly directive structures might be resisted. Successful BE interventions balance guidance with perceived autonomy, ensuring that learners feel supported rather than controlled.

Globally, a single design principle of the path of least resistance in making the desired educational behavior whether enrolling in essential modules, engaging with critical content, or maintaining consistent study habits must be used. Appropriate choice architecture guided technology augments this effect by applying nudges into regular learning interactions.

16.3.2 Motivation, Engagement, and Lifelong Learning

In medical education settings due to competing demands, long working hours, fatigue, and working shifts, to keep students motivated is highly challenging. In this regard, BE by aligning incentives with cognitive tendencies provides strategies that make ongoing engagement more likely [9].

Using social norms and loss framing to encourage participation such as digital reminders or dashboards comparing individual progress to the cohort median leverage competition and the desire to avoid loss is a common strategy [10].

Gamification elements, such as leaderboards, streak counters (a tool to encourage users to consistently complete a basic amount of repetitive daily action), and visual progress bars, maintain engagement by making progress visible and socially contextualized. This reflects Thaler and Sunstein's insight that salience and public visibility of performance can shape long-term behavior [2].

16.3.3 Clinical Decision-Making Training

In medical education clinical decision-making is crucial; however, diagnostic and treatment errors often happen due to cognitive biases (e.g., anchoring, availability, and overconfidence) [9, 10]. In this context BE strategies support students to overcome these biases and avoid medical errors by reflective evidence-based decision-making.

Simulation-based training is particularly effective when combined with BE techniques. Varying the framing of identical cases; for example, presenting outcomes as survival rates in one version and mortality rates in another, can reveal how framing effects influence clinical choices [9]. As Thaler and Sunstein highlight, reframing options can shift decisions without altering the underlying facts, providing a powerful tool for bias awareness [2].

Evidence demonstrates the added value of BE elements in simulation-based medical education (SBME). Incorporating commitment devices, structured reflection, and choice framing led to significantly greater improvements in residents' coping skills and self-efficacy compared to SBME alone [4, 9]. Similarly, addressing therapeutic inertia in complex conditions such as multiple sclerosis can involve defaulting learners into more challenging simulation scenarios, reducing avoidance of uncertainty [11].

From the Nudge perspective, the path of better decision-making aligns the path of least resistance [2]. For example, in medical settings, medical students must optimally perform in highly challenging real clinical situations, which requires immediate feedback from educators and actual engagement with reality.

16.3.4 Training Educators in Behavioral Economics

For BE interventions to be implemented effectively, medical educators and administrators must understand BE principles and be skilled in applying them [3]. Although clinician-educators are mostly clinical field experts, their formal curriculum lack training on choice architecture, framing, and commitment concepts.

Faculty development programs such as webinars, short courses, workshops, integrated training modules, etc. and structured curricula and toolkits in designing, delivering, and evaluating nudges for specific educational contexts [3] they include practical exercises, such as reordering learning materials for salience, setting beneficial defaults in course registration, and embedding feedback systems into daily teaching practice that fill the gap. Following feedback, reflection leads to in-depth rapid learning. As medical education evidence indicates continuous deep reflection as a characteristic that is emphasized in the path of Scholarship of Teaching and Learning transforms medical teacher to medical teacher scholar [12].

In Nudge, Thaler and Sunstein highlight that choice architecture is most effective when implemented by those who understand its nuances and ethical considerations [2]. Training should therefore include the "how," "when," and "why" of nudging ensuring interventions enhance autonomy. It is important to consider cultural norms that affect perception of nudges. Other priorities include faculty awareness of factors such as stereotype threat, scarcity mindset, and decision fatigue to be incorporated into BE training and practical "nudge checklists" for educators covering defaults, framing, feedback, and workload perception [13].

Accrediting bodies could integrate BE competency into teaching excellence standards, and grants could support pilot interventions and faculty training initiatives. Over time, BE-informed pedagogy should become as routine as evidence-based medicine and just as clinicians continually update their clinical skills, educators should regularly update their behavioral design skills [2].

16.4 Ethical and Contextual Considerations

There are numerous benefits to applying BE in medical education; however, ethical and contextual challenges play a significant role in their application. As Thaler and Sunstein emphasize, influencing behavior through choice architecture must be done transparently, respect autonomy, and align with learners' own goals [2].

Four key considerations for ethically sound BE implementation are:

16.4.1 Transparency and Autonomy

Nudges shape behavior without explicit instruction. This can be problematic if learners are unaware of their influence or feel unable to opt out. Two types of nudges have been described: (1) automatic default that act at a subconscious level, (2) informational prompts that invite conscious reflection. Across cultures, surveys show a preference for transparent informational prompts [1]. For example, showing comparative quiz scores with a note such as "Your peers scored higher—consider reviewing this topic" preserves autonomy, whereas unannounced enrollment in additional modules may feel coercive.

Even overt prompts such as emails recommending review sessions may not be recognized as persuasive by some learners [1]. To ensure ethical practice, educators should explain why they choose a specific strategy ("We recommend this review because data show repetition improves retention") and ensure that students have freedom of choice, their participation is voluntary and there is no fear of penalty for their choices. In other words, their autonomy is respected.

16.4.2 Cultural Context

Cultural contexts have a crucial influence on perception and acceptance of nudges. Therefore, in traditional systems, professors are at the top of teaching and learning hierarchy, and their orders must be obeyed by students. While in individualistic cultures, learners may resist perceived overreach. BE interventions must be context-specific, highlighting cohort norms may work in collectivist settings, while stressing individual achievement might be more persuasive in individualistic contexts [14]. From a nudge perspective, the ethical "middle path" lies in designing culturally sensitive choice architectures that preserve both respect and relevance [2].

16.4.3 Equity and Access

Not all learners have equal access to technology or resources. In addition, language and framing must also avoid cultural bias to prevent alienation of minority students. Moreover, nudges remind faculties to apply assessment standards that support fairness in evaluation, and in BE training of educators all interventions must be to the advantage of all groups with no discrimination.

16.4.4 Evaluation and Long-Term Impact

A nudge may change behaviors promptly without producing long-lasting learning or professional growth and does not guarantee improved competence or clinical judgment. Ethical evaluation therefore requires longitudinal monitoring and alignment with strategies that engage learners in the reasoning process. Moreover, individual differences and demographics such as gender or personal life situations influence how people responds to nudges [9]. Finally, in high-pressure environments such as emergency care, BE strategies should be designed to counteract "herding" behaviors, encouraging deliberate decision-making supported by visual aids and simplified frameworks. Neuroimaging evidence suggests such aids activate brain regions linked to self-control and reflection, providing a neurobiological rationale for nudges that slow automatic, potentially biased choices [15].

16.5 Case Studies from Diverse Contexts

Globally, across diverse situations, BE principles have been applied in medical education settings. In this regard, the following table (Table 16.2) indicates BE principles and their corresponding strategies that focus on specific medical education domains [2, 10, 11, 15].

This structure allows us to examine not only *what* interventions are being implemented, but also *why* they work and *how* they can be adapted across contexts.

Table 16.2 BE principles and their corresponding strategies that focus on specific medical education domains

Domain	Focus	Illustrative strategies	Key BE principles
Curriculum and technology-enabled choice architecture	Structuring curricula and integrating digital tools to guide learners	Default learning paths, sequencing modules, LMS reminders	Choice architecture, default effect, salience
Motivation, engagement, and lifelong learning	Sustaining learner effort during and after training	Gamification, social comparison, loss-framed reminders	Social norms, loss aversion, commitment devices
Clinical decision-making training, and reflective critic	Enhancing diagnostic reasoning and reducing biases	Framing variations, simulation design, checklists, and interactive meetings	Framing effect, debiasing strategies
Training educators in behavioral economics	Preparing faculty to design and implement BE interventions	Faculty workshops, nudge toolkits, inclusive design	Choice architecture, stereotype threat reduction

16.6 Long-Term Impacts of Behavioral Nudges in Medical Education

BE interventions have demonstrated notable short-term benefits such as increased quiz participation, improved module completion, and enhanced engagement but their long-term influence on professional competence, decision-making, and patient outcomes remains less well understood. As Thaler and Sunstein emphasize, the true value of behavioral intervention lies in whether it produces persistent habit change and aligns with learners' intrinsic goals over time [2].

16.6.1 Evidence of Long-Term Effects

Some studies suggest that nudges can generate durable changes when designed to reinforce habits or reshape attitudes. Immersive nudges combined with reflective debriefing have been shown to maintain positive attitudinal shifts, especially in sensitive domains such as mental health [15].

In large-scale "mega-studies," it is found that repeated prompts such as regular reminders to study can establish habit loops that persist even after the intervention ends. In medical education, this may translate into sustained study routines, consistent clinical skill practice, and ongoing professional development [10].

In another study, residents exposed to BE-informed simulation training aimed at reducing biases such as overconfidence and anchoring maintained a 20% improvement in diagnostic accuracy 1 year post-intervention [15]. Similarly, a residency program that introduced peer leaderboards for continuing medical education (CME) indicated a 40% increase in module completion rates that carried over into the following academic year [10]. These findings align with Thaler and Sunstein's view that social norms and timely feedback can sustain engagement well beyond initial exposure [2].

16.6.2 Challenges and Research Gaps

Despite encouraging evidence available about BE, longitudinal research in this area remains limited. Most published work focuses on short-term metrics (attendance, quiz scores) and lacks follow-up to assess whether improvements translate into better clinical judgment, reduced burnout, or improved patient outcomes [11, 14].

Potential challenges include [14]:

- Nudge fatigue: Providing repeated prompts over time, desensitize learners and decrease their impact.
- Dependence on external cues: self-regulation may be inhibited by excessive dependence on nudge reminders.
- Equity concerns: Technology may not be available to all learners and therefore those with limited access will be excluded.

Ethical considerations: To support autonomy, nudge must be accompanied by transparent optional withdrawal mechanisms [2]. Moreover, the effectiveness of BE strategies is under the influence of financial strain, stereotype threat, and limited advising access that must be addressed simultaneously.

16.6.2.1 Future Potential and Recommendations

Smart nudges are supported by advances in new technologies of AI and learning analytics where prompts are given according to the learners' progress, context of study and students' readiness. For example, an AI-powered LMS could track and deliver targeted reminders for refreshers and reflective practice.

To increase the impact of nudges, pairing nudges with feedback tools is suggested. This improves self-reflection and mastery-oriented goals. In addition, using defaults and social norms to prompt action and normalizing lifelong learning behaviors is a must. Conducting multi-center studies over time to assess the effectiveness of BE strategies on patient safety, competence, and career satisfaction and embedding equity considerations to make nudges available to all learners is recommended.

As Thaler and Sunstein emphasize, when designed for habit formation, reflective engagement, and inclusivity, behavioral interventions can extend their influence far beyond the classroom, shaping clinicians who remain adaptive, motivated, and patient-focused throughout their careers [2].

16.7 Conclusion

To nudge medical students and physicians toward better understanding and educational outcomes rich, evidence-based framework presented by BE is a solution. To help learners stay motivated, think critically and study effectively, careful curriculum design, using modern technology and understanding cognitive biases, by educators is critically important to support students' learning. Diverse nudge elements (defaults, framing, and feedback) shape learners' behavior by decreasing cognitive overload, counteracting biases, and creating the path of least resistance.

Transparent, culturally sensitive, and easy to withdraw BE strategies are effective and trustworthy. Since dependency on external prompts may create nudge fatigue, to encourage intrinsic motivation is suggested. Availability of nudges dependent on technology, cultural concerns, and available resources must be equal for all learners.

Personalized learning interventions dependent on learners' needs over time are available via AI and learning analytics. Therefore, adaptive, data-driven nudging is the next step in using BE in medical education. In this regard, international collaborations provide shared evidence related to best practices across contexts. Medical educators, by creating effective humane training environments, can close the gap between what learners do and what they aspire to do. The challenge is about evaluation, ethical refinement, and sustainable integration of the proposed approaches to shape the next generation of students and physicians. All these interventions will nudge better doctors of the future.

References

1. Weijers RJ, de Koning BB, Paas F. Nudging in education: from theory towards guidelines for successful implementation. Eur J Psychol Educ. 2021;36(3):883–902.
2. Thaler RH, Sunstein CR. Nudge: improving decisions about health, wealth, and happiness. Penguin; 2009.
3. Thirumurthy H, First-of-its-Kind HIV. "Nudge unit" to be established in South Africa: Department of Medical Ethics and Health Policy. University of Pennsylvania; 2020. Available from: https://medicalethicshealthpolicy.med.upenn.edu/events/in-the-news/first-of-its-kind-hiv-nudge-unit-to-be-established-in-south-africa.
4. Liu C, Liu W, Jiao M, Li Y, Zhang G, Wei L, et al. A combined behavioural economics-and simulation-based medical education to promote effectiveness among medical residents in coping with workplace violence in Northern China: a quasi-experimental study. BMC Public Health. 2022;22(1):1090.
5. Chang TP, Raymond T, Dewan M, MacKinnon R, Whitfill T, Harwayne-Gidansky I, et al. The effect of an international competitive leaderboard on self-motivated simulation-based CPR practice among healthcare professionals: a randomized control trial. Resuscitation. 2019;138:273–81.
6. Neckermann S, Turmunkh U, van Dolder D, Wang TV. Nudging student participation in online evaluations of teaching: evidence from a field experiment. Eur Econ Rev. 2022;141:104001.
7. Hallsworth M, Chadborn T, Sallis A, Sanders M, Berry D, Greaves F, et al. Provision of social norm feedback to high prescribers of antibiotics in general practice: a pragmatic national randomised controlled trial. Lancet. 2016;387(10029):1743–52.

8. Joachim S, Forkan ARM, Jayaraman PP, Morshed A, Wickramasinghe N. A nudge-inspired AI-driven health platform for self-management of diabetes. Sensors. 2022;22(12):4620.
9. Dewi RM. Development of learning material in behavioral economics for higher education. Pegem J Educ Instr. 2024;14(3):192–9.
10. Milkman KL, Gromet D, Ho H, Kay JS, Lee TW, Pandiloski P, et al. Megastudies improve the impact of applied behavioural science. Nature. 2021;600(7889):478–83.
11. Lavecchia AM, Liu H, Oreopoulos P. Behavioral economics of education: progress and possibilities. In: Handbook of the economics of education, vol. 5. Elsevier; 2016. p. 1–74.
12. Mirhosseini F, Mehrdad N, Bigdeli S, Peyravi H, Khoddam H. Exploring the concept of scholarship of teaching and learning (SoTL): concept analysis. Med J Islam Repub Iran. 2018;32:96.
13. Barton AL, Tweed SR, Chesley CG. The currency of studenthood: behavioral economics in the higher education classroom. In J Teach Learn High Educ. 2020;32(3):476–85.
14. Loewenstein G, Chater N. Putting nudges in perspective. Behav Public Policy. 2017;1(1):26–53.
15. Saposnik G. Applying behavioral economics and neuroeconomics to medical education and clinical care. Can J Neurol Sci. 2019;46(1):35–7.

Understanding the Future's Purpose and Possibilities

17

Reimagining Medical Education: Challenges and Imperatives from the Past, the Present, and the Future

Madalena Patricio

Key Points

- Recognizing medical education's past, present, and future challenges helps us anticipate and shape future transformations.
- Technological advances must be integrated critically, ensuring they enhance—not replace—the human dimensions of care and learning.
- The future doctor must be educated not only as a competent clinician but also as a socially accountable, adaptive, and ethically grounded professional.
- Guiding principles for futuristic medical education must balance innovation with ethics, technology with humanity, and global imperatives with local realities.
- From the very first day of training, students should be regarded as "doctors of tomorrow," not merely as "students of today."

17.1 Introduction

17.1.1 The Call to Reimagine Health Professions Education

Medical education is not only about teaching and training to produce competent doctors—it is also about preparing professionals who can respond to human needs with care, empathy, and integrity. As the world faces rapid transformation, the question is not whether medical education should change but how courageously and urgently it will do so [1].

The twenty-first-century healthcare landscape is characterized by volatility, uncertainty, complexity, and ambiguity. The exponential growth of biomedical

M. Patricio (✉)
Department of Medical Education, Faculdade de Medicina, Universidade de Lisboa, Lisbon, Portugal
e-mail: patricio@medicina.ulisboa.pt

J. Sandars et al. (eds.), *Modern Medical Education*,
https://doi.org/10.1007/978-3-032-27958-3_17

knowledge, the integration of artificial intelligence (AI) into clinical decision-making, the global crisis of climate change, and the growing diversity of both patients and students are reshaping the terrain on which medical education stands. Yet, alongside these innovations and disruptions lies a quieter but equally urgent crisis—burnout, moral distress, depersonalization, and inequities in access to care—that technology alone cannot resolve.

If medical education is to remain relevant and meaningful, it must move beyond the transfer of knowledge to a more profound role: shaping professionals who are not only technically competent but also ethically grounded, socially accountable, and capable of leading change.

This chapter integrates institutional lessons from the Faculdade de Medicina da Universidade de Lisboa (FMUL), where since 1995 more than 350 first-year students annually have engaged in community-based experiential learning with vulnerable populations. These insights, combined with reflections shared in international conferences, anchor the arguments developed here.

Our task is threefold: (1) to evaluate the shaping forces of the past, (2) to critically examine the urgent challenges of the present, and (3) to articulate the imperatives that must guide the future.

What emerges thereafter is a vision of medical education not merely as the transmission/acquisition of knowledge but also as the formation of professional identity, the cultivation of ethical engagement, the humanization of medicine, and the advancement of societal and technological transformation.

17.2 The Past: Forces and Challenges that Have Shaped Medical Education

Medical education has always faced significant challenges, but now it will face one of its most challenging and exciting times due to the complexity of its challenges, which have repercussions on healthcare. Its story is one of continual adaptations. Although the pace of change has accelerated in recent decades, the profession has long been shaped by external pressures, scientific discoveries, social movements, political contexts, and shifting conceptions of what it means "to be a doctor."

Understanding the root causes discussed in the following paragraphs is not only a nostalgic exercise but also a road map to guide us in choosing a path in the present as well as the future times.

17.2.1 Globalization of Healthcare and Education

Medical education has never been purely local. The movement of students and faculty, international accreditation frameworks, and the global demand for health professionals have created increasingly interconnected systems of training. The World Federation for Medical Education (WFME) and similar bodies have sought to harmonize standards across countries, while student migration has raised questions about accreditation, workforce distribution, and cultural competence. Globalization with new frontiers, opportunities, and mobility for doctors and student has also exposed deep inequities: while some countries export trained professionals, others face critical shortages. These dynamics continue to challenge educators to think beyond national borders and prepare graduates who can act in global, as well as local, contexts [2]. For a "global world," we need a "global doctor, with skills to work in an international context, deep knowledge of global issues, and the values of a global citizen," as stated by Jenny Lunn in 2008 [3].

17.2.2 Explosion of Knowledge and Technology

Exponential growth of medical knowledge—once estimated at every 50 years in 1950, every 7 years by 1980, and now every 73 days in some domains—has profoundly challenged curricula. Genomics, imaging, minimally invasive surgery, and AI-driven diagnostics have stretched curricular boundaries to breaking points [1].

With medical knowledge exploding at unprecedented rates, curricula must prioritize core learning and critical appraisal over rote memorization. The rise of genomic medicine, imaging technologies, and interdisciplinary specialties has stretched curricular boundaries. What matters now is not only what to teach but also how students learn, unlearn, and adapt over a lifetime. Above all, what matters most is that students acquire the trait of critical thinking [4, 5].

17.2.3 The Emergence of Patients' New Requests, New Rights, and Expectations

The twentieth century saw a profound shift in the doctor-patient relationship. The paternalistic model of medicine gave way in the twentieth century, with the emergence of patients' new requests, new rights, and new expectations, to a new ethic of patient autonomy, informed consent, and shared decision-making. Landmark frameworks—from the Nuremberg Code (1947) to the Declaration of Helsinki (1964)—reshaped medical ethics and demanded accountability and human dignity.

The integration of bioethics into curricula embedded with reflections on norms, values, justice, and rights is inseparable from professional competence.

17.2.4 Shifting Student Profiles and Expectations

Today's learners are more diverse in culture, gender, and background and bring digital fluency, global connectedness, and strong social (*sometimes political*) agendas. They seek not only technical expertise but also meaning, purpose, and balance [6].

They expect education to prepare them as change agents and collaborators in interprofessional teams. Professionalism cannot be cultivated simply by having medical students attend lectures and plenary sessions alongside nurses and other healthcare professionals. This is why medical faculties must therefore rethink education, mentorship, and curriculum.

Many students, having lived through financial crises and the COVID-19 pandemic, carry a strong social agenda: they expect education to prepare them not just as clinicians but also as advocates and collaborators in interprofessional teams.

17.2.5 Social Accountability of Medical Schools

Perhaps one of the most significant shifts is the recognition that medical schools are accountable to society. The WHO framework of 1995 emphasized that institutions must respond to the priority health needs of communities, especially the most vulnerable. From 10 to 13 October 2010, the author had the privilege of being one of the 65 delegates from medical educational and accrediting bodies around the world who met in East London, South Africa, to finalize the Global Consensus on Social Accountability of Medical Schools (GCSA), a document to guide the schools in this area. Social accountability reframes education from professional reproduction to social contract—training doctors not for prestige but for service.

17.2.5.1 The Present: Transformations and Gaps

If the history records archives of change over time, the present is marked by unprecedented acceleration. Medical schools stand at the crossroads of technological innovation, shifting health needs, and cultural transformation [7]. The COVID-19 pandemic acted as a catalyst, exposing vulnerabilities and forcing rapid adaptation and collaboration among all healthcare professionals.

17.2.6 Demographic and Epidemiological Shifts

Portugal, like many other countries, faces an aging population with multiple chronic conditions. Lisbon's hospitals increasingly care for patients who are not acutely ill but chronically vulnerable. All around the world, chronic and multiple conditions require integrated, long-term, person-centered care.

Doctors must be trained not only as clinicians but also as system agents who can balance individual- and population-level priorities, integrate healthcare across settings, and collaborate with nurses, pharmacists, social workers, and other healthcare professions; in other words, practice interprofessional education.

Training must consider the following domains:

1. *Diversity, Equity, and Inclusion*

Cultural diversity and systemic inequities demand education that cultivates equity-oriented practice, cultural humility, and cultural empathy. Beyond representation, equity requires structural change: admissions policies that widen access, curricula that critically address health disparities, and institutional cultures that promote inclusion [7].

Increasingly, the patients are bringing cultural and linguistic diversity into the consulting rooms. Therefore, institutions must dismantle barriers, address health disparities, and foster belonging.

2. *Climate Crisis and Planetary Health*

Portugal's fires, floods, and heat waves as indeed in many other parts of the world remind us that planetary health is not abstract. The climate crisis magnifies inequalities and health risks. Preparing doctors for planetary health is a curricular priority, demanding interdisciplinary engagement and sustainable practices in healthcare systems. It is no longer optional: it is now a moral imperative.

3. *Technological Integration*

AI, telemedicine, and precision medicine offer a promise but raise concerns of bias, depersonalization, and misuse. Virtual and augmented reality tools are revolutionizing learning, [4, 5] but while digital tools can enrich clinical decision-making, an overreliance on data risks fragmenting the patient into isolated metrics. When care becomes driven primarily by numbers, the person's narrative, values, and lived experience may be overshadowed. Preserving human connection is essential to prevent technology from depersonalizing care.

Around the world, students train with simulation mannequins and virtual reality anatomy labs, but they also worry about medicine being reduced to data points. AI in particular demands critical and ethical integration with schools debating how to teach AI critically: not as an unquestionable tool with enormous potential but as a sociotechnical system rife with biases, limitations, and ethical dilemmas. What we need is competent doctors not only in their use but also knowing their limitations [4].

4. *Persistent Gaps in Medical Schools*

The challenges outlined above reveal a growing gap in medical education, with schools debating the following curricular options:

- Rigid curricula vs. the need for flexibility.
- Biomedical emphasis vs. the need for humanistic and digital competencies.
- Siloed training vs. the need for interprofessional collaboration.
- Major focus on technical assessment and evaluation vs. the need for assessment and evaluation of values and ethics.
- Hesitant approaches to AI with insufficient curricular guidance vs. the need to embrace its power responsibly (preventing cheating and other problems while taking advantage of its enormous potential). At the same time, medical education faces crises of burnout, moral distress, and depersonalization. Moral distress arises when doctors feel unable to act according to their values, eroding integrity and personal well-being.

Education must therefore respond not only with resilience training but also with structural changes that humanize learning environments. Addressing these situations requires not only conducting resilience workshops but inculcating structural changes to humanize learning environments.

Without a strong curricular reform, medical schools risk irrelevance in the face of the transformative change.

17.3 Lessons Learned from Teaching in the Community Over the Last 30 Years at the Faculdade de Medicina da Universidade de Lisboa (FMUL)

17.3.1 Origins of the Program

In 1995, the FMUL introduced a new curricular area, *Introduction to Medicine*, created by Prof. João Gomes-Pedro. Since then, more than 10,000 students (approximately 350 each year) have engaged in community-based experiences, visiting institutions and organizations that care for vulnerable populations. These include prisons, nursing and retirement homes, centers for migrants and minority groups, gypsy communities, and even mobile units offering support to sex workers at night, among others.

This program was born of a clear conviction: to truly serve society, doctors must not only care for those at its center but also deliberately engage with those at its edges—the marginalized, vulnerable, and often invisible populations. Today, it has evolved into *Module III-I Clinical Medicine: The Doctor, the Patient, and the Person*, not as an adjunct to medical training but as one of its foundations.

17.3.2 Educational Objectives

Recognize vulnerability and value the difference.
Critically reconstruct perspectives on society.
Prepare doctors as agents of social change.

17.3.3 Educational Strategies

Methods include weekly *plenary seminars* to discuss equity, diversity, ethical dilemmas, end-of-life care, etc., reminding students that medicine is always a moral practice; *student visits to vulnerable institutions outside FMUL* in small groups; *individual students' interviews* with users, technicians, or families at one of the visited institutions; and a *final seminar* where each group share the most important message they took away from the visits to improve society, as future doctors.

Students are intentionally "deconstructed" through immersion in vulnerability during the visits, discuss ethical dilemmas during plenaries, etc.

They are asked to do things, feel, think, and elaborate individually and in groups. Reflection sessions, facilitated by teachers, transform experience into insight. The institutions were selected because they exemplify excellence in serving vulnerable populations, offering models of dignity and resilience.

Students' deconstruction of prior assumptions is particularly relevant in medicine, as the highly competitive admission process drives them to spend their secondary school years solely focused on gaining entry. Selection based on top grades and rigorous entrance exams often leads them to become isolated from the world, with many being overprotected by parents (often physicians themselves) and sacrificing nearly everything in pursuit of academic success.

17.3.4 The Impact of the Program

Students often recall these community experiences as defining moments in their education, shaping professional identity and anchoring empathy.

This immersion illustrates how experiential learning cultivates not only clinical skills but also core values, showing how education can shape doctors into true agents of change [8].

Some excerpts from the anonymous open-ended evaluations, conducted at the end of *Module III-I Clinical Medicine: The Doctor, the Patient, and the Person*, reaffirm this perspective, through the following comment:

We discovered that we must be doctors of people and not doctors of bodies.
We realized real situations that we had not valued before.
We could never have imagined situations like these just 2 km from my home.

17.4 Learning Framework to Support the Above Proposed Change

Module III-I is grounded in the three-level learning model first proposed in the landmark 2010 *Lancet Report* "Health professionals for a new century: transforming education to strengthen health systems in an interdependent world." [9].

This model was recently reaffirmed by Julio Frenk, the first author of the *Lancet Report*, during the opening plenary of the 2025 WFME Conference "Health for All Through Quality Medical Education" (Bangkok, May 25–28). It underscores three progressive levels of learning:

1. *Informative learning*—acquisition of knowledge and skills → *forming experts.*
2. *Formative learning*—socialization around values → *forming professionals.*
3. *Transformative learning*—cultivation of leadership → *forming enlightened agents of societal change.*

17.5 The Future: Looking Ahead, Ethical Imperatives, and Future Directions

The future of medical education is not only about anticipating technological innovations but also about asking deeper questions of purpose. Healthcare systems face crises of sustainability, inequity, and trust. The education of future doctors must be reimagined as a moral and societal project.

17.5.1 Rehumanizing Medicine

One of the paradoxes of modern healthcare is that while we have more advanced technologies than ever before, many patients report feeling unseen or dehumanized. The future must reclaim the centrality of human connection. Narrative medicine, reflective practice, and empathy training are not luxuries but imperatives.

17.5.2 Equity, Diversity, and Inclusion

Futuristic medical education cannot succeed without embedding equity at every level from admissions that widen access to curricula that critically address social determinants of health to institutional cultures that celebrate belonging. Structural barriers must be reduced, and curricula must address social determinants of health.

17.5.3 Planetary Health and Sustainability

Medical education must integrate planetary health into curricula, preparing doctors to act as agents of both patients and ecosystems.

17.5.4 Beyond the Biomedical Model

Holistic care requires integration of social sciences, humanities, and systems thinking [10]. The future doctor must bridge the precision of science with the wisdom of human experience.

17.5.5 Identity Formation and Professionalism

At its core, medical education is all about who the doctors become. Identity formation must be intentional, reflective, and inclusive, shaped through mentorship, ethical dialogue, and resilience-building.

17.5.6 Preparing for Uncertainty

Future must develop adaptive expertise, capable of navigating pandemics, technological disruptions, and global crises. Critical thinking, collaboration, and creativity are essential.

17.5.7 The Ethical Imperative

Across all futures runs the need for an ethical and moral compass. Medical schools must cope with ethical challenges, namely, by providing a strong foundational understanding of ethical principles and real-world applications and engaging students with ethical dilemmas. Innovation without ethics risks inequity; efficiency without compassion risks trust; progress without sustainability risks health itself.

17.6 Guiding Principles for the Future

These directions echo Harden's (2018) vision of defining features of the future medical school [11].

Humanization at the core—Empathy, communication skills, and relational care must remain central.

Equity, diversity, and inclusion as foundations—Structural change in admissions criteria, curricula, and institutional culture is essential.

Alignment with planetary and societal health—Preparing doctors as stewards of both human and environmental well-being.

Integration of technology with wisdom—AI and digital tools must enhance, not erode, humanistic practice.

Doctors as agents of change for a better society—Embracing their role as leaders and change agents who confront injustice, promote social responsibility, and work toward a healthier, fairer world.

Embedding these principles requires structural alignment: assessment, faculty development, and institutional culture must reinforce these values. Changing a culture takes time, demands the collective effort of all stakeholders (dean, faculty, students, administrative staff, etc.), and above all requires commitment, passion, and a sense of ownership.

17.7 Conclusion

Medical education faces unprecedented challenges stretching from knowledge transmission to transformation, shaped by global forces, technological advancement, and urgent societal needs. The lessons of the past, the challenges of the present, and the imperatives of the future converge call for bold, ethical, and human-centered transformation.

Ultimately, the purpose of medical education is not simply to produce competent practitioners only but to form doctors who are adaptable, empathetic, and socially accountable. Rehumanizing care, addressing inequities, integrating planetary health, balancing technology with wisdom, and nurturing professional identity are not optional ideals; they are imperatives.

The task before us is clear: to prepare doctors who not only know but also care and who not only practice but also lead change. The responsibility lies with all of us—teachers, students, institutions, and societies. The question is no longer whether transformation is necessary but whether we will act with courage and urgency to realize it.

As Fernando Pessoa (1888–1935), one of Portugal's greatest poets, once wrote:"There comes a time when we must abandon the worn clothes that already have the shape of our body, and forget the paths that always lead us to the same places. It is the time of crossing; and if we do not dare to do it, we will remain forever at the margin of ourselves."

Medical education stands at crossroads. If we fail to change, we will remain forever at the margins, not only of ourselves but also of the societies we serve.

The future will not wait. Let us build it together.

Acknowledgments I used ChatGPT to support the preparation of my chapter, specifically to translate the text from Portuguese into English and to improve readability, grammar, and formatting. I carefully reviewed, modified, and verified all suggestions provided, and I therefore take full responsibility for the content of this chapter. The version I used was OpenAI's ChatGPT (GPT-4-level model available at the time I wrote the chapter in September 2025).

References

1. Sklar DP. Looking ahead: futures planning for medical education. Acad Med. 2019;94(10):1401–3.
2. Jogerst K, Callender B, Adams V, et al. Identifying interprofessional global health competencies for 21st-century health professionals. Ann Glob Health. 2015;81(2):239–47.
3. Jenny L. Global perspectives in higher education: taking the agenda forward in the United Kingdom. J Stud Int Educ. 2008;12(3):231–54.
4. Ellaway RH, Topps D, Pusic M. Data, big and small: emerging challenges to medical education scholarship. Acad Med. 2019;94(1):31–6.
5. Barry DS, Marzouk F, Chulak-Oglu K, Bennett D, Tierney P, O'Keeffe GW. Anatomy education for the YouTube generation. Anat Sci Educ. 2016;9(1):90–6.
6. Cook DA, Artino AR. Motivation to learn: an overview of contemporary theories. Med Educ. 2016;50(10):997–1014.
7. Thibault GE. The future of health professions education: emerging trends in the United States. FASEB BioAdv. 2020;2(12):685–94.
8. Gruppen LD, Irby DM, Durning SJ, Maggio LA. Conceptualizing learning environments in the health professions. Acad Med. 2019;94(7):969–74.

9. Frenk J, Chen L, Bhutta ZA, Cohen J, Crisp N, Evans T, et al. Health professionals for a new century: transforming education to strengthen health systems in an interdependent world. Lancet. 2010;376(9756):1923–58.
10. Hodges BD, Lingard L, editors. The question of competence: reconsidering medical education in the twenty-first century. New York/Ithaca: Cornell University Press; 2012.
11. Harden RM. Ten key features of the future medical school—not an impossible dream. Med Teach. 2018;40(10):1010–5.

Challenges in Medical Education and Future Directions: A Forward-Looking Approach

18

Tabassum Zehra and Nadia Al Wardy

Key Points

- Medical education curricula must adapt to diverse healthcare settings, integrating digital health technologies and meeting the needs of digitally fluent, interconnected learners.
- Robust and unified "Faculty Development Framework" grounded in theoretical perspective is essential for empowering twenty-first century faculty educators.
- Re-defining "Quality" for health care and health professions education is imperative in the modern era.
- Regulatory standards of Continuous Quality Improvement (CQI) in healthcare education need to be established that are aligned with competency framework.
- A shared vision is crucial to collaborate between medical educators, institutions, and policymakers to respond to educational and health system priorities.

18.1 Introduction

Medical education in twenty-first century is at a crossroad. On one hand there is an increasing demand to ensure healthcare professionals are more capable of meeting the demands of those they care for and the wider population. On the other hand, there is rapid transformation in healthcare delivery, education and training due to advancements in technology, globalization, and shifting student expectations. The shift is driven by changing healthcare contexts, evolving physician roles, societal demands, scientific advances, and innovative educational methods [1].

T. Zehra (✉) · N. Al Wardy
Medical Education and Informatics Department, College of Medicine and Health Sciences, Sultan Qaboos University, Muscat, Oman
e-mail: z.tabassum@squ.edu.om; naiwardi@squ.edu.om

J. Sandars et al. (eds.), *Modern Medical Education*,
https://doi.org/10.1007/978-3-032-27958-3_18

The traditional system that used to focus primarily on treating illness has now evolved into a more complex system putting emphasis on prevention, patient engagement, and coordinated care. There is an intentional move to restructure health care systems and service delivery to enhance equity, quality, and patient outcomes. Healthcare organizations have shifted from episodic treatment of acute illnesses to delivering coordinated services that emphasize chronic disease management, prevention, and continuity of care. Medical educators face the critical challenge of preparing students to navigate and excel in health systems that will continue to evolve over the coming decades [2].

Globally, the effectiveness of medical education systems varies. Two primary educational models prevail: the traditional model, which emphasizes theoretical knowledge acquisition, and the innovative model, which prioritizes hands-on, integrated, community based, practical competency-based training. Grounded in scientific principles, Medical Education provides a robust foundation for learning. These principles are translated into practical and experiential skills that healthcare professionals need. Ultimately, this learning framework enhances patient care and promotes public health [3].

A century after the Flexner Report, medical education experts reflected and recognized the need for another transformation in medical education to meet the demands of twenty-first-century patients and student learning. They emphasized standardized outcomes, personalized learner pathways, integration across traditional disciplines, and the development of professional identity. There was a need to respond to the increasing disconnect between the healthcare system's requirements and the capabilities of the healthcare professionals produced by current educational systems. Today medical education is being shaped by several key factors, including rapid technological advancements, growing healthcare demands, and the continuous evolution of competency-based frameworks [1]. These influences call for a rethinking of both teaching, learning and assessment strategies and practices. In 2010, the Lancet Commission on Education of Health Professionals for the twenty-first Century published a landmark report advocating a thorough and authoritative reassessment of health professional education [4]. Coping with the challenges requires an understanding of the broader medical education landscape. This chapter looks holistically at the landscape of medical education, provides evidence-based description of the main pillars of medical education, and analyzes the challenges related to each pillar, providing forward thinking strategies to overcome the challenges.

18.2 Broader Landscape of Medical Education

Today, medical education is increasingly recognized as a continuum of lifelong learning, encompassing undergraduate, graduate medical education as well as continuing professional development. There is a growing emphasis on reflective practice, social accountability, and the cultivation of relevant professional competencies [4]. The Lancet Commission on Medical Education reported a mismatch in professional competencies and societal needs. The COVID-19 pandemic acted as a potent catalyst for change, profoundly transforming medical education and prompting rapid and substantial adaptations in teaching, learning and assessment methods and educational frameworks [4].

With the evolving landscape of medical education, the challenges faced revolve around the four main pillars, namely:

1. Curriculum Design
2. Learning Environment
3. Faculty Development
4. Socio-Structural

18.2.1 Curriculum Design

During the early nineteenth and twentieth centuries, medical students were expected to memorize long lists of diseases, symptoms, and treatments. This rigid curriculum reflected a knowledge-heavy model that valued individual study over teamwork and gave little importance to communication or emotional intelligence. Although traditional teaching methods provided a structured foundation for learning medical theories, they inadequately address the development of practical skills and innovative thinking, and remain insufficient in responding to the dynamic challenges of emerging diseases and evolving educational requirements [1, 3].

The future of medical education curricula revolves around four integrated themes:

1. Humanistic, patient-centered clinical experiences
2. Community-based learning beyond hospitals
3. Active, student-driven, tech-enhanced learning
4. Personalized, socially engaging education

Existing curricula increasingly fall short of meeting the evolving demands of both teaching and clinical practice, resulting in a widening gap between educational approaches and real-world healthcare needs [1, 3].

18.2.1.1 Curriculum Challenges: Aligning, Integrating, and Adapting Content for Modern Education

Content alignment in curriculum design ensures that medical education is structured. It ensures objectives, teaching approaches, and assessments work together, with explicit clarity on what students should learn and how they will be able to demonstrate their understanding and application of the concepts and skills learnt [5]. Despite its benefits, achieving curriculum alignment remains a major challenge. Today electronic mapping tools are available that can map the curriculum to highlight gaps and redundancies and align learning with assessments. However, successful curriculum implementation depends on curricular alignment that involves coordination among multiple stakeholders, effective integration of content and adaptability to the evolving needs which requires substantial faculty training and committed leadership. It is anticipated that Artificial intelligence will reduce the efforts required by future healthcare professionals. However, the humanistic approach to patient safety remains a priority in curriculum design with early learning experiences allowing students to interact with patients and collaborate with health professionals in their clinical practice to ensure patient safety [5].

The adoption of integrated curricula has reshaped medical education, moving away from isolated discipline-based structures toward a more interconnected and cohesive approach to learning. This demands educational institutions to transform student learning "in a contextual manner across traditional disciplines, integrating information, improving retention, and facilitating application to clinical practice." Medical schools face challenges including limited resources, the need to balance research and curriculum requirements, and the importance of cultivating a research-oriented institutional culture while implementing strategies that involve vertically and horizontally integrating research methodology throughout the undergraduate curriculum [6].

With the complexity of integration, successful implementation faces multiple practical barriers. There remains a lack of clarity regarding standardized definitions, best practices for implementation, and criteria for successful curriculum integration. This hampers institutions' ability to achieve their integration goals effectively [6, 7].

Additionally, due to slow revision processes, traditional medical curricula often lack medical breakthroughs and technological advancements in teaching and learning, leaving students with limited exposure to new paradigms. The technical demands of adaptability pose considerable challenges for medical institutions. Educational teams often struggle to navigate multiple online learning platforms and to stay abreast of their features while remaining flexible in response to evolving educational technologies [8].

18.2.1.2 The Digital Shift: Opportunities and Hurdles in Health Professions Education

In medical education, the shift towards technology-enhanced learning presents multiple challenges. Beyond technical and institutional hurdles, adaptability is constrained by limited resources, competing priorities, and varying faculty readiness. Compounding these challenges, a global digital divide persists, shaped by cultural and socioeconomic factors that influence the adoption and effective implementation of new technologies. Key barriers include restricted access to digital tools, inadequate or poorly maintained ICT infrastructure, costly and unreliable internet connectivity, rural and underserved outreach and generational differences among learners and educators (generations X, Y, Z). Addressing these factors is critical to ensuring equitable, effective, and sustainable integration of technology in medical education curricula [8, 9].

18.2.1.3 Recommendations

There is a need to revolutionize curriculum design and delivery. The use of Bloom's Taxonomy by healthcare educators in construction of outcomes and objectives seems redundant. Conversely, Flink's Taxonomy of Significant Learning goes beyond thinking to also include feelings, personal growth, and learning how to learn. Constructing outcomes and objectives that combine the use of Bloom's

Taxonomy and Flink's Taxonomy of Significant Learning would help keep pace with the evolving medical educational landscape.

Successful adaptability requires engaging stakeholders in continuous improvement, incorporating their knowledge and perspectives to maintain a flexible curriculum that can respond to rapidly changing demands. To remain relevant, medical education curricula must respond to varied healthcare environments, incorporating digital health technologies and addressing the expectations of digitally fluent learners in an interconnected world [6].

18.2.2 Learning Environment

The Macy Foundation defines the learning environment as the social, cultural, structural, physical, and virtual factors that shape learners' experiences and outcomes. The clinical learning environment (CLE) is a pivotal element of healthcare education, providing the context in which learners bridge theoretical knowledge with practical application in real-world healthcare settings. The essential components that shape the learning environment include infrastructure, social and psychological well-being, organizational culture, teaching and learning opportunities and educational resources. The scope of the learning environment in medical education has expanded into the wider community, surpassing the traditional boundaries of teaching hospitals. Consequently, future physicians will be required to address increasingly complex societal health challenges and manage the needs of diverse patient populations [1, 10].

Adequate and meaningful learning opportunities are essential for learners to apply theoretical learning, develop clinical reasoning, and assume greater responsibility as they progress in their learning. Effective role modeling and attitudes toward teaching and patient care are considered as fundamental aspects of the learning environment in healthcare education. It influences learners to internalize professional behaviors, ethical standards, and communication practices through observation and guided participation. Moreover, faculty attitudes toward both clinical teaching and approach to patients strongly shape the hidden curriculum, conveying implicit messages about the value of education, empathy, and professionalism. When these elements align positively, they not only enhance clinical competence but also foster learner motivation, psychological well-being, and satisfaction with education and training. Conversely, inadequate opportunities, poor role modeling, or negative attitudes can undermine confidence, professional growth, and overall learning outcomes [10].

18.2.2.1 Healthcare Learning Environments: Confronting Challenges and Embracing Change

Modern learning approaches in the healthcare education learning environment differ significantly from traditional methods. The rapid transition to online medical education underscored substantial technical and infrastructural deficiencies that constrained effective educational delivery. Main challenges that emerged across the globe, particularly in Lower Middle-Income Countries (LMICs) that affected the learning environments, included urban and rural socio-economic disparity and lack of unreliable internet connectivity. Furthermore, incompatibility of online platforms with institutional learning management systems enhanced the digital divide. Faculty preparation emerged as a major obstacle, with many educators lacking the technical skills necessary for effective online teaching [10].

Facilitating the professional development of medical students in high-demand clinical environments presented significant challenges, as experiential learning opportunities involving direct patient contact steadily declined. Meanwhile, structured simulation-based educational interventions outside of clinical settings gained increasing prominence. Furthermore, the historic disruption in delivery of education caused by COVID 19 challenged not only simple course delivery but also challenged the existing clinical education models. Traditional bedside teaching was replaced by virtual patient interviews, telemedicine clinics, and live-streamed surgeries, while clinical rotations were urgently canceled and replaced with virtual alternatives.

Medical education curricula are structured to enable learners to adapt rapidly to evolving clinical contexts, for instance through rotation blocks across multiple specialties that cultivate their capacity to respond to changing demands of varied healthcare settings. Within this framework, the concept of a learning organization is central, highlighting that both individual self-directed learning and collaborative, team-based learning are important for addressing institutional challenges and achieving high-quality educational and clinical outcomes [10, 11].

Post COVID 19, healthcare education has embraced diversity and inclusivity. The notion of "Education with no borders" is gaining popularity. Similarly, the responsibility of educational leaders has increased to promote classroom diversity as an organizational culture at the same time fostering genuinely inclusive learning environment where learners feel valued, included, and able to contribute in meaningful and authentic ways. Curriculum developers should include cross-culture content in healthcare education and instructional strategies that focus on ensuring every learner can clearly understand and engage in meaningful learning opportunities [11].

18.2.2.2 Recommendations

A shared long-term vision is inevitable for sustainable healthcare education, adapting to emerging global health trends, advances in research, and rapidly changing healthcare delivery models. Only through fostering learning environments that value adaptability can medical educators ensure that their programs remain relevant, effective, and capable of preparing learners to meet the evolving demands of healthcare delivery.

18.2.3 Faculty Development

Faculty development in healthcare education has grown increasingly important in response to rising demands in the field. The need for comprehensive faculty development arises from expectations of the society of healthcare graduates. Rapid advances in medical and information technology, increasing commercialization, rising ethical and litigation concerns, and the exponential expansion of medical knowledge have reshaped what communities expect from healthcare providers. Today, healthcare requires professionals to go beyond clinical expertise to effective educators and communicators, collaborative team members, competent leaders, dedicated scholars, ethical and socially accountable professionals, and proactive health advocates. The driving factors to shape innovative faculty development initiatives include increasing sense of accountability in medical education, the pursuit of excellence in education and training outcomes, and the ongoing professionalization of medical education [11, 12].

Technology enhanced learning has highlighted significant competency gaps that demand urgent attention. Similarly, the changing landscape of healthcare delivery from the rise of precision medicine to well-being and team care has implications for educating and training healthcare professionals [12].

Developing faculty skills in online teaching, designing and sharing digital learning resources, and implementing effective online assessments has become essential. Faculty development is crucial to equip medical educators with the competencies needed to fulfill their evolving roles in technology-enhanced learning environments [13, 14].

18.2.3.1 Navigating Barriers: Faculty Development in Health Professions Education

Faculty development challenges may vary across healthcare educational systems, programs and contexts. Cultural norms and hierarchical structures may further create distinct challenges, particularly in many developing contexts.

Across the globe, the development of competency frameworks in undergraduate and postgraduate medical education, as well as in nursing and allied health programs during the 1970s and 1980s, facilitated the integration of technology and innovative approaches into health professionals' education. Building on this, integration of Artificial Intelligence (AI) now enables personalized student learning experiences and adaptive assessments. However, many institutions (particularly in Lower Middle-Income Countries) find it challenging to keep up with fast-moving AI developments, underscoring the need for focused faculty capacity development to help educators develop learners' digital skills, ethical understanding, and ability to use technology effectively in clinical practice [13].

Despite these developments and need to enhance digital skills of the learner, there is a conceptual divide in literature with respect to the expected competence of a medical graduate. There is a growing debate and emphasis on Digital Skills Competence or Health Informatics competence as an outcome [13–15].

Digital competence refers to the fundamental skills needed to navigate and engage with the digital world, while health informatics is a specialized discipline focused on designing, implementing, and utilizing technology to enhance patient care. This distinction is important: digital competence provides a foundational skill set for all healthcare professionals, whereas informatics involves the advanced application and management of healthcare technologies. Medical educators need to develop a clear understanding of the two terminologies and their applications in curriculum [15].

Several competency frameworks have been developed to guide digital health skills in healthcare education. A review of 30 such frameworks, in the study conducted by Nazeha, N et al. in 2020, identified 28 key digital health competency areas. The most common areas reported were basic Information Technology (IT) skills, managing health information, digital communication, understanding ethical and legal responsibilities, and ensuring data privacy and security. It is reported that these varied frameworks help standardize the digital skills expected of medical students and healthcare professionals. However, the scope of competencies varies significantly between frameworks and programs. Hence, there is a need to target the specific needs of healthcare professionals based on their role, seniority, setting, and context, in defining digital and informatics competencies rather than covering all areas from comprehensive frameworks. Evolving competency framework broadens the scope of expected competencies necessitates a corresponding evolution in how medical educators are prepared and supported [11].

Additionally, the underlying theoretical construction of faculty development activities is essential. To foster higher-order thinking and deep learning in healthcare educators, Faculty Development Activities (FDA) need to be aligned with a sound theoretical perspective and expected competency and outcome. This involves application of established learning theories, such as constructive alignment, designing the objectives, content, instructional methods, and assessments in a consistent and cohesive way [13].

18.2.3.2 Recommendations

Faculty development should go beyond improving teaching skills to also include learning in the context and workplace. Institutions and medical educators need to design faculty development activities based on sound theoretical principles. There is a need for a comprehensive 'Faculty Competency Framework' inclusive of digital and informatics competence in healthcare education for twenty-first century educators. Faculty developers must be creative in making faculty development programs meaningful, joyful, and interesting while considering potential future trends to ensure program relevance.

The future of faculty development in medical education demands innovative approaches that address rapidly changing educational landscapes and emerging healthcare priorities.

18.2.4 Socio-structural Dynamics in Medical Education

Academic institutions have a higher responsibility to uphold the professional education and training of the educators for better fulfillment of their roles and to safeguard their well-being. Socio-structural factors play a significant role in effective faculty development programs that can transform educators by enhancing the attitudes, values, and skills that enable them to contribute to the organizational educational landscape. This includes institutional culture, educational resource allocation, leadership support, workload demands, interpersonal relationships, organizational policies, academic environment, and the accreditation standards [8].

18.2.4.1 The Hidden Hurdles: Institutional Barriers to Educational Transformation

Medical education faces complex and systemic institutional challenges. In today's rapidly changing medical education landscape, programs are expected to manage cultural, financial, and curricular challenges within constraints of limited time, resources, and faculty capacity. These challenges are compounded by deep rooted institutional values, intrinsic resistance to change, and strict accreditation requirements [8, 11].

The shift to digital methods in medical education presents challenges, including modifying professional identity standards, uneven student engagement and disparities in technology access, digital role modeling, ethical and legal implications (informed consent etc). Addressing these issues requires institutions to adopt comprehensive policies in use of digital strategies that strengthen infrastructure and enhance educators' technological competencies. It is essential to devise strategic approaches that not only address these challenges but also safeguard the quality of education, ensure alignment with accreditation standards, and promote sustainable improvement in teaching and learning practices.

18.2.4.2 Accreditation Pressures and the Future of Medical Education

The accreditation landscape in medical education has evolved considerably in recent years. There has been a move towards more progressive models that emphasize balance between quality assurance and continuous quality improvement (CQI). Accreditation standards are no longer seen as the only tool for guaranteeing minimum requirements; rather, the aim is to integrate the protection of established educational standards with the promotion of emerging trends and innovation in medical education. The three globally renowned bodies with global accreditation standards include World Federation for Medical Education (WFME), Liaison Committee on Medical Education (LCME), Accreditation Council for Graduate Medical Education (ACGME). The published standards are used as an international benchmark globally. Little attention has been paid to the factors influencing compliance with quality regulations. Understanding these determinants can enhance regulatory processes and provide valuable insights for quality improvement initiatives led by service providers and policymakers [14, 15].

Competency-based Medical Education (CBME) has created avenues to better align undergraduate and postgraduate training. The use of Entrustable Professional Activities (EPAs) and defined milestones further enables linking undergraduate preparation with residency performance and outcomes. Promoting well-being and ensuring inclusivity have become essential elements of accreditation, especially within postgraduate training.

Regulatory bodies play a pivotal role in determining quality regulatory standards. The nature of agreement and understanding between the regulatory body and the regulatee is essential for effective compliance. Additionally, their role is to encourage collaborative governance, develop data-driven accreditation and innovation strategies, and adapt to a changing healthcare landscape that requires healthcare professionals (undergraduate and postgraduate levels) to possess skills beyond traditional clinical practice. However, literature has reported variability in compliance with regulations across the globe [14]. Continuous Quality Improvement measures should be able to (i) guide institutions and curricula, (ii) develop support systems and inclusive learning environment, (iii) remain inclined with emerging trends and competency-based requirements, (iv) ensure accountability driven by complexity of healthcare system, and (v) measure impact of faculty development activities [15].

With the growing use of technology and AI in instruction and assessments, the need to relook at the accreditation standards is taking a toll. The rising concerns of learner and faculty tech-burnout are in debate. When and where to support technology in clinical practice, when to withdraw technology in clinical supervision of postgraduate students is not been defined by these accreditation standards. The required hours under technology-driven supervision are also a growing concern which seems to be overlooked by the accreditation bodies [14, 16].

Broad overarching areas as future challenges in accreditation include [13–15, 16]:

- *Alignment*: Monitoring and evaluation of institutions by regulatory bodies to ensure alignment of training programs and learning environments to effectively promote CBME.
- *Redesign*: Redesigning accreditation standards and link technology driven reforms in medical education and clinical service delivery.
- *Expectations*: Outlining clear expectations for learners, programs, institutions, and healthcare systems to enable systematic evaluation of performance.
- *Culture*: Fostering a culture of shared responsibility to achieve the agreed-upon outcomes.

18.2.4.3 Recommendations

The re-assessment of quality standards, conceptual, operationalized, and integrated definition of "quality of medical care" is essential. Regulatory frameworks need to incorporate support systems to address the significant academic pressures and mental health concerns faced by students. Expected standards must be consistent and aligned across the entire learning continuum, from undergraduate to postgraduate and professional practice, to ensure a cohesive competency-based learning environment.

Future medical education curricula must address challenges such as aligning undergraduate and postgraduate competency and regulatory standards, integrating digital technologies, promoting lifelong learning, and delivering competency-based education that meets diverse public health needs. A unified curriculum framework from undergraduate to postgraduate training, and even professional practice, is needed to provide clarity and efficiency.

There is a need for medical educators and policy makers to work collaboratively.

18.3 Conclusion

Modern medical education requires a forward-looking approach that emphasizes advanced technological literacy, humanistic values, and a global perspective to develop adaptable, empathetic, and innovation-driven healthcare professionals and educators.

References

1. Zeren Q, Zeng Y, Zhang J, Yang J. Flexner's legacy and the future of medical education: embracing challenge and opportunity. World J Clin Cases. 2024;12:6650–4.
2. Han ER, Yeo S, Kim MJ, Lee YH, Park KH, Roh H. Medical education trends for future physicians in the era of advanced technology and artificial intelligence: an integrative review. BMC Med Educ. 2019;19(1):460.
3. Reddi S, Javidi D. A critical narrative review of medical school curricula: teaching methods, assessment strategies, and technological integration. Cureus. 2025;17.
4. Skochelak SE, Lomis KD, Andrews JS, Hammoud MM, Mejicano GC, Byerley J. Realizing the vision of the Lancet Commission on Education of Health Professionals for the 21st Century: transforming medical education through the accelerating change in medical education consortium. Med Teach. 2021;43(sup2):S1–6.
5. Kim K. Moving forward: embracing challenges as opportunities to improve medical education in the post-COVID era. Humanit Soc Sci Commun. 2022;9:419.
6. Tolkacheva IV. Modern challenges of medical education and their reflection in the curriculum. 2023. Vestnik of Kostroma State University. Series: Pedagogy. Psychology. Sociokinetics.
7. Miguez-Pinto JP, Garcia-Rosa BS, Maggitti-Bezerril M, Ramalho C, Garcia SL, Pustilnik HN, Boczar D, Avena KM, Andrade BB. The medical student of the future: redefining competencies in a transformative era. Front Med. 2025;12:1593685.
8. Ahn DS. Current trend of accreditation within medical education. J Educ Eval Health Prof. 2020;17:30.
9. Farzaneh M, Faghihi E, Sanagoo A, Jouybari L. You won't learn until you want to: medical students' experiences of the educational nature of the clinical environment. BMC Med Educ. 2025;25:661.
10. Surapaneni KM. ABC's of creating a modern clinical learning environment to support learner growth. South-East Asian J Med Educ. 2025;18(2):70–5.
11. Nazeha N, Pavagadhi D, Kyaw BM, Car J, Jiménez G, Tudor Car L. A digitally competent health workforce: scoping review of educational frameworks. J Med Internet Res. 2020;22:e22706.
12. Rafi A, Anwar MI. Challenges for implementing WFME standards for accreditation in health professions education in low and middle-income countries: a scoping review. J Pak Med Assoc. 2021;71(3):966.
13. Salajegheh M, Sandars J, Mirzazadeh A, et al. Understanding the capacity development of faculty development programs: a sequential explanatory mixed methods study. BMC Med Educ. 2024;24:744. https://doi.org/10.1186/s12909-024-05715-5.
14. Robertson ML, Cofrancesco J Jr, Levine RB. Transforming individuals and institutions through competency-based faculty development. Front Med. 2025;12:1621376.
15. Dunbar P, Browne JP, O'Connor L. Determinants of regulatory compliance in health and social care services: a systematic review protocol. HRB Open Res. 2021;4:13.
16. Han ER, Yeo S, Kim MJ, Lee YH, Park KH, & Roh H. Medical education trends for future physicians in the era of advanced technology and artificial intelligence: an integrative review. BMC medical education. 2019;19(1):460.

Future of Medical Education in Resource-Constrained Settings

19

Saniya Sabzwari, Syed Moin Ali, and Sara Shakil

Key Points

- Medical education in RCS is currently encountering complex challenges.
- Technology has the potential to bridge educational gaps and enhance learning accessibility.
- Curriculum reform focusing on ensuring the acquisition of locally and globally relevant core and "soft" skills is crucial for preparing an effective healthcare workforce.
- The emphasis on the development of core clinical skills has to be fused with emerging competencies in medical curricula.
- In RCS, progress towards access to quality education and training have to have long-term partnerships involving financial support, political commitment, and capacity building.

19.1 Introduction

19.1.1 Background

Medical education serves as the scaffold for a vigorous and dynamic healthcare system, responsible for building a skilled and compassionate workforce capable of addressing the complex health needs of its populace. The importance of medical education is especially remarkable in the context of global health, where differences in health outcomes are dependent on the availability and quality of healthcare providers [1].

S. Sabzwari (✉) · S. M. Ali · S. Shakil
Aga Khan University, Karachi, Pakistan
e-mail: saniya.sabzwari@aku.edu; syedmoin.ali@aku.edu; sara.shakil@aku.edu

J. Sandars et al. (eds.), *Modern Medical Education*,
https://doi.org/10.1007/978-3-032-27958-3_19

The relevance and importance of medical education is particularly evident in the context of global health, where disparities in patient outcomes are dependent on the presence and efficient functioning of the attending physicians1. Effective clinical training has a direct impact on the health care providers' competences to prevent diseases, treat them, and promote overall community well-being. Therefore, ensuring top quality, affordable, and contextual medical education training is not just a theoretical rhetoric but also a key contributing factor of societal health and development.

When medical education is implemented as per pedagogical principles and includes the key stakeholders in its design and execution, it is bound to positively impact disease outcomes, improve disease prevention measures and overall community health. Thus efforts for high quality education and training translate into societal development. The 2010 Lancet Commission Report on education of health professionals [2] emphasizes the integral role of education in impacting health care delivery. The UN Sustainable Developmental Goals have targeted "Good Health and Well-Being," "Quality Education" and "Partnership for the Goals" as among the 17 goals for 2030. These, and many other publications, call for an urgent action for earnestly considering the direction in which medical education should be moving, especially in resource-constrained settings.

19.1.2 Resource-Constrained Settings: Definition and Impact

Resource constrained settings (RCS) are characterized by significant dearth of economic, human, and infrastructural resources. This gravely affects the ability to provide key academic and healthcare facilities. Such dire scenarios are prevalent not only in low and middle-incomes countries (LMICs) but also in underserved regions within high income nations [3].

19.1.3 Purpose of the Chapter

This chapter aims to provide an exploration of the existing features and future path of medical education while contributing to the current discourse on bracing international medical education and fostering health equity. The authors aspire to articulate a vision for an equitable, resilient, and effective medical education system in RCS, capable of producing healthcare professionals adept at dealing with distinctive demands and health priorities of their communities.

19.2 Challenges in Medical Education in Resource-Constrained Settings

Medical education in RCS faces a series of deeply endemic barriers that collectively hinder the productive physician training and are worsened by socio-politico-economic factors, creating an intricate and complex environment for educational reform.

19.2.1 Infrastructure and Resource Limitations

The paucity of physical and technological resources is a universal challenge in RCS. Many institutions function below the minimum essential requirements of infrastructure and medical equipment. In medical colleges this scarcity would include the presence of only a few models, mannequins, laboratory instruments and diagnostic facilities, grossly insufficient to cater to the ever-burgeoning number of class size. Such shriveled academic conditions impact effective skills development. Furthermore, limited access to internet connectivity and a dearth of computing devices restrict extensive use of e-learning platforms. This alienates a significant proportion of learners from the internationally available medical databases. Economic limitations, at the heart of many of these deficiencies, cause persistent underfunding for academic activities and technological upgrades [4].

19.2.2 Faculty and Workforce Shortages

The shortage of qualified medical faculty is a huge impediment in RCS. Migration to wealthier regions by skilled healthcare providers and faculty members causes a significant 'brain drain' and a resultant vacuum that takes time to fill. Toyin-Thomas et al. [5] divided the reasons for this migration into macro (remuneration and security concerns) and meso-level concerns (career prospects and positive working environment). This results in high student-to-faculty ratios, resulting in superficial learning, inefficient supervision and assessment during clinical training. Moreover, there are limited opportunities for professional capacity building and research. Coupled with these are issues of inadequate financial incentives and inflexible administrative policies. These factors further stagnate the delivery of high-quality medical education and make it difficult to build and sustain a pool of forward-looking and engaged faculty members. The struggle between service provision and scholarship thus becomes harder for faculty members in RCS, impacting motivation and retention. With the balance almost always tipping in favor of service, it is academic work, like developing engaging learning experiences or contextually-focused assessment strategies that get jeopardized.

19.2.3 Curricular Deficiencies and Relevance

Training in medical skills has undergone a sporadic evolution from the traditional apprenticeship-model curriculum to a more structured, competence-based one. Curricula in many RCS medical schools often suffer from being antiquated and inadequately focused around the prevailing community health needs and disease prevalence. Traditional, teacher-centered pedagogical practices persist, that fail to encourage student engagement to foster critical thinking and problem-solving. There is frequently a lack of emphasis on community health, primary care, and the development of professional behavior, despite these being the most pressing health challenges in these settings. The disconnect between curriculum content/delivery and local health priorities can lead to a workforce that is ill-equipped to address the specific health disparities they will encounter [6].

The training of health care providers in most RCS by and large occurs in tertiary care hospitals, although community health care problems and the role of family physicians have been emphasized for decades. This lack of emphasis on community health, primary care and the development of professional behavior has created a disconnect between curriculum delivery and local health priorities. This has resulted in graduating physicians who are ill-equipped to address the specific health disparities they will encounter. The dire sequelae of not "doing the thing right" and not "doing the right thing" has directly impacted not only on health statistics but also on community satisfaction with the services and service providers.

19.2.4 Impact of Global Events

The existing vulnerabilities of the medical education system in RCS are easily prone to enter a negative cycle due to climate change related calamities such as infection pandemics, floodings, or droughts. During the COVID-19 pandemic, many institutions suffered due to almost non-existent internet facilities and rampant digital illiteracy among both students and faculty [7]. Power outages and fluctuations are occurrences that trouble LMICs and delay technological processes. Such grim situations reduce the number of working days and produce a cascade of uncontrollable obstructions to effective health care delivery in an already resource-choked situation. These barriers underscore the pressing need for adaptable and sustainable educational models that can withstand emerging global challenges and ensure continuity of learning.

The challenge that medical educationists must now face, and counter, is to integrate the impact of climate change on disease manifestations, prevention and health care delivery while continuing with the quantum of time and effort expended on the development of core skills and competencies.

19.3 Innovations and Strategies for Medical Education

Institutions in RCS need to analyze their growth from multiple angles. In this section, the authors endeavor to present an overview of how technology, curricular reform and faculty development and partnerships can create an overall system that can improve the quality of physicians, ready to effectively serve their communities as well as capable of practicing safely in diverse global contexts.

19.3.1 Technology and Digital Learning

Technology can now easily be used to narrow the digital disparities among the resource-rich and resource constrained academic communities due to the availability of low- cost e-learning platforms and mobile learning initiatives. Students, previously deprived of recent technological advances, have better access to online, asynchronous lectures, interactive courses, synchronous discussions and assessments. Learning through virtual patients and virtual clinics and support clinical reasoning and decision making thereby overcoming limitations in local clinical sites and faculty supervision. Simulation-based training (SBT) offers safe environments for students to practice clinical skills without necessarily requiring expensive equipment. Procuring low-fidelity mannequins can bolster learner confidence and safeguard patients from unnecessary harm. Also, SBT standardizes training, ensuring a relatively more homogenously skilled workforce. The integration of Artificial Intelligence (AI) in medical education holds significant promise, from personalized learning pathways and intelligent tutoring systems to AI-powered diagnostic tools for training and assessment, potentially leveling the playing field across institutions [9]. The challenge here is the ethical use of Large Language Models due to the absence of such guidelines. This provides an opportunity for institutions to collaborate for the development of ethical guidelines for AI use which may be adapted from the 2021 WHO guidelines on the same [8].

The fast (and often furiously-paced) evolution of technology impacting education and health-care delivery has mandated the incorporation of "life-long learning," "digital fluency," and "e-health proficiency" as key competencies in medical curricula. If institutions wish their graduates to adapt to a rapidly evolving healthcare milieu, these competencies must be treated at par with those of "management skills" and "clinical reasoning," for example. As the world embraces AI in all aspects of medicine, medical education must consider it a strategic ally of the present and the future.

19.3.2 Curriculum Reform and Contextualization

Curricular success depends on its relevance to local needs and the prevailing statutes. Institutional decision-making must weigh its own vision and realities, against benefits and challenges of introducing innovative content, pedagogies and assessment practices. Technologies, attractive as they are, will benefit the academic system if they can be sustained and provided consistently to the end-users.

Curricula in RCS, apart from being contemporary, have to cater to the emerging local health conditions. Competency-based Medical Education (CBME), a pedagogical framework focusing on outcomes, needs to be leveraged in letter and spirit to ensure that graduating physicians possess the requisite knowledge, skills, and attitudes to effectively cater to the community health needs. Incorporating prevalent diseases, cultural practices, and healthcare delivery models along with fostering Interprofessional Education (IPE) are now recommended components of locally relevant academic programs. Furthermore, the evolving requirements of health care delivery necessitate that due importance be given to public health, preventive medicine, and primary care. Such integrated and helical curricular designs should foster teamwork and communication skills that are crucial for collaborative, culturally sensitive, patient care. The tilting of curricula towards such issues should result in a workforce of healthcare providers adept at being effective agents of change within their communities. Leadership, as one of the competencies, must be inculcated, and assessed in medical education.

Curricula, relevant to the community, must include dynamic and emerging population demographics and trends. As an example, within the next 25 years, South Asia's existing youth bulge will be coupled with a rapidly growing older population. Most African nations also show similar patterns [9].

In addition, with urban migration and inter-provincial resettling, cultural competence is now a necessary adjunct skill to be built into the operational curricula. Furthermore, modern curricula need to explicitly address issues relevant to marginalized communities, instead of shying away and shifting sensitive topics to the hidden curriculum. Graduates must be adept at providing safe and efficient health care to addicts, HIV+ patients and those generally shunned by society without feeling awkward or at a loss. Providing unconditional positive regard, even in the face of inner conflict, is the hallmark of a professional health care provider. Preparing such high caliber workforce is a realistic target even in constraint-ridden situations; a diverse simulated-patient bank, real and/or virtual, capable of providing practice and feedback in a safe environment should diffuse the traumatic transfer of such skills to real-life vagaries.

The authors consider that yet another major variable for curricular success in RCS is the creation of a locally feasible balance between teacher- and student-centered methods of teaching. To be labelled as "progressive" and "innovative," some institutions adopt resource-intensive pedagogies like Problem-Based Learning, online teaching, high-fidelity simulation labs etc. Institutions need to carefully and critically consider whether their available resources will suffice to sustain the innovation or utilize resource-efficient pedagogies like Team-Based Learning. While pedagogy is important, curricula will have to be flexible to cater to new generation learners who will not want to sit in traditional learning spaces but rather learn in their own space and time.

19.3.3 Faculty Development and Capacity Building

Faculty development (FD) can be viewed from two perspectives: institutional and individual. Any academic activity that faculty members undertake to improve their own knowledge, skills, and behaviors aimed at improving their professional responsibilities may be termed as FD. On the other hand, programs and activities meant to bring organizational change and influence its culture also come under the ambit of FD [10].

The importance of leveraging the role of medical faculty in RCS cannot be overemphasized. FD programs must be developed and implemented to bear in mind the current level of skills of the recipients. As an example, as technology is increasingly utilized by learners, FD programs to enhance digital literacy and comfort must be offered to allow them to step into the world of virtuality and remote learning. Faculty development programs should focus on modern pedagogical techniques, the development and implementation of locally relevant curricula and attainment of competencies that help foster, technological dexterity and student-centered approach to content delivery. Opportunities, locally supported or externally funded, must be leveraged for faculty exchanges, joint research projects, and advanced training opportunities [10].

As the move towards global health education becomes stronger, the need to forge collaborations among institutions opens pathways for faculty and expertise exchange that can easily assuage the dearth of subject expertise for faculty development. Such curated programs improve faculty satisfaction and provide them with a sense of achievement; faculty retention and the percolation of the newly acquired skills to students is a strong reason for institutions to fight for these activities.

Building a sustainable and high- impact teaching workforce is dependent on recruiting *and* retaining faculty that feels empowered to become leaders in medical education. Such a cohort of teachers would be a natural consequence of a need-based and institutionally owned continuous professional development program.

19.3.4 Collaborative Models and Partnerships

Regional and global collaborations and partnerships can bolster several educational projects and fill the existing void for institutions desirous of academic upliftment and progress. Institutions in the developing countries can share human resources and expertise and offer solutions that might otherwise be unique for the West. Cooperation between resource-rich and resource constrained institutions can be of value with regard to technical support and research collaborations. Mutual benefits must, however, be given due considerations in these collaborations with emphasis on nurturing independence rather than excessive reliance.

Non-Governmental Organizations (NGOs) and international organizations play a significant role in establishing academic connections among institutions by ensuring access to funds, technical support, and novel yet realistic academic initiatives. These alliances should construct a shared responsibility for improving education at a macro level.

Another emerging partner in medical education is the learner, a key stakeholder who can co-create content and support in its delivery. This emerging concept must be embraced by RCS as global health moves not only precision medicine but also precision learning [11].

19.4 Medical Education in Resource-Constrained Settings: The Path Forward

The path forward for medical education in RCS direly warrants reform and redesign. Clarity of vision, pragmatism of strategic planning and politico-economic commitment must be the key elements that are taken into account during planning. The focus of this planning must target the development of sustainable and contextually relevant academia along with incorporation of innovation to counter traditional limitations [2].

19.4.1 Towards Equitable and Inclusive Education

A core principle for future medical education in RCS must be the pursuit of fairness and inclusivity. This would require institutions at the government and local levels to solve problems by lateral thinking while cautiously experimenting with novel solutions. Initiatives to provide easily affordable and accessible technology and educational resources that work offline are crucial.

Inclusive education is not merely designing curricula that encourage cultural sensitivity, but also promoting an ethos of embracing student and faculty diversity. Institutions are socially accountable to engage with relevant stakeholders from multiple geo-politico-economic backgrounds where everyone learns and practices tolerance along with acceptance of those who may be different from oneself. Such institutions would successfully play their role in dealing with health inequities and empowering learners. The definitive target is to form a learning environment where quality medical education isn't a luxury, but an accessible right. The education system must foster a diverse and representative healthcare workforce capable of efficiently providing services in resource-depleted and often nebulous conditions, definitive.

19.4.2 Sustainable Models and Funding

Political will and commitment, at macro- and micro-levels, must be well established and dependable for any innovation to have lasting impact [12]. The future warrants the establishment of long-lasting financing mechanisms beyond the traditional donor-dependent models. Such processes must explore public-private collaborations, local government dedication, and philanthropic commitment. Long-term investment in medical education infrastructure, faculty development, and curriculum reform would be impossible with the firm backing from governments, academic institutions, healthcare providers, and communities. The key to the longevity and impact of such programs would base on their ability to either generate revenue or bank on broader national resources.

19.4.3 Decolonizing the Curricula and Embracing Similarities

Decolonization in the higher academia would entail actively identifying and teasing out policies and practices that were inherited and have sustained regardless of their utility in the existing culture. This would include Eurocentric perspectives and policies in the curriculum and institutional hierarchies. The incorporation of local factors into the system should foster a more inclusive and equitable learning environment.

These reforms would require learning from institutions in settings similar to one's own and adopting and adapting what works. Decolonization does not forbid looking at and studying the best global practices; it simply guards us against blind submission to and adoption of policies and practices that resource-rich institutions promote. The future of medical education in RCS is not to re-focus our vision to ourselves, but to broaden it to make it more inclusive to seriously consider building short-hop bridges while continuing our journey on long haul ones [13].

19.4.4 Globalization vs. Localization of Healthcare Providers

The dilemma of graduating healthcare providers fit for the local community versus those capable of working "sans frontiers" is definitely a tight-rope walk. In order to produce doctors who qualify highly reputed international examinations like the PLAB, USMLE or the AMC-WPBA medical schools are prone to follow patterns in their curricula that inadvertently and ultimately foster health force migration.

Doctors now are clearly expected to be more than treatment providers; CanMed competencies stated this explicitly [14] and have adapted by many countries. The challenge of including newly identified, essential competencies of Professionalism, Health Advocacy, Scholar etc. along with the traditional competency of Medical Expert has to be carefully addressed and contextualized. Each RCS must carefully consider competencies relevant to its own settings and *how* it will implement them to retain a substantial proportion of these health care providers without stopping doctor migration.

19.4.5 Preparing the Future Healthcare Workforce

In the current tumultuous and nebulous environment, with financial shackles and political whips, adding content for the nouveau physician to learn is a daunting task. Concepts of Health Equity, Climate Change and principles of disaster management, Ethical AI use, well-being and Geriatrics are necessary additions that will compete for time. Institutions in RCS have to endeavor to come up with out-of-box solutions to ensure effective graduate competence.

Tomorrow's healthcare providers will have to be incredibly adaptable, resilient, and equipped with a wide range of skills to effectively deal with complex and nebulous health scenarios. Along with due emphasis on the development of clinical expertise, medical education will have to provide opportunities for the attainment of competencies of reasoning abilities, ethical and culturally sensitive communication, and inter-professionalism. Training will then have to develop a workforce that can be advocates and leaders in their communities, capable of putting evidence-based practices work in local contexts. Ethical considerations for adopting new technologies, especially AI, will also become increasingly important. Future curricula must inculcate ethical use of AI in learning and clinical practice without compromising the development of higher cognitive functions. The aim is to cultivate a workforce that is clinically skilled and socially dedicated to improving health outcomes in their amorphous and blurred environments.

19.5 Conclusion

Medical education in RCS faces a tangled set of challenges, ranging from acute infrastructural and economic constraints to severe dearth of qualified and experienced human resources to archaic curricula. These significantly restrict the development of an adequate number of members of a competent healthcare workforce, promote health disparities, and harm the provision of health equity. Contrary to this, the situation offers opportunities for sustainable progress.

The future of medical education in this context pivots around an effort to promote equitable and evolving learning environments and systems, balanced on long-term financial support and stakeholder commitment. By embracing fostering South-South and North-South partnerships and investing in strategic faculty development, RCS can build resilient educational systems in order to prepare healthcare providers who are clinically proficient, adaptable, socially conscious and committed to addressing the health needs of their communities. The journey ahead demands strategic investment and robust collaboration to offer quality medical education which is a universal right and not a privilege.

References

1. Datta V, Shukla A, Meena JL. Improving the quality of healthcare in resource-constrained settings: is improving undergraduate medical education quality the way out? BMJ Open Qual. 2023;12(Suppl 3):e002582.
2. Frenk J, Chen L, Bhutta ZA, Cohen J, Crisp N, Evans T, et al. Health professionals for a new century: transforming education to strengthen health systems in an interdependent world. Lancet. 2010;376(9756):1923–58.
3. United Nations, Department of Economic and Social Affairs, Division for Sustainable Development Goals. The 17 Goals. New York (NY): United Nations; [cited 2025 Oct 01]. Available from: https://sdgs.un.org/goals.
4. Amin Z, Hoon Eng K, Gwee M, Dow Rhoon K, Chay HT. Medical education in Southeast Asia: emerging issues, challenges and opportunities. Med Educ. 2005;39(8):829–32.
5. Toyin-Thomas P, Ikhurionan P, Omoyibo EE, Iwegim C, Ukueku AO, Okpere J, Nnawuihe UC, Atat J, Otakhoigbogie U, Orikpete EV, Erhiawarie F. Drivers of health workers' migration, intention to migrate and non-migration from low/middle-income countries, 1970–2022: a systematic review. BMJ Glob Health. 2023;8(5):e012338.
6. Saliu F, Behera SK, Qadeer A. Healthcare analytics in resource-constrained settings: opportunities and challenges. J Adv Analytics Healthc Manage. 2022;6:1–8.
7. Sarfaraz S, Ali SK, Khurshid Z, Aly SM. A journey toward online teaching: lessons learnt. Eur J Gen Dent. 2022;11(02):137–40.
8. World Health Organization. Ethics and governance of artificial intelligence for health. Geneva: World Health Organization; 2021. [cited 2025 Oct 10]. Available from: https://www.who.int/publications/i/item/9789240029200.
9. United Nations, Department of Economic and Social Affairs, Population Division. World Population Prospects. New York (NY): United Nations; [cited 2025 Oct 01]. Available from: https://population.un.org/wpp/.
10. Steinert Y, Macdonald ME, Boillat M, Elizov M, Meterissian S, Razack S, Ouellet MN, McLeod PJ. Faculty development: if you build it, they will come. Med Educ. 2010;44(9):900–7.
11. Geraghty JR, Young AN, Berkel TDM, et al. Empowering medical students as agents of curricular change: a value-added approach to student engagement in medical education. Perspect Med Educ. 2020;9:60–5. https://doi.org/10.1007/s40037-019-00547-2.
12. Baig LA, Ali SK, Sarfaraz S. Role of politics, guilds and pedagogy in defining policies in medical education: the Pakistan scenario. Pak J Med Sci. 2022;38(6):1708.
13. Shahjahan RA, Estera AL, Surla KL, Edwards KT. "Decolonizing" curriculum and pedagogy: a comparative review across disciplines and global higher education contexts. Rev Educ Res. 2022;92(1):73–113.
14. Royal College of Physicians and Surgeons of Canada. (n.d.). CanMEDS Framework. Retrieved October 1, 2025, from https://www.royalcollege.ca/en/standards-and-accreditation/canmeds.html.

Providing Sustainable Health Professions Education

20

Farzana Mahdi, Anuja Bhargava, Sucheta Dandekar, and Nirmala Rege

Key Points

- The three main pillars of sustainability in healthcare are social implications, economic demands, and environmental effect. Additionally, they establish the foundation for long-term healthcare education.
- Making sure that the training of health professionals is sustainable in and of itself, meaning that it lowers the long-term financial, social, and environmental costs of education while remaining resilient and equitable.
- A call for a more thorough incorporation of social justice, planetary health, and global equality into curricula is necessary to really "future-proof" health education.
- By reorienting the educational focus toward preventive and the underlying determinants of health, health professional education can support patient-centred, equity-driven care.
- It is advised to develop inclusive curricula that address local contexts and global injustices, cultivate environmentally conscious institutional leadership, and incorporate sustainable healthcare education into accrediting criteria.

20.1 Defining Sustainable Healthcare

Sustainable healthcare involves delivering healthcare in a way that not only supports individual and public health but also protects the environment, remains economically feasible, and promotes fairness across populations, both today and in the years to come. Sustainable healthcare encompasses three fundamental dimensions: Environmental, economic, and social sustainability.

F. Mahdi (✉) · A. Bhargava · S. Dandekar · N. Rege
Eras Lucknow Medical College, Era University, Lucknow, Uttar Pradesh, India

J. Sandars et al. (eds.), *Modern Medical Education*,
https://doi.org/10.1007/978-3-032-27958-3_20

- *Environmental sustainability*: Protecting environment, e.g., by reducing the carbon footprint of healthcare operations.
- *Economic sustainability*: Using finances responsibly, e.g., by ensuring affordability and efficient resource use.
- *Social sustainability*: Promoting health equity and comprehensive access to care while taking socioeconomic implications into account [1].

20.2 Environmental Sustainability in Healthcare

The environmental crisis is among our most pressing problems. It is impossible to isolate the damage to our planet from the colonization and extraction businesses that continue to influence the state of world health today. Movements such as "degrowth" encourage us to envision an alternative future in which people's well-being is more important than unrelenting economic growth. Environmental justice guarantees that all communities have equitable access to environmental policies and practices. That concept directly affects healthcare. Professionals need to think not only about treating disease but about the conditions that create and worsen it, especially in underrepresented communities [1].

Economic Sustainability in Healthcare The economic dimension needs to be looked at objectively. Over time, health outcomes have been shaped by systems that often benefit a few at the expense of many. This connection between economic forces and health has to addressed. While discussions about the social determinants of health are becoming more common in healthcare education, economic policy remains relatively left out. Growing inequalities and environmental harm can be traced back to systems that place profit over people. For future healthcare professionals, it is essential to develop an understanding of how global economic forces such as trade practices, job conditions, and resource allocation can shape the health of the communities they serve.

Social Sustainability in Healthcare
Sustainability also demands that we broaden our perspective from treating individuals to addressing deeper social systems. Healthcare that respects dignity across generations and communities is the need of the hour. Advocacy and justice are now drawing new understanding to the day-to-day lives of the healthcare provider. Equity has now begun to appear more often in course content. Sending students into underserved areas is not enough unless institutions also reflect on whether their own systems inadvertently favor inequality [1].

Before proceeding to sustainable health professions education, it is essential to understand various models of sustainability.

20.3 Overview of Sustainability Models

Table 20.1 shows how each model offers unique insights while addressing limitations of earlier approaches.

Table 20.1 Comparison of sustainability models [2, 3]

Framework	Type	Key characteristics	Limitations/challenges
Global reporting initiative (GRI)	Sustainability reporting framework	Provides detailed indicators for sustainability reporting	Voluntary use, varies among companies, challenging comparability, large number of KPIs difficult to implement in developing countries
Triple bottom line (TBL)	Sustainability measurement framework	Covers economic, environmental, and social aspects	Voluntary adoption, effectiveness concerns, used mainly for published sustainability reports
OECD manufacturing toolkit	Manufacturing sustainability framework	Provides indicators for manufacturing sector sustainability	Voluntary use, comparability challenges
Sustainable development goals (SDGs)	Global sustainability framework	UN framework for sustainable development	2030 agenda for sustainable development with 17 SDGs
Life cycle assessment (LCA)	Product sustainability assessment	Focuses on sustainable products and life cycle methods	Favors environmental/ economic aspects over others
Organizational life cycle assessment (UNEP)	Comprehensive disclosure framework	Organizational-level sustainability assessment	Comprehensive but not focused on performance measurement
Eco-efficiency model	Economic sustainability assessment	Monetary valuation of sustainability contributions through cost-benefit analysis	Cost-benefit focused, may not capture all sustainability dimensions
7E model	Performance measurement tool	Developed in this research, covers seven operational areas, provides company sustainability score (CSS)	Helps identify savings, explore greener materials and energy choices. Allows ranking and comparison of companies using a sustainability index.

20.4 Development of Sustainable Healthcare Education Program

Sustainability frameworks, evolving from the traditional three-pillar model to multidimensional approaches, now encompass the delivery of education by emphasizing adaptive, inclusive, and resilient teaching practices that reduce environmental impact, promote equity, and prepare health professionals for complex, real-world challenges. In order to develop sustainable healthcare education programme, it is better to integrate aspects from the various models that suit each situation, rather than adopt a single framework. This should involve:

- Maintaining environmental boundaries as non-negotiable limits.
- Addressing social equity and economic viability within those limits.
- Considering institutional, cultural, and ethical contexts.
- Engaging participant values and worldviews.
- Leveraging appropriate technologies for scale and impact.

This evolution toward multi-dimensional models suggests that effective sustainability requires both, systems thinking and values-based approaches. Future frameworks will need to integrate technical, social, and ethical dimensions while maintaining clear priorities for decision-making.

The progression from Triple Bottom Line model to multi-dimensional models reflects deeper understanding of sustainability's complexity while highlighting the ongoing challenge of translating comprehensive frameworks into practical, implementable programs, for both sustainable healthcare and its education, that drive meaningful change [4].

20.5 Making These Ideas Work [5–7]

It is not simple to put these ideas into practice. Social and political movements, poverty, global economic inequality, social injustice, and climate change are examples of recent global changes. Illnesses linked to climate change are increasing. Natural resource depletion and changing populations are putting further strain on health systems around the world. Teaching clinical skills is one aspect of preparing the next generation of healthcare professionals in such circumstances; another is assisting them in comprehending the wider implications of healthcare, such as the carbon footprint of hospital systems and the disparities in access that may have an influence on their lives. Professionals need to have a systemic mindset, understanding how their daily choices, interventions, and regulations can either improve or worsen the social structures and ecosystems, in which they operate. Sustainable healthcare education will go a long way to prepare health professionals for the future through curricula that integrate the concepts of the core pillars of sustainable healthcare. It empowers healthcare workers to lead the transformation—grounded in principles of equity, stewardship, and long-term resilience [8].

Understanding the Basics of Sustainability It is essential to have a clear understanding of the basics of sustainability, to prepare healthcare workers to what they will face in the future. This means helping learners to see how hospitals and clinics affect the environment. Energy use is no doubt important, but they need to understand how much waste is produced and how resources are managed. For example, when students discover that operating theatres are responsible for the bulk of hospital waste—up to 70%—they begin to understand just how much room there is for change. That awareness can be a powerful motivator.

Climate Change and the relation to Patient Care Environmental changes can show up in examination rooms and emergency departments. Training needs to reflect that. Students should learn how rising temperatures can lead to heatstroke, or how poor air quality worsens respiratory conditions like asthma. Diseases like malaria are now appearing in regions that never used to worry about them. These shifts can help to understand and anticipate how a changing climate can influence daily practice.

Making Sustainability Part of the Job To become environmentally conscious, everyday alternatives on the job can be itemised and included. This means learning to prescribe only what their patients need, or choosing equipment they can reuse after taking proper precautions and only when it is perfectly safe to do so. Using washable blood pressure cuffs for routine check-ups, when there is no infection risk, can reduce the single-use plastic that hospitals throw away every day. When we teach these habits from the very beginning, we shape healthcare professionals to see sustainability not as another burden simply as part of caring for patients the right way.

Working Together Across Specialties Real change in healthcare sustainability happens when everyone comes together. It takes doctors, nurses, pharmacists, and environmental specialists all pulling in the same direction to make a difference that matters. Take the example of the fight against antibiotic resistance—it requires entire teams sitting down together to create prescribing guidelines that protect patients while also preventing the waste of precious medications that might not even help. When different experts combine their knowledge and experience, they can solve problems that no single profession could tackle alone.

Focussing on Prevention Prevention of illness is better than trying to cure it. Public health should get involved here. Students can be taught how vaccines, good nutrition, and tackling social inequalities play a big role in keeping people healthy and out of the hospital. Imagine a public health student designing a local campaign that helps people make better food choices—it is a simple idea with major long-term benefits for both health and healthcare costs.

Policy and Advocacy Involvement Future healthcare professionals they can be changemakers besides being caregivers. By engaging in promotions, students begin to influence the bigger systems that affect health. This could be pushing for clean energy in hospitals or supporting bike-friendly city planning. These actions have ripple effects. Some students even help organize medicine take-back programs to cut down on unused drugs ending up in landfills or waterways.

Environmental Thinking as Everyday Integration Rather than treating climate and environment as separate topics, the idea is to make them part of every health discussion. If heart disease is taught, one should also understand how air pollution plays a role. Study of infectious disease can include how warming temperatures affect disease patterns. This way, students begin to see the environment not as a separate issue, but as central to every part of healthcare.

Supporting Faculty and Eco-Ethical Leadership Building a sustainable healthcare education system starts with the educators. There is a tendency for educators to make sustainability-issues-checklists. Faculty development helps instructors bring sustainability into their teaching, not just in theory, but in action. Educators can lead by example, citing choices that are environmentally and ethically sound. For instance, a faculty member might rework clinical rotations so that students not only treat patients but also learn to consider the environmental impact of different treatment options. Space needs to be created for students to wrestle with the hard questions. This needs leadership that is authentic, not performative. It also means collaboration across fields, disciplines as mentioned above and actual experiences. Most importantly, we must remain humble about what we do not know while acting on what we do understand [8].

Using Technology to Reduce Our Footprint Technology will help to incorporate remote simulations, online classrooms, and virtual conferences by allowing learners to connect without the carbon footprint of constant travel. By using virtual reality to practice or perform procedures, critical skills can be mastered without generating the waste that comes with traditional training equipment. Hands-on experience can be achieved, leaving barely a trace behind. Developing state of art simulation laboratories should be a goal to achieve sustainable HPE; albeit a start can be made with low cost simulators for resource constraint settings.

Learning Through Global and Local Lenses True sustainability education means opening minds to wisdom from all cultures and acknowledging the mistakes of the past. It means recognizing that indigenous communities have been living in harmony with their environments for generations, developing health practices that naturally emphasize balance and conservation rather than consumption. When students and teachers sit down as equals with these communities, really listening and learning together, they can discover solutions that work not just on paper, but in real life, respecting the deep traditions and knowledge that each culture brings to the table. This kind of collaboration creates approaches that heal both people and the planet.

Helping Patients Understand and Act Health literacy plays a huge role in making healthcare more sustainable. When patients understand their health better, they can take preventive steps, manage medications properly, and reduce unnecessary treatments. Providers also learn how to explain these things in clear, meaningful ways. For example, a pharmacist could explain to a patient safe way to store and dispose of medications, thus protecting both their health and the environment in the process.

Table 20.2 provides summary of education delivery themes that can be introduced in healthcare education to make it sustainable, their implementation strategies, strengths, and challenges likely to be faced [5, 9, 10]. These themes if implemented can safeguard and address emerging healthcare needs.

Table 20.2 Sustainable healthcare education delivery themes, implementation strategies, strengths, and challenges

Sr No.	Theme	Implementation strategy	Strengths	Challenges
1.	Adaptable and inclusive integrated curriculum	Embed sustainability across existing courses as a cross-cutting theme.	Builds relevance across disciplines; supports systems thinking.	Limited curriculum space; competing priorities.
2.	Teaching methods	Use case studies, simulations, and online modules.	Engages learners actively; models real-world complexity.	Requires instructional design support and digital infrastructure.
3.	Resource repository	Develop centralized repositories for teaching materials.	Reduces duplication; improves access and quality.	Requires collaboration and ongoing maintenance.
4.	Assessment strategies	Incorporate sustainability in OSCEs, reflective portfolios, and problem-based exams.	Links theory to clinical reasoning; reinforces values.	Lack of validated tools; assessment fatigue.
5.	Technology and innovation	Use telehealth, AI, and electronic records to reduce environmental impact.	Improves access and efficiency; promotes eco-friendly delivery.	Digital divide; need for training and infrastructure.
6.	Learning environment	Encourage experiential and active learning. Foster collaboration among stakeholders. Promote systems approach. Also emphasize on reflective practices.	Breaks silos and cultivates interprofessional team work	Hierarchical and cultural barriers, resource constraints and lack of faculty preparedness
7.	Global and Decolonial perspectives	Include equity, history, and indigenous knowledge in curriculum design.	Promotes inclusion and global relevance; challenges dominant narratives.	Institutional inertia; lack of representation in leadership.

(continued)

Table 20.2 (continued)

Sr No.	Theme	Implementation strategy	Strengths	Challenges
8.	Health literacy	Integrate environmental health literacy into curricula.	Empowers patients and communities; supports all sustainability pillars.	Requires multi-sectoral collaboration and targeted training.
9.	Accreditation and policy	Align program accreditation with SHE principles.	Provides systemic incentive for integration.	Varying accreditation standards across regions.
10.	Faculty development	Upskill educators through training and co-learning with students.	Enhances faculty confidence; fosters innovation.	Lack of existing faculty expertise; time constraints.
11.	Student partnership	Involve students in curriculum co-creation and advocacy efforts.	Promotes learner engagement; supports mutual learning.	Institutional resistance to student-led change.
12.	Postgraduate integration	Extend SHE principles into residency and continuing medical education.	Translates theory into clinical application; long-term practice change.	Currently underdeveloped; unclear delivery strategies.

20.6 Transforming Health Professions Education Through a Global Lens on Sustainability

Sustainability in HPE should be approached from a truly global, decolonized perspective. International academic conferences play a significant role in shaping what is valued as legitimate knowledge. These conferences often reflect a narrow worldview, dominated by experts and ideas from the Global North. A case study revealed that discussions around sustainability, especially economic fairness, were notably scarce, underscoring the imbalance in whose voices are heard and which issues are prioritized.

For meaningful "future-proof" health education, deeper integration of social justice, planetary health, and global equity into curricula must be attempted. On a happy note, many institutions are already incorporating topics like health disparities and rural health experiences. However, for systemic change, HPE must intentionally challenge lingering colonial influences and broaden its narratives to include diverse, global perspectives.

On the other hand, Global South differs from Global North with regards to different domains of sustainable healthcare education as shown in Table 20.3. However, Global South has its own strengths and challenges. The latter can be overcome using appropriate solutions or strategies. These are also depicted in Table 20.3.

Table 20.3 Comparison of global north and global south with respect to domains of sustainable healthcare education, strengths and challenges of global south and possible solutions [12]

Domain	Global North	Global South	Strengths	Challenges	Solutions/strategies
Policy & governance	Advanced climate-health policies, but often fragmented.	Policies exist but are underfunded or poorly implemented.	Strong public health institutions.	Limited enforcement, political instability.	Global policy frameworks; WHO guidance; regional cooperation.
Infrastructure	Green hospital initiatives gaining ground.	Many facilities lack basic infrastructure.	Access to technology and innovation.	Power and water shortages; lack of waste management.	Invest in low-resource, high-impact sustainable models (e.g., solar clinics).
Workforce training	Some medical schools include planetary health topics.	Sustainability rarely integrated into health curricula.	Educational technology and faculty capacity.	Faculty shortages; limited resources for curriculum reform.	Open-source modules; interinstitutional mentorship (global north–south collaboration).
Waste management	More regulated systems for disposal of hazardous waste.	High levels of unmanaged medical waste.	Regulatory infrastructure in place.	Informal waste disposal; lack of training in sustainable practices.	Community-based waste initiatives; mobile incinerators; education.
Technology & Innovation	Low-carbon tech being piloted; AI for efficiency.	Rapid mobile health (mHealth) uptake due to low-cost access.	Innovation hubs and funding.	Digital divide; data privacy gaps.	Localized tech development; cross-border innovation transfer.
Equity & Access	Universal healthcare coverage in some countries.	Unequal access persists, especially in rural areas.	Community health worker networks.	Inequity across regions; funding gaps.	Scale task-sharing models; invest in community-based care.

Ultimately, transforming HPE means moving beyond Eurocentric models and embracing sustainability as a guiding principle for building fairer, more inclusive, and ecologically responsible healthcare education systems worldwide [11]. To achieve these, certain recommendations have been proposed below.

20.7 Recommendations for Action

For the Global North

- Lead in research and funding for sustainability innovations.
- Share open-access education modules and resources globally.
- Decarbonize healthcare by 2040 in line with planetary boundaries.

For the Global South

- Embed sustainability in national health policies.
- Strengthen health systems through South-South collaboration.
- Prioritize community participation in sustainable solutions.

20.8 Faculty Development for a Sustainable Health Future

As healthcare systems started reflecting on their environmental impact, there increased a growing awareness that delivering high-quality care must go hand in hand with responsibility toward the planet. The health sector is a major contributor to global carbon emissions, yet many healthcare workers are not equipped with the frameworks or tools needed to shift toward more sustainable practices—economically, socially, and environmentally [13, 14].

It takes a new set of values and skills to prepare future health professionals for this reality, in addition to clinical and technological proficiency. These include having solid ethical underpinnings, being able to advocate for others, and using systems thinking to promote health justice and environmental sustainability. Therefore, faculty readiness is required first.

A study by Brand, et al (2021) explored how educators in 13 health professions programs engage with social and environmental health (SHE) through a planetary health lens. They assessed educators' understanding, teaching practices, and self-confidence, and identified structural factors that either enable or hinder integration of; SHE content [15].

The above study highlights that although most healthcare educators have a grasp of social and environmental health concepts, there remains a disconnect when it comes to teaching these ideas in ways that stick. Many admit that they feel unprepared to bring these topics to life in the classroom or to spark the kind of passion in their students that leads to real change. Institutional red tape, entrenched professional habits, and rigid accreditation requirements often determine whether these crucial topics ever make it into the curriculum at all. These gaps demand action on multiple fronts.

We need leaders at every level—from department heads to deans to accrediting bodies—all pushing in the same direction. Healthcare disciplines need to stop working in isolation and start collaborating, while students should be invited in as partners in designing their own learning experiences, not just passive recipients of information. The path forward requires concrete steps: (1) creating clear curriculum frameworks that put sustainability at the centre, (2) investing in faculty development that focuses on how to teach these concepts effectively, and (3) building shared resource materials that any educator can adapt and use. Most critically, accreditation standards must evolve to reflect these priorities, ensuring that sustainability becomes non-negotiable rather than optional. The role of faculty to put these steps into action is invaluable. Hence faculty training programs need to be instituted. Such programs should focus not only on sustainability concept and global priorities but also should equip the faculty with necessary skills required to institute various above-mentioned delivery themes. Inculcating skills for effective leadership and scholarship is a must. The faculty should be aware of various research methods, especially action research, that can generate appropriate evidences to current and future innovative practices. Training for evaluation of educational programs and reflective practices become an integral part of faculty development programs.

The AMEE Consensus Statement (2021) presents a global blueprint for training healthcare professionals who can champion sustainability and planetary health [14].

20.9 Conclusion

With climate goals demanding nearly 50% emission cuts by 2030 and carbon neutrality by 2050, it warns that current education models are failing to prepare graduates for these urgent challenges.

The AMEE Consensus Statement demands comprehensive reform across all health professions education, making sustainability a foundational principle rather than an add-on. The recommendations include integrating sustainable healthcare education into accreditation standards, fostering eco-conscious institutional leadership, and creating inclusive curricula that address global inequities and local contexts. Developed through collaboration between educators, practitioners, and students via the Association for Medical Education in Europe, this roadmap aims to align health education with the Sustainable Development Goals by 2030. By implementing these changes, health professions education can prepare graduates who are not only clinically competent but also equipped to serve both human health and planetary wellbeing [14].

References

1. Zanobini P, Del Riccio M, Lorini C, Bonaccorsi G. Empowering sustainable healthcare: The role of health literacy. Sustainability. 2024;16(10):3964. https://doi.org/10.3390/su16103964. Accessed on 26th July 2025.

2. Silva DN, Wehrmeyer W, Murphy R. Development of a holistic framework for sustainability measurement: a case study of the tea sector. Clean Prod Lett. 2024;7:100072. https://doi.org/10.1016/j.clpl.2024.100072. Accessed on 28th July 2025.
3. Correia MS. Sustainability: An overview of the triple bottom line and sustainability implementation. Int J Strateg Eng. 2019;2(1):29–38.
4. Olawade DB, Popoola TT, Egbon E, David-Olawade AC. Sustainable healthcare practices: pathways to a carbon-neutral future for the medical industry. Sustain Futures. 2025;9:100783. https://doi.org/10.1016/j.sftr.2025.100783. Accessed on 28th July 2025.
5. Aronsson J, Nichols A, Warwick P, Elf M. Nursing students' and educators' perspectives on sustainability and climate change: an integrative review. J Adv Nurs. 2024;80(8):3072–85.
6. McKimm J, McLean M. Rethinking health professions' education leadership: developing 'eco-ethical' leaders for a more sustainable world and future. Med Teach. 2020;42(8):855–60.
7. Lee J, Kim H, Kron F. Virtual education strategies in the context of sustainable health care and medical education: a topic modelling analysis of four decades of research. Med Educ. 2024;58(1):47–62.
8. Wanyenze RK, Alfvén T, Ndejjo R, Viberg N, Båge K, Batte C, et al. Sustainable health—a call to action. BMC Global and Public Health. 2023;1(1):3. https://doi.org/10.1186/s44263-023-00007-4. Accessed on 20th July 2025.
9. Gandhi V, Al-Hadithy N, Göpfert A, Knight K, van Hove M, Hockey P. Integrating sustainability into postgraduate medical education. Future Healthc J. 2020;7(2):102–4.
10. Teherani A, Nicastro T, Clair MS, Nordby JC, Nikjoo A, Collins S, et al. Faculty development for education for sustainable health care: a university system-wide initiative to transform health professional education. Acad Med. 2023;98(6):680–7.
11. Naidu T, Ramani S. Transforming global health professions education for sustainability. Med Educ. 2024;58(1):129–35.
12. Hameed K, Naha R, Hameed F. Digital transformation for sustainable health and well-being: a review and future research directions. Discov Sustain. 2024;5(1):104. https://doi.org/10.1007/s43621-024-00273-8. Accessed on 26th July 2025.
13. Zolo Y, Demissie MA, Echengi EM, Davis B, Ornella PF, Sichimba D, et al. Assessing the presence of sustainability education in the curriculum of medical students and surgical trainees in Africa: a cross-sectional study. Health Sci Rep. 2024;7(7):e2246. https://doi.org/10.1002/hsr2.2246. PMID: 39006152. Accessed on 26th July 2025.
14. Shaw E, Walpole S, McLean M, Alvarez-Nieto C, Barna S, Bazin K, et al. AMEE consensus statement: planetary health and education for sustainable healthcare. Med Teach. 2021;43(3):272–86.
15. Brand G, Collins J, Bedi G, Bonnamy J, Barbour L, Ilangakoon C, et al. "I teach it because it is the biggest threat to health": integrating sustainable healthcare into health professions education. Med Teach. 2021;43(3):325–33.

21 Faculty Development in the Future Perspective of Medical Education

Shahid Hassan, Hasnain Zafar Baloch, and Gauhar Hassan

Key Points

- The future of medical education depends on adaptive, innovative, and community-aligned faculty who are ever-ready to lead learning.
- Faculty development must evolve from isolated workshops into strategic, immersive, and measurable professional growth pathways.
- Rapid shifts in pedagogy, technology, accreditation, and healthcare complexity demand faculty who can teach, inspire, and continuously adapt.
- Effective faculty training requires needs-based planning, alignment with institutional goals, and readiness for challenges such as Emergency Remote Teaching.
- Long-term faculty competence must be demonstrated through authentic evaluation models that show sustained impact and achievement of measurable objectives.

S. Hassan (✉)
School of Medicine, American University of Barbados, Bridgetown, Barbados

H. Z. Baloch
Digital Learning, Teaching and Learning, MILA University, Nilai, Malaysia

Medical Education and Emerging Technologies, Smart University of Medical Sciences, Tehran, Iran
e-mail: hasnainzafar@imu.edu.my

G. Hassan
Department of Anatomy, School of Medicine, American University of Barbados, Bridgetown, Barbados

J. Sandars et al. (eds.), *Modern Medical Education*,
https://doi.org/10.1007/978-3-032-27958-3_21

21.1 Introduction

Medical education is undergoing a transformative evolution, driven by shifting paradigms in pedagogy, rapid technological advancements, increasing emphasis on accreditation standards [7] and the growing complexity of healthcare needs. The faculty, as frontline agents of this transformation, not only needs updated knowledge and skills but also a mindset for future vision rendered through faculty development program on regular basis. The landscape of medical education is rapidly transformed during and after the Covid-19 pandemic, shaped by advances in technology, shifts in educational philosophy and health systems, with growing emphasis on social accountability and accreditation standards [2, 24].

Table 21.1 The comparison between faculty training and faculty development activities

Aspect	Faculty training	Faculty development
Scope	Narrow, task-specific	Broad, holistic
Focus	Immediate skill acquisition	Long-term professional growth
Duration	Short-term workshops	Ongoing, iterative process
Examples	LMS training, OSCE checklist use	Curriculum design, mentoring, educational research
Outcome	Competence in specific task	Growth as an educator, leader, and scholar

Faculty development is a structured process of enhancing the knowledge, skills, attitudes, and professional growth of educators to improve their effectiveness in teaching, research, leadership, and service within an academic institution. Faculty development is a structured process of empowering educators with the skills, knowledge, and mindset needed to enhance teaching, scholarship, leadership, and service in medical education. While faculty training focuses on specific competence of immediate effect, faculty development encompasses a broader, ongoing process aimed at long-term professional growth and educational excellence (see Table 21.1).

Faculty development in this new landscape must transcend faculty training offered through workshops and short-term courses. Faculty development activities are determined via need assessment surveys, institutional goals, strategically integrated training design, and its implementation [5]. Imperative to this are immediate short- and long-term impact monitored through evaluation for continuing quality improvement (see Fig. 21.1). The areas of faculty training should focus on curriculum innovations for design typically incorporated with technological, pedagogical, and content knowledge known as TPACK [18], personalized learner diversity, outcome-based education competency, and programmatic assessment with institutional support (see Fig. 21.2). Faculty, as the cornerstone of this transformation, must be equipped with the competencies not just to teach but to lead, inspire, and adapt to new challenges [16].

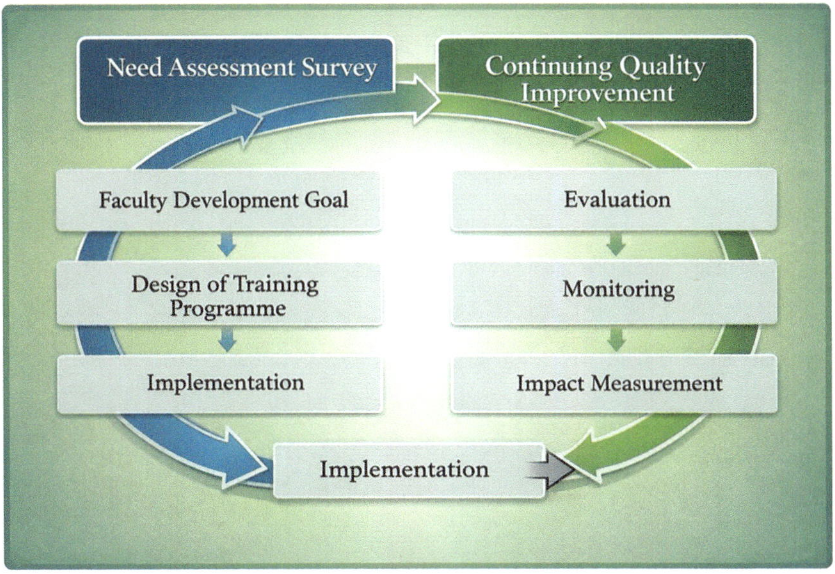

Fig. 21.1 The structured framework of faculty development in future perspective

Fig. 21.2 Some of the relevant features of faculty development explained for future practice

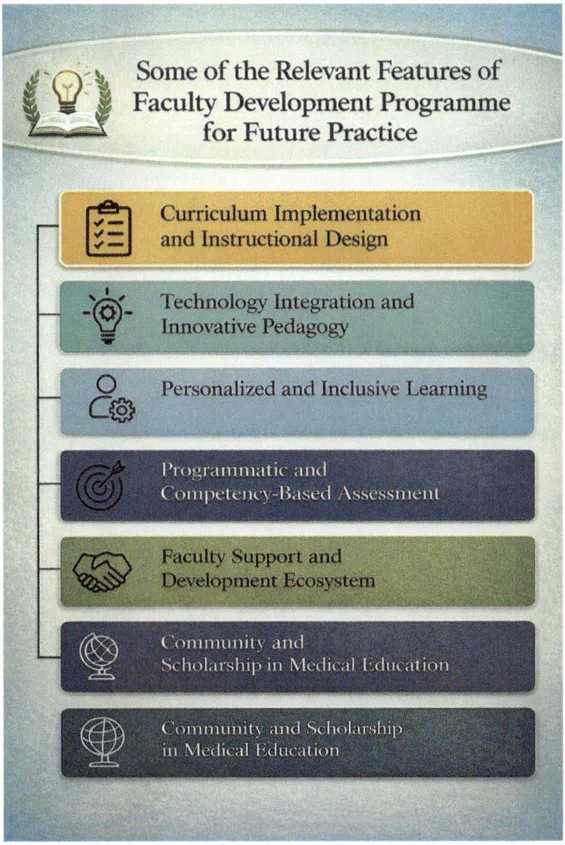

Table 21.2 The thematic clusters of faculty development in future and the associated concepts

No	Thematic clusters	Inclusive concepts
1	Curriculum implementation and instructional design	Curriculum alignment
		Instructional design
		Student-centred learning
		Student engagement
2	Technology integration and innovative pedagogy	Technology integration (TPACK)
		Autonomy in teaching
		Certified educator pathways
3	Personalized and inclusive learning	Learning needs assessment
		Disability accommodation
		Decelerated programs
4	Programmatic and competency-based assessment	Programmatic assessment
		Graduate-fit training
		Retention-oriented training
5	Faculty support and development ecosystem	Faculty resilience
		Impact measurement
		Continuous quality improvement
6	Community and scholarship in medical education	Community-based training
		Educational research
		Societal relevance

Table 21.3 Future-oriented faculty development training workshops and the expected outcome

Focus area	Development strategy	Expected outcome
Curriculum alignment	Workshops on accreditation standards and curriculum mapping	Compliance with curriculum claims and standards
Student-centerer learning	Training on facilitating SDL, mentorship models	Self-motivated and responsible learners
Student engagement	Interactive learning design, active strategies	Higher engagement and learning outcomes
Technology integration (TPACK)	TPACK modules, LMS and EdTech hands-on	Meaningful use of technology in teaching
Instructional design	Backward design, constructive alignment training	Structured and outcome-aligned instruction
Faculty resilience	Stress management, peer support programs	Healthy and sustained faculty performance
Disability accommodation	Training on Universal Design for Learning	Inclusive and equitable learning environment
Learning needs assessment	Diagnostic teaching and learning analytics	Personalized and efficient teaching approaches
Decelerated programs	Competency-based mentorship for slow learners	Flexibility and personalized progression
Programmatic assessment	Multiple low-stakes assessments, rubrics, feedback	Continuous and holistic learner assessment
Graduate-fit training	Curriculum design for real-world competencies	Work-ready and community-responsive graduates

(continued)

Table 21.3 (continued)

Focus area	Development strategy	Expected outcome
Community-based training	Participatory community needs analysis	Locally-relevant and socially-accountable curriculum
Impact measurement	Key performance indicator (KPI) development, tracking outcomes of FDA	Evidence-based development decisions
Retention-oriented training	Longitudinal booster sessions, micro-credentials	Sustained knowledge and skill retention
Certified educator pathways	Institutional certification/fellowship programs	Recognition and motivation for teaching roles
Autonomy in teaching	Innovation grants and peer sharing platforms	Innovative and contextualized teaching and learning methods
Educational research	Training on education research and publishing	

The current chapter explores the multifaceted features of future-oriented faculty development, laying out a comprehensive model for cultivating competent, adaptive, and forward-thinking educators in medical schools. A clustered and cohesive narrative of future-ready faculty development may best be practiced with some core and multiple sub-core domains (see Table 21.2). Faculty development, therefore, must evolve from sporadic workshops into a structured, strategic, and evidence-informed ecosystem based on expected outcomes (see Table 21.3). Faculty should be prepared to implement student-centred, self-directed learning integrated with technology using TPACK approach, and instructional design models that are responsive to the dynamic needs of learners and society as under.

21.2 Accreditation, Curriculum Implementation, and Instructional Design

Faculty development must begin with a strong foundation in understanding, aligning, and implementing accreditation-driven curricula [14]. Faculty should be trained to translate curriculum blueprints into practical learning friendly environment, which is structured, aligned, and measurable [17]. Faculty should have clear concepts of curriculum goals and learning outcomes outlined by accrediting bodies and institutional vision. Workshops on curriculum mapping, constructive alignment, and program learning outcomes are vital. Faculty training in adult learning principles, learning taxonomies, and principles of effective instruction are imperative. This can be achieved through designing sessions that scaffold knowledge and skills using blended and spiral approaches. The shift from didactic to learner-centred models require faculty in facilitators role. Faculty should be promote self-directed learning (SDL), flipped classrooms, and guided inquiry with active, participatory sessions that cultivate critical thinking and collaboration [20]. These sessions involved group dynamic methods of case-based learning (CBL), problem-based learning (PBL) and team based learning (TBL) that foster.

21.2.1 Alignment with Accreditation Standards in Curriculum Implementation

Faculty development must reinforce the authentic implementation of curricula that meet accreditation standards [8]. Faculty should support curricular claims, such as student-centerer learning (SCL), SDL, integrated competencies, and interprofessional education into real-world instructional practices.

Key Element Workshops and mentoring sessions focusing on interpreting accreditation standards into teachable moments, course design, and assessment planning.

21.2.2 Instructional Design and Analytical Problem-Solving

Faculty should know the principles of instructional design for content and pedagogy, backward curriculum design, constructive alignment, and spiral curriculum [23]. They also require training in analytical and diagnostic reasoning to solve real-time teaching and assessment issues.

Key Element Faculty design clinics and case-based discussions on solving pedagogical challenges.

21.2.3 Student-Centered and Self-Directed Learning Implementation

A shift in faculty role from information deliverers to learning facilitators is foundational. This includes nurturing their ability to guide SCL/SDL, where learners take ownership of their learning goals, resources, and self/peer-assessment.

Key Element Faculty workshops on facilitating SCL/SDL, coaching, and reflective practices.

21.2.4 Enhancing Student Engagement and Active Learning Strategies

Student engagement is important for effective learning. Faculty need tools to design learners engaging environment using active learning strategies like flipped classrooms (TBL), problem-based learning (PBL/CBL), and think-pair-share approaches.

Key Element Faculty skill-building in designing student-led discussions, simulations, and collaborative learning.

21.2.5 Technology Integration and Innovative Pedagogy

Post-COVID education increasingly shaped by digital tools, require faculty training to integrate technology meaningfully into pedagogy. Faculty development activities should focus on TPACK framework, enabling educators to select and use tools aligning not simply substituting content and pedagogy. Institutions should empower educators to experience new instructional formats and learning environments. This will foster autonomy of innovation and contextual responsiveness. A medical school should incentivize teaching excellence by developing in-house or externally accredited certification programs in medical education, enabling faculty to grow professionally and gain recognition in areas of curriculum review and accreditation as under.

21.2.5.1 Technology Integration Through the TPACK Framework

A major highlight of future-ready faculty development particularly for emergency remote teaching (ERT) is the integration of technology, pedagogy, and content knowledge (TPACK). Faculty must be adept at selecting and using digital tools purposefully to support learning objectives.

Key Element TPACK-based modular training, hands-on with platforms Learning Management System (LMS), Artificial Intelligence (AR), Virtual Reality (VR), simulation, and AI tools) mapped to curriculum goals.

21.2.5.2 Innovation Autonomy and Teaching Freedom

Faculty should be trusted with autonomy to innovate with indigenous research in teaching and assessments. Institutions must foster a culture of experimentation, peer review, and scholarly discussion.

Key Element Innovation grants, sabbaticals for educational research, and teaching excellence awards.

21.2.5.3 Certified Medical Educators and Faculty Recognition

This will establish a pathway for faculty recognition as trained educators, either through institutional certification or professional fellowships in order to motivate and legitimize their role being educator.

Key Element Structured medical education certification programs or linkage to national/international recognition (e.g., FAIMER, AMEE).

21.3 Personalized and Inclusive Learning

Faculty must be equipped to meet the diverse needs and learning styles of learners, reckoning that one-size-fits-all approaches are no longer acceptable in modern medical education. Faculty development should include, the use of diagnostic tools to assess learners' prior knowledge, learning preferences, and skill gaps. Adaptive teaching strategies and data-informed feedback loops as assessment evaluation report (AER) and course monitoring report (CMR) culture must be introduced. Universal Design for Learning (UDL) recommended by the accreditation standards, inclusive of assessment practices, and legal/ethical responsibilities toward learners with disabilities to accommodate should be part of institution policy matters. Universal Design Learning (UDL) is an educational framework that provides flexible curriculum design principles to ensure equal learning opportunities for all students, including those with disabilities [21].

The rise of individualized learning pathways on their own pace is becoming imperative in curriculum developed with probation and decelerated programme options. Faculty should feel comfortable in mentoring students on variable timelines, including competency-based progression models. The key elements of faculty training should therefore accommodate the following.

21.3.1 Learner Needs Assessment and Learning Style-Aware Teaching

Modern medical education calls for learner-centred and self-directed learning diagnostics. Faculty must explore learner needs and styles, prior knowledge, and preferences to personalize learning during the orientation and thereafter as necessary.

Key Element Training on diagnostic tools, learning analytics, and adaptive teaching methods.

21.3.2 Decelerated and Flexible Academic Pathways

As personalization grows among the learners, decelerated programs should be in place to allow students to learn at their own pace. Faculty must be trained to mentor and assess students who follow non-linear pathways.

Key Element Faculty workshops on competency-based progression and mentoring slow-paced learners.

21.3.3 Accommodating Learner Diversity and Disabilities

Inclusive education is an ethical and legal imperative and accommodating disabilities is standard accreditation requirement. Faculty must be equipped to recognize and respond to diverse learning needs and disabilities with sensitivity and evidence-based approaches worked through.

Key Element Sensitization training on Universal Design for Learning (UDL), accommodations, and equitable assessment.

21.4 Programmatic and Competency-Based Assessment

The boundaries between formative and summative assessment are dissolving, making way for a more holistic and continuous evaluation approach and faculty should view assessment as a continuum. This refers to designing of multiple low-stakes assessments, feedback and reflective practice, and portfolio evidence to support learners' growth. Faculty training should ensure learning activities and assessments preparing students not for examinations, but for real-world practice. Competency frameworks and workplace-based assessment tools (e.g., ACGME and CanMed Core Competencies, EPAs) should be emphasized. Knowledge decays over time without reinforcement and faculty development should incorporate strategies for iteratively done workshops and modules, and longitudinal assessments that reinforce durable learning adopting to following principles.

21.4.1 Programmatic Assessment and Blurring Formative-Summative Divide

Faculty must move beyond single-point assessments currently practiced to programmatic assessment, using continuous data from multiple low-stakes assessments to informed decisions.

Key Element Training on writing high-quality rubrics, giving feedback, and using learning portfolios.

21.4.2 Graduate-Fit Training for Workforce and Community

Faculty development should prepare educators to shape graduates who are fit-for-purpose, i.e., competent, ethical, community-oriented, and ready for complex health systems. The curriculum assessment must ensure to produce fit to practice graduates.

Key Element Curriculum mapping and faculty dialogue with healthcare stakeholders and communities.

21.4.3 Long-Term Retention and Iterative Skill-Building

Learning decays without practice and to address this faculty development must include reflective practice, booster sessions, micro-credentialing, and longitudinal support to ensure transfer of knowledge to long-term memories.

Key Element Faculty academies, digital learning portfolios, and iterative skill refreshers.

21.5 Faculty Development Support Learning Environment

For sustainable educational innovation, institutions should invest in faculty wellness and competence attainment, and data analytic-informed faculty development systems. Faculty development should include well-being programs, mindfulness, peer mentoring, and emotional intelligence training. Institutions must track the outcomes of faculty development initiatives through KPIs, student evaluations, peer feedback, and workshop impact studies using an evaluation method. To ensure the effectiveness of faculty development program, evaluation methods must be strategically selected. The Kirkpatrick Four-Level Model is one of the most widely used frameworks for evaluating training programs. It consists of four levels that measure the effectiveness and impact of faculty development program (see Table 21.4). The ADDIE (Analysis, Design, Development, Implementation and Evaluation) model also serves as another effective framework for developing faculty in educational programme across diverse context. The model has also proven valuable in faculty development programme, where it is facilitating training need analysis and evaluation of 100 participants using ICT tools [4].

This indigenous data informed evaluation ensures continuing quality improvement. A good practiced faculty development ensures feedback-driven modifications brought to routine teaching and learning practice as under.

Table 21.4 The four levels of Kirkpatrick evaluation of faculty development program

Level	Features specified	Action	Evaluation methods
Level 1	Measures participants' initial reactions to the training and whether they found it engaging and relevant	Reaction	Feedback forms, surveys, or smile sheets
Level 2	Assesses the degree to which participants acquired the intended knowledge, skills, and attitudes based on their participation in the training	Learning	Pre- and post-tests, quizzes, demonstrations, and assessments.
Level 3	Examines whether the participants apply what they learned and determines change in workplace behavior	Behavior	Observations, follow-up surveys, interviews, and performance appraisals
Level 4	Evaluates the final results of the training, such as improved quality, increased productivity, or client satisfaction	Result	Return of investment analysis, outcome metrics, and key performance indicators

21.5.1 Building Resilience and Well-Being for Faculty

Sustainable faculty development performance demonstrates emotional resilience, stress management, and work-life balance [10]. With increased teaching loads, administrative and research responsibilities, burnout is often a real threat.

Key Element Well-being programs, peer support groups, and time management training.

21.5.2 Faculty Development with Measurable Impact

There is growing pressure to demonstrate short and long-terms impact of faculty development initiatives on student learning, faculty performance, and institutional quality [13].

Key Element Development of KPIs, follow-up assessments, feedback loops, and scholarly dissemination of outcome.

21.5.3 Continuous Quality Improvement

Continuous Quality Improvement in a faculty development programme is a structured and ongoing process aimed at enhancing the effectiveness, relevance, and impact of faculty training initiatives. It ensures professional development activities aligned with institutional goals and mission, accreditation standards, and medical educators needs.

Key Element Needs-based planning, feedback and evaluation, iterative improvement, outcome-oriented**,** stakeholder engagement and documentation and monitoring:

21.6 Community and Faculty Scholarship in Medical Education

Faculty are not just deliverers of knowledge; they are scholars, collaborators, and community advocates role models. Faculty engagement with communities through their leaders allows curriculum developed with local health needs [6]. Community immersion and service-learning pedagogy must be upheld by an institution. Faculty development activities should support surveys and research addressing community needs assessment and sharing of those innovations at scholarly forums. Faculty development training should emphasize equity, diversity, and inclusion (EDI), social determinants of health, and the moral obligation of educators to serve societal health priorities as under.

21.6.1 Community-Based Education and Curriculum Relevance

Understanding and addressing community needs must be embedded in medical education [12]. Faculty must be engaged in developing curriculum content that resonates with local and global health priorities.

Key Element Community immersion experiences and needs-assessment participatory projects for faculty.

21.6.2 Research in Medical Education and Scholarship Support

Training in medical education research often a shortcoming of faculty seeking to propose a research design, grant and manuscript writing. A faculty development activity in this area may elevate faculty from consumers to contributors of educational scholarship.

Key Element Journal clubs, mentorship in publishing, and seed funding for education research.

21.6.3 Societal Relevance and Community Responsiveness

A faculty development activity in future must equip educators with the skills to align teaching and curriculum with the evolving health needs of the communities they serve. Societal relevance emphasizes the design and delivery of education that addresses public health priorities, health equity, underserved populations, and global health challenges. Faculty should demonstrate their responsibilities in fostering long-term health improvements and social justice. Faculty members as the change agents are not only clinically competent but also socially accountable and ready to serve their communities effectively.

Key Element Community need assessment, service-learning integration, health advocacy training, Cultural and Contextual Competence and sustainability and Social Accountability.

21.7 Role of TPACK in Faculty Development Program

In the wake of the COVID-19 pandemic, education systems around the world faced an unprecedented shift. Classrooms moved online almost overnight, forcing us to rethink how we teach, what we teach, and the tools we use. This disruption challenged our comfort zones but it also offered an opportunity to revamp our teaching and learning and assessment we practice. This chapter will not be complete without a discussion, how the Covid-19 pandemic impacted curriculum delivery and how hybrid formats incorporating technology became not just optional, but essential subject of faculty development programme in medical education. Many of us realized that simply moving content online wasn't enough. What was truly needed was a thoughtful integration of content, pedagogy, and technology and that's where the TPACK framework becomes so relevant. TPACK defines the three knowledge domains as content, pedagogy, and technology and explains why balancing all three is crucial. TPACK framework can be best explained by a Venn diagram (see Fig. 21.3) and consider the three domains becoming dynamic by their overlaps resulting in four zones of interaction. The resulting three domains are Pedagogical Content Knowledge (PCK), Technological Content Knowledge (TPK), Technological Pedagogical Knowledge (TCK), and where all three meet—the sweet spot of TPACK [15]. Post-COVID teaching and learning adjustments revealed our vulnerability in education delivery and an urgency for flexible and personalized teaching models and imperative faculty training for hybrid learning and assessment integrated with TPACK.

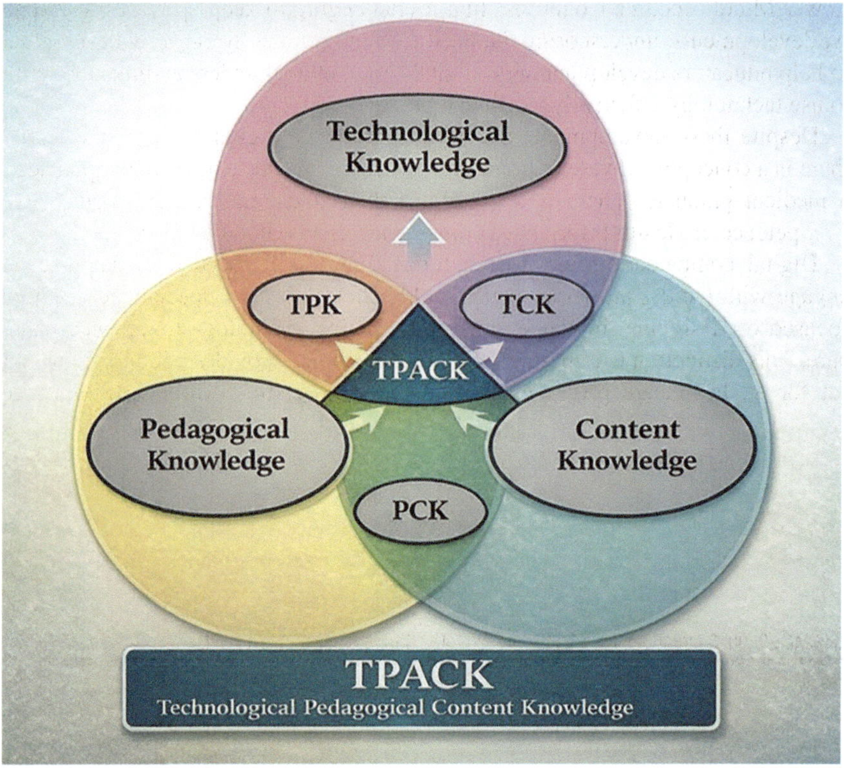

Fig. 21.3 The Venn diagram of TPACK components of content knowledge (CK)), pedagogical knowledge (PK) and technological knowledge (TK)

Table 21.5 Application of theoretical models to a lesson planning incorporating TPACK, Instructional Design and delivery methodology with cognitive reasoning and metacognition

Theory/model	Linked to	Reason for use
TPACK	Lesson planning and tool selection	Integrates content, pedagogy and technology for online teaching
Gagné's 9 events	Instructional structure of online lessons	Step-by-step guide for lesson transformation
HD reasoning	Case-based/problem-solving sessions	Mimics real-world thinking in disciplines like medicine
Think-aloud	Microteaching, reflection, student engagement	Promotes metacognition, transparency, and reflection
Microteaching (strategy)	Application of all above in practice	Practice + feedback loop in a safe learning environment

Faculty may resist change and to overcome this a support systems in terms of mentorship, workshops, and technology help desks will essentially be required. Institutional leaders must institutionalize support with generous investments in terms of grant schemes, integrated technology expert teams, and faculty recognition for innovation as part and parcel of faculty development programme [1, 3].

TPACK serves as the overarching framework for designing lesson plans suitable with digital instruction to helps faculty in balancing the technology use with pedagogical methods and subject content. In the design of a training sessions that guide how to choose the right digital tools (Zoom, Padlet, LMS, etc.) based on content and teaching strategy [11]. In assignments of lesson for faculty in training to redesign and reflect on right selection of tools in teaching and learning can be a good hand-on training workshop mandatory for faculty development in technology incorporating with content and pedagogical knowledge and skills. Faculty often know content well but struggle with aligning pedagogy and technology and TPACK bridges that gap by promoting pedagogical reasoning about tool selection in context [19] TPACK is not just a theory—it's a practical guide for educators designing digital instruction. It emphasizes the integration of Technology, Pedagogy, and Content Knowledge, helping faculty members strike the right balance. Instead of adding tech as an afterthought, TPACK encourages us to think critically. Instead of adding technology as an afterthought, TPACK encourages us to think; what content are we teaching? what pedagogical strategy fits best? and what technological tool will enhance this combination? TPACK under a bigger umbrella provide integration between technology, pedagogy, and content knowledge to strike a balance between what, how and why we need technology in teaching and learning (see Table 21.5). Let's take a closer look at, how the theoretically TPACK framework serves as a foundation in course lesson planning, particularly in a digitally supported environments. Three types of knowledge educator brings when planning to integrate technology into a lesson planning (see Fig. 21.3). Content knowledge (CK), pedagogical knowledge (PK), and technological knowledge (TK). CK in this model is the subject area knowledge what an educator brings to the classroom in any given discipline. PK is about arts and science of teaching, how educator teaches, and involves learning theories to instructional design. TK is about the technological tools as how to select, use, and integrate technology into the curriculum.

Pedagogical content knowledge (PCK) was coined by Lee Shulman in 1980s to emphasize subject matter knowledge. It's about teaching strategies a teacher needs to effectively deliver the content from his areas of expertise. Added to this was another knowledge domain by Runya Mishra and Mathew Koehler from Michigan State University [15]. The added new component was to meet the requirement of twenty-first century teaching called the technological knowledge [22]. Apart from faculty training in TPACK, their training in instructional design and teaching and learning strategies to the extent to equip them in designing and developing their course lesson plan has become new norms for a certified teacher and any faculty training must address these components of a good practiced medical education (see Table 21.5). Instructional Design (ID) is the systematic development of instructional materials and experiences. ID ensures content is effectively structured to support learning outcomes guided by learning theories, educational psychology, and pedagogical principles. Popular models: ADDIE [4] Gagné's Nine Events Instructional Model [9]. Besides ID an authentic teaching strategies equally compatible for physical classroom and online hybrid delivery, in author opinion would be hypothetico-deductive and think aloud approaches.

21.8 Conclusion

The future of medical education relies on future-ready faculty and competent educators who are adaptive, innovative, inclusive, and aligned with both institutional vision and community needs. Faculty development must shift from episodic events to strategic, measurable, and immersive experiences. Empowered with technological fluency, pedagogical strength, and emotional resilience, such faculty will not only implement transformative curricula but will also inspire and sustain a new generation of competent, ethical, and reflective healthcare professionals. By institutionalizing comprehensive, evidence-informed, and forward-looking faculty development practices, medical schools can ensure that their faculty evolve into leaders of learning, architects of change, and advocates of equity in healthcare education.

References

1. Alhassan AI. Implementing faculty development programs in medical education utilizing Kirkpatrick's model. Adv Med Educ Pract. 2022;13:945–54. https://doi.org/10.2147/AMEP.S372652.
2. Armstrong S, Rispel L. Social accountability and nursing education in South Africa. Glob Health Action. 2015;8:27879. https://doi.org/10.3402/gha.v8.27879.
3. Baker VL, Lunsford LG, Pifer MJ. Systems alignment for comprehensive faculty development in liberal arts colleges. J Educ Dev. 2015;34(1–2) https://doi.org/10.1002/tia2.20029.
4. Bamrara A. Applying Addie model to evaluate faculty development program. Issues Ideas Educ. 2018;6(1) https://doi.org/10.15415/iie.2018.61001.
5. Behar-Horenstein LS, Garvan CW, Catalanotto FA, Hudson-Vassell CN. The role of needs assessment for faculty development initiatives. J Fac Dev. 2014;28:75–86. https://api.semanticscholar.org/CorpusID:141583162.
6. Bullcock K, Jackson BR, Lee J. Engaging communities to enhance and strengthen medical education: rationale and summary of experience. World Med Health Policy (WMHP). 2014;6(2):133–48. https://doi.org/10.1002/wmh3.94.
7. CAAM-HP Standards. 2024. https://caam-hp.org/https://caam. Standards for Medicine, Sections 1–5.
8. Denoya LE. Accreditation, curriculum model, and academic audit strategies for quality improvement in higher education. In: 2005 6th International Conference on Information Technology Based Higher Education and Training, Santo Domingo, Dominican Republic; 2005. p. F2B/7–12. https://doi.org/10.1109/ITHET.2005.1560271.
9. Gagne RM, Wager WW, Golas KC, Keller JM. Principles of instructional design. 5th ed. Belmont: Wadsworth; 2005. https://doi.org/10.1002/pfi.4140440211.
10. Ghosh P, Kaur C, Yu L. Faculty resilience: the mediating roles of work engagement and affective commitment. J Hosp Tour Educ. 2024; 1–13. https://doi.org/10.1080/10963758.2436587
11. Harris J, Mishra P, Koehler M. Teachers' technological, pedagogical content knowledge and learning activity types: curriculum-based technology integration reframed. J Res Technol Educ. 2009;41(4):393–416. https://doi.org/10.1080/15391523.2009.10782536.
12. Hassan S. Commitment of medical graduates educated with and without community-based medical education towards community health care–a study from Malaysia. Educ Med J. 2013;5(4):2013. https://doi.org/10.5959/eimj.v5i4.152.
13. Hassan S, Venkateswaran SP, Nadarajah VD. Evaluation of immediate impact of faculty development programme using a pretest–post-test study design format. Innov Educ. 2021;3:1. https://doi.org/10.1186/s42862-021-00009-9.

14. Jolly BC. Faculty development for curricular implementation. In: Norman GR, et al., editors. International handbook of research in medical education. Springer international handbooks of education, vol. 7. Dordrecht: Springer; 2002. https://doi.org/10.1007/978-94-010-0462-6_35.
15. Koehler MJ, Mishra P. What happens when teachers design educational technology? The development of technological pedagogical content knowledge. J Educ Comput Res. 2005;32(2):131–52. https://doi.org/10.2190/0EW7-01WB-BKHL-QDYV.
16. Magaña-Valladares L, Penniecook T. The future of public health education: the post Covid-19 era. Salud Publica Mex. 2022;64:550–5. https://doi.org/10.21149/13949
17. Moye JN. Chapter 3: Differentiating the dimensions of the curriculum. In: Learning differentiated curriculum design in higher education. Emerald Publishing Limited; 2019. https://doi.org/10.1108/978-1-83867-114-320191006.
18. Niess ML. Investigating TPACK: knowledge growth in teaching with technology. J Educ Comput Res. 2011;44(3):299–317. https://doi.org/10.2190/EC.44.3.c.
19. Nilufer F, Gottlieb M, Löffler A, Utesch MC, Krcmar H. State-of-the-Art to Measure the TPACK Level of Trainees in Higher Education to Increase the Learnability of the Train-The-Trainer (TTT) Sessions. In: 2019 IEEE Global Engineering Education Conference (EDUCON), Dubai, UAE; 2019. p. 384–91. https://doi.org/10.1109/EDUCON.2019.8725056.
20. Nordquist J, Sundberg K, Laing A. Aligning physical learning space with the curriculum: AMEE Guide No. 107. Med Teach. 2016;38(8):755–68. https://doi.org//10.3109/0142159X.2016.1147541
21. Robinson DE, Wizer D. Universal Design for Learning and the quality matters guidelines for the design and implementation of online learning events. Int J Technol Teach Learn. 2016;12(1):17–32. https://api.semanticscholar.org/CorpusID:198322466.
22. Shafie NH, Ismail IS. Technological pedagogical content knowledge (TPACK) in teaching 21st century skills in the 21st century classroom. Asian J Univ Educ. 2019;15(3):24–33. https://doi.org/10.24191/ajue.v15i3.7818.
23. Shah V, Kumar A, Smart K. Moving forward by looking backward: embracing pedagogical principles to develop an innovative MSIS program. Journal of Information. 2018;29:139–56. https://api.semanticscholar.org/CorpusID:69822882.
24. Ventres W, Boelen C, Haq C. Time for action: key considerations for implementing social accountability in the education of health professionals. Adv Health Sci Educ. 2018;23:853–62. https://doi.org/10.1007/s10459-017-9792-z.

Leadership Competency in Futuristic Medical Education

22

Tabassum Zehra and Jacqueline Maria Dias

Key Points

- Globalization has necessitated future physicians to be prepared to lead within complex systems.
- Leadership is not static or one size fits all but is dynamic and is recognized as both an individual skill set and a collective process.
- Contemporary medical education demands that faculty become futuristic leaders.
- The growing focus on interprofessional education (IPE) and systems thinking has led healthcare leaders to rethink leadership competencies.
- The *VITAL Leadership Competency Framework for Healthcare Education* serves as a valuable guide for educators in designing leadership curricula and training programs for the modern era.

22.1 Introduction

Leadership has been interpreted in many ways in the literature. Essentially, it is the process of influencing groups to achieve common goals, drawing on interconnected skills in leadership, management, and followership. Leadership, from a social perspective, is co-constructed through dynamic interactions between leaders and followers as tasks are carried out. Although definitions vary widely, the concept remains consistent within healthcare education, rooted in personal conscience (who

T. Zehra (✉)
Medical Education and Informatics Department, College of Medicine and Health Sciences, Sultan Qaboos University, Muscat, Oman
e-mail: z.tabassum@squ.edu.om

J. M. Dias
Department of Nursing, College of Health Sciences, University of Sharjah, Sharjah, UAE
e-mail: jdias@sharjah.ac.ae

J. Sandars et al. (eds.), *Modern Medical Education*,
https://doi.org/10.1007/978-3-032-27958-3_22

I am) and self-determination (what I choose to do) and guided by values such as patience, accountability in patient care, respect for human dignity, humility, and resilience in relationships [1].

Leaders are said to possess certain abilities to shape the values of their followers. In the era of rapid technological transformation in healthcare education and changing paradigms in healthcare delivery, leadership competencies need to be relooked and redefined. The theories that evolve around the competency frameworks need to be viewed through the lens of futuristic practice of medical education, not solely relying on what is currently available [1].

Healthcare settings are changing shapes with the advent of artificial intelligence and advanced technology, especially robotics. The medical education landscape is also changing paradigms and evolving. Hence, there is a need to redefine leadership competency and the frameworks aligning to the rapidly evolving landscape.

The authors holistically investigate the evolving landscape of medical education and the need to redefine leadership competency for futuristic medical education.

22.2 Understanding Leadership Competency: Definitions and Debates

Leadership has puzzled researchers and educators in healthcare for decades. Most leadership theories and definitions stem from business settings and are then adapted to healthcare and human services. Educational leadership research has identified multiple competing definitions and approaches. One review found 23 different leadership definitions or conceptualizations in medical education alone [2, 3].

Leadership in healthcare today is no longer just the responsibility of people with formal titles or administrative authority. In the complex reality of modern clinical practice—where care depends on interprofessional teams and is centered on the needs of patients—leadership has become a skill expected of every health professional. But what exactly does "leadership competency" mean?

In today's era, one of the strongest forces reshaping how we think about leadership is the rapid rise of digital technologies, which demand new ways of guiding teams and making decisions. Over time, the idea of leadership has shifted from early trait-based models, which focused on inherent personal qualities, to more modern competency-based frameworks that emphasize skills, behaviors, and collective capacity.

This section explores the ongoing debate between individual and shared leadership and examines how medical education frameworks such as *CanMEDS* and the Accreditation Council for Graduate Medical Education (*ACGME*) have worked to define leadership competencies. Finally, it looks ahead to how these frameworks might continue to evolve in preparing future health professionals for the realities of practice.

22.2.1 Competency-Based Approaches: The KSA Model

The move toward competency-based education has changed the way we think about leadership. Instead of being seen as an abstract set of personal traits, leadership is now understood as a collection of knowledge, skills, and abilities (KSAs) that can be taught, observed, and measured. This shift reflects a larger trend in health professions education ensuring accountability, standardization, and evidence-based training are paramount [4].

In the KSA model, leadership is no longer about whether someone has the capability to perform. The emphasis lies on how they perform in real-world situations, for instance, imagine a trainee faced with a patient who is rapidly deteriorating. Their ability to call and coordinate a code blue demonstrates much more than medical expertise. It shows how well they can communicate with a diverse team, stay aware of the bigger picture, and act decisively under pressure. Those are the KSAs of leadership in action [5].

22.2.2 Relational Leadership

In the past, leadership was often seen as the job of a single person of authority. Today, the focus has undergone change. Leadership is viewed as teamwork and relationships. It is something that happens between people, in a particular situation with a common goal.

This means leadership is not always tied to hierarchy. A junior doctor speaking up to improve discharge safety and a nurse championing a quality improvement project are both clear examples of leadership in action. In healthcare—where patient outcomes depend on many disciplines working in sync—leadership often looks like building consensus, creating trust, and empowering others to contribute their best. Seeing leadership as a shared, socially constructed responsibility not only matches the reality of modern clinical practice but also ensures that influence, initiative, and innovation can come from anyone, at any level of the team [4].

22.2.3 Dynamic Relationship of Leadership and Followership

The relationship between leadership and followership in healthcare is shifting from traditional hierarchical models to dynamic, collaborative partnerships. Contemporary literature emphasizes that leaders and followers co-create interactive relationships, particularly in clinical settings. While earlier studies (1993–2010) depicted followers as largely subordinate, current perspectives position them as active contributors within interprofessional teams, where shared leadership predominates. Although healthcare education has traditionally focused on leadership, followership is increasingly recognized as essential for effective team functioning. Integrating formal followership training into curricula can equip trainees with critical communication, teamwork, and relational skills, preparing them to navigate hierarchical and collaborative dynamics [5].

22.2.4 Leadership in Medical Education Frameworks: CanMEDS and ACGME

In 2015, the CanMEDS Physician Competency Framework made a vital move, thereby replacing the role of "manager" with "leader" [6, 7]. This change reflected a recognition that leadership in healthcare is not just about managing tasks; it is about actively shaping everyday clinical practice and contributing to system-level improvements. CanMEDS highlights leadership in areas such as quality improvement, wise use of resources, and health advocacy, for example, when residents are taught to lead morbidity and mortality conferences, the goal is not only to review cases—it is to foster reflective practice and promote learning that strengthens the system.

The Accreditation Council for Graduate Medical Education (ACGME) takes a slightly different approach. Instead of treating leadership as a standalone competency, it weaves leadership development into multiple domains like professionalism, systems-based practice, and communication. In practice, this might look like a resident leading a cross-departmental initiative to reduce hospital readmission rates—drawing on teamwork, ethical reasoning, and system awareness to achieve meaningful change [7].

What both frameworks make clear is that leadership in healthcare is essential—and it is complex. Competency-based models give us useful structures for teaching and assessing leadership, but they also remind us that leadership is not static or one-size-fits-all. It is dynamic, relational, and deeply context-dependent. Preparing future health professionals, therefore, means recognizing leadership as both an individual skill set and a collective process. And it also requires approaches that are adaptable, culturally sensitive, and grounded in the realities of practice.

22.3 Emerging Trends Impacting Medical Education

Medical education is undergoing transformation with rapid advances in technology and are reshaping how we teach and learn while healthcare itself is evolving in ways that demand new approaches to preparing future professionals. Tools such as artificial intelligence (AI), virtual and augmented reality (VR/AR), and even robotics are no longer futuristic concepts—they are already changing how students gain knowledge and practice clinical skills [6].

Furthermore, traditional models are giving way to competency-based approaches that focus on what learners can do in real-world situations. The focus is on working together across professions, thinking beyond individual roles to see the bigger healthcare system, and keeping the patient's needs at the very center of everything we do ensuring evidence-based practice. Furthermore, care is digitally mediated, requiring graduates to be not only clinically skilled but also adept at navigating technology-rich environments. This section explores these emerging trends, highlighting both the opportunities and challenges they pose to learners, educators, and institutions.

22.3.1 Technological Advancements in Medical Education

New technologies like artificial intelligence (AI), augmented and virtual reality (AR/VR), and robotics are changing the way future doctors and nurses learn, practice, and are assessed, for instance, AI tools can now track how students perform in real time and suggest personalized learning plans. Intelligent tutoring systems adapt the material to a student's pace, while language-based AI can even coach learners in writing clinical notes [8].

Artificial intelligence (AI) takes learning one step further by immersing students in realistic, high-pressure clinical scenarios—without putting patients at risk [8]. A medical student can step into a virtual operating room, repeat a procedure as many times as needed, and gain confidence before ever working with a real patient. Robotics is also becoming part of the learning journey, whether through surgical simulations or demonstrations that mirror the latest clinical workflows.

In supervision, AI-powered diagnostic tools and virtual patient avatars give educators a unique window into how trainees make decisions and communicate [8]. These innovations do not just make learning more engaging; they also help standardize training, make it more widely accessible, and ensure it can be scaled to meet the growing demands of modern healthcare education.

22.3.2 Shifts in Educational Paradigms

One of the biggest changes in medical education today is the shift toward Competency-Based Medical Education (CBME). Unlike the older, time-based training models, CBME is not about how many hours a student spends in class or on the wards—it's about whether they can demonstrate the skills, attitudes, and clinical reasoning needed in real practice. This approach allows learners to progress at their own pace and ensures that when they graduate they are truly ready to meet the complex demands of modern healthcare [9].

Another important development is the growing focus on interprofessional education (IPE) and systems thinking. Healthcare today is rarely a solo effort—it is a team sport. That means students need to learn how different professionals work together and how to see patient care in the bigger context of the health system. Activities like joint simulations, shared courses across disciplines, and case studies that highlight integrated care help learners build the skills they will need to collaborate effectively once they are in practice.

Finally, the rise of patient-centered and digitally mediated care is reshaping both the curriculum and the core values of medicine. Future doctors must learn not only how to deliver compassionate care in person but also how to do so through telemedicine platforms. They will need to interpret data from wearable devices, manage digital health records, and engage with patients who are increasingly informed, empowered, and tech-savvy. The role of the physician is shifting from being the sole authority to being a partner in care—someone who co-creates health solutions with patients in a digital age [10].

22.3.3 Challenges and Opportunities

Integrating new technologies into existing curricula comes with a price. Faculty development is paramount to ensure that educators can effectively utilize digital literacy. While Competency-Based Medical Education offers personalized progression, it raises concerns about assessment reliability. Moreover, interprofessional education brings multiple challenges including structural barriers, such as misaligned schedules, institutional silos, and varied accreditation standards among health professions.

Furthermore, reliance on digital tools risks widening the digital divide among learners with unequal access to high-speed internet or advanced devices. Other challenges include ethical considerations such as data privacy and AI bias.

By embracing innovation with thoughtful pedagogy and robust governance, medical education can be more responsive, equitable, and future-oriented.

22.4 Rethinking Leadership Competency in the Future Context

The recognition of leadership as competency in medical practice has grown significantly, with competency frameworks identifying it as key to building high-quality healthcare systems. However, these competency frameworks lack strong evidence-based foundations. Lack of dedicated training programs for academic medicine leadership represents a further challenge.

Globalization has greatly influenced healthcare education, necessitating future physicians to be prepared to lead within complex systems. There is a growing emphasis in medical education on alleviating systems, policy awareness, and global health leadership. Leaders in health professions education today face unprecedented challenges that demand acquiring new levels of competencies, knowledge upgradation, unprecedented combination of skills, and managing diverse healthcare teams with changing values and relationships. Essential skills and competencies include digital skills, adaptability, emotional intelligence, strong communication, and critical thinking. Leaders in health professions education are expected to be visionary and demonstrate ethical integrity, resilience, and the capability of innovation through cross-sector collaboration and inclusive engagement. Despite recognition of these skill set, leadership in health professions education suffers from a critical lack of longitudinal assessment and skill reinforcement [9].

Established leadership theories that formed the foundation of competency frameworks are now considered inadequate for modern era realities and rapidly changing paradigms. The twenty-first-century leadership in health professions education landscape requires leaders who can comprehend emerging paradigms, apply novel strategies to bring change, adapt leadership styles according to situations, foster collective culture, have information dynamics, are knowledge-driven, and cultivate a culture of continuous learning and self-management prowess.

22.4.1 Missing Competency Areas in Current Competency Frameworks

Context-specific healthcare leadership challenges reveal the limitations of competency frameworks in addressing specialized educational environments. Researchers have discovered gaps in the literature on developing healthcare leaders who oversee longitudinal or integrated healthcare education curricula [10]. Hence, there is a need for new frameworks and shared mental models, as existing models cannot be applied effectively to address the interconnected challenges of longitudinal integrated curricula. Important areas identified as gaps in existing leadership competency frameworks in healthcare education include [9–11] the following:

- *Conscious Leadership*: Current competency frameworks fail to incorporate competencies specific to conscious leaders that are essential for modern healthcare contexts.
- *Equity, Diversity, and Inclusion (EDI) Leadership*: Healthcare education curricula lack to address EDI principles adequately. These principles should be foundational rather than peripheral. In healthcare education, leaders need to benefit from the diversity of workforce. They need to acquire competencies in intercultural sensitivity and diversity transforming systemic power structures, further demanding longitudinal assessments. Current competency frameworks fail to address this important leadership competency.
- *Digital Literacy and Adaptive Leadership*: Use of AI is changing how we need to lead healthcare organizations. Adaptive leadership is the new normal in healthcare leaders. Rapid digitalization has caused a paradigm shift, requiring leaders to continuously adapt and possess digital skills for sustainable performance. Evolution and complexity of these technological changes create unique leadership challenges that traditional models cannot address. The revolution of technology demands "a more human-centered form of leadership" capable of balancing AI with human judgment, ethical responsibility, and emotional intelligence.
- *Socially Accountable Leadership*: Social accountability has emerged as a core leadership competency for healthcare leaders to exemplify as a role model. This includes specific competencies like cultural competency, advocacy, stewardship, and professional accountability to enable leaders to address social determinants of health while maintaining ethical standards.

The literature highlights a new form of leadership characterized by the ability to balance autonomy with accountability, promote effective teamwork, and place priority on improving patient outcomes. There is a need to relook at the current competency frameworks considering the expected competencies of the twenty-first-century healthcare education leader.

22.5 Proposed Framework for Futuristic Leadership Competency in Medical

Health professions educators reported to have difficulty incorporating leadership into curricula at both undergraduate and postgraduate levels. Numerous studies published between 1991 and 2017 report that the leadership curriculum is diversified and limited in its effectiveness.

Healthcare education requires a leadership competency framework that prepares future healthcare professionals for value-based healthcare delivery through highly functioning interprofessional teams.

22.5.1 VITAL Leadership Competency Framework for Healthcare Education

The authors propose the *VITAL Leadership Competency Framework for Healthcare Education* for educators to base curricula and training programs on leadership in healthcare education. The framework is anchored in leadership competencies that are essential today, sustaining for tomorrow, and future-ready [11, 12].

22.5.1.1 Visioning (Transformative Visioning)

Definition: Transformational leaders are those who are persuasive (inspirational communicator), forward-thinking (visionary), empathetic (demonstrate emotional intelligence), supportive (provide guidance and support in personal and professional development), relational (relationship building), motivational, and adaptive to change.

Transformative leaders have a purpose and direction; they challenge status quo, encourage new ideas, and function as a change agent. With shared vision and strategy, transformative leaders and their teams are inspired and committed to a shared goal [12]. Carefully planned leadership development training programs help cultivate forward-looking (visionary) mindsets and improve strategic planning abilities in learners. Table 22.1 presents the expected behaviors and outcome.

22.5.1.2 Influence (Collaborative Influence)

Definition: Collaborative influence is defined as the ability to build trust and develop partnerships to take collective cross-disciplinary action for advancement of healthcare education and delivery [13].

Table 22.1 Expected behaviors and outcomes as transformational visionary leader

Expected behavior(s)	Expected outcome and impact
Articulates and shares clear and inspirational vision with the team	Leaders steer institutions with effective, sustainable, future-focused strategies to advance and enhance healthcare education
Analyzes opportunities and challenges in healthcare education and proposes evidence-based solutions	
Transforms leadership style with evolving trends and context	
Encourages innovation and creativity in problem-solving	
Inspires others to embrace change and adopt forward-looking strategies	

Table 22.2 Expected behaviors and outcomes as a leader with collaborative influence

Expected behavior(s)	Expected outcome and impact
Promotes respectful relationships with stakeholders	Leaders mobilize interdisciplinary teams, strengthen partnerships, and enhance the quality and impact of healthcare education
Communicates effectively, a shared vision to align team efforts toward common goals	
Uses evidence-based approach to influence decisions and motivate action	
Values diverse viewpoints and approach disagreements with a constructive attitude	
Encourages collaboration and fosters collective ownership	

The Canadian College of Health Leaders (CCHL) and the Canadian Certified Physician Executive provide "LEADS" framework as a tool for fostering the development of future health leaders and developing collaborative influence as a leadership competency. It has five main pillars: (i) lead self, (ii) engage others, (iii) achieve results, (iv) develop coalitions, and (v) system transformation. Table 22.2 presents the expected behaviors and outcomes.

22.5.1.3 Technological Agility (Digital Agility)

Definition: The capacity to leverage digital technologies, adapt to the twenty-first-century technological advancements, and integrate them effectively into educational practice [12, 13].

At the intersection of technological agility and healthcare leadership, leaders can harness and apply technological capabilities to enhance organizational performance and outcomes. This involves exploring how healthcare leaders can drive innovation,

Table 22.3 Expected behaviors and outcomes as a leader with technological agility

Expected behavior(s)	Expected outcome and impact
Demonstrates proficiency with digital tools relevant to healthcare education	Leaders enhance learning efficiency, innovation, and accessibility through the agile use of technology
Adapts and integrates new technologies to enhance learning	
Promotes a culture of digital literacy among learners and colleagues	
Evaluates innovative technology solutions to improve healthcare education outcomes	

Table 22.4 Expected behaviors and outcomes as a leader with sense of accountability

Expected behaviors	Expected outcome and impact
Upholds highest ethical standards, models integrity and trust in decision-making	As a role model, leaders foster trust, equity, and socially responsible practices in educational environments
Ensures fairness, inclusivity, and respect for diversity	
Promotes policies and practices that prioritize social responsibility	
Reflects on the impact of decisions on learners, patients, and society	

manage technological change, and cultivate a culture of adaptability to emerging technologies within their organizations. Table 22.3 presents the expected behaviors and outcomes.

22.5.1.4 Accountability (Ethical and Social)

Definition: Commitment to ethical practice, social responsibility, ensuring equity and integrity in healthcare education.

Social obligation was at the highest level of social accountability described by the World Health Organization (WHO) in 1995. According to the WHO, academic and healthcare organizations should assess the impact of expected graduate performance on community well-being and population health outcomes. These should be evaluated in alignment with principles of quality, equity, relevance, and cost-effectiveness [11]. Table 22.4 presents the expected behaviors and outcomes.

22.5.1.5 Learning Stewardship (Systems)

Definition: The capacity to manage, sustain, and improve learning systems in alignment with institutional goals and learner needs.

Stewardship is one of the key competencies in leadership alongside others. Healthcare leaders who demonstrate stewardship are more accountable. Systems-based practice is one of the required competencies and performance measures in

Table 22.5 Expected behaviors and outcomes as a leader with learning stewardship

Expected behaviors	Expected outcome and impact
Develops educational systems that support effective learning	Academic leaders ensure adaptable educational environments and systems that support self-directed lifelong learning and institutional excellence
Review, monitor, and evaluate educational programs for quality assurance	
Encourages reflection, continuous quality improvement through data-driven decision-making	
Allocates resources sensibly to optimize learning outcomes	
Mentors' faculty and learners to enhance system-based learning capabilities	

Accreditation Council for Graduate Medical Education (ACGME) competency framework for a healthcare professional [12, 13]. Table 22.5 presents the expected behaviors and outcomes.

Applying the VITAL Leadership Competency Framework can help healthcare educators design leadership competencies for healthcare professionals at undergraduate and postgraduate training programs and curricula.

22.6 Implications for Faculty Development and Policy

In today's landscape of medical education, governed by technological integration, competency-based curricula and patient-centered digital care are paramount for faculty development.

22.6.1 Faculty Development for Futuristic Leadership

Traditional faculty development focused on teaching techniques and content delivery. However, contemporary medical education demands that faculty become futuristic leaders. In this case, the individuals receiving faculty development must be technologically literate and capable of cultivating innovation, inclusivity, and interprofessional collaboration. Development programs must therefore extend beyond pedagogy and include modules on AI integration in education, digital professionalism, telemedicine supervision, interdisciplinary collaboration, and change management [12], for instance, equipping faculty with skills to interpret AI-generated learning analytics or guide students through virtual reality (VR) simulations ensures that they can effectively navigate new educational modalities while maintaining pedagogical integrity.

Another point which needs special mention is mentoring. Mentorship programs should focus on reflective leadership and peer-coaching models to facilitate faculty in developing self-awareness and adaptability [13].

22.6.2 Aligning Faculty Roles with Evolving Competency Frameworks

As medical education increasingly adopts competency-based and interprofessional models, faculty must realign roles and assessment measures. In today's world, teaching excellence is no longer limited to content mastery but is equally measured by a faculty member's ability to facilitate the development of entrustable professional activities (EPAs), critical thinking, and collaborative practice [14].

Faculty development must therefore focus on performance-based assessment, multisource feedback, coaching for competence, and narrative assessment methods. In contexts like CanMEDS and ACGME, where leadership, advocacy, and systems-based practice are recognized competencies, educators need to evaluate them in routine teaching and feedback processes.

Today's students are learning through digitally mediated care environments. It is imperative that faculty are skilled in assessing virtual clinical interactions, including telehealth and e-consult platforms.

22.6.3 Institutional and Policy-Level Enablers

Institutional commitment and policy-level support are mandatory. Faculty development activities should include strategic plans, protected time, recognition, and funding for ensuring educational leadership roles. Incentives for faculty to engage in educational innovation and scholarships are the impetus for change. Furthermore, policy frameworks at national and accreditation levels play an important role. Accrediting bodies must align expectations around faculty competencies for emerging educational technologies and pedagogies. Institutional policies that promote equity, digital infrastructure, and cross-disciplinary collaboration will ensure faculty growth.

In summary, faculty development in the era of transformative medical education is evolving and will continue to build momentum for futuristic leadership. In this way, educators can effectively lead the next generation of health professionals.

22.7 Conclusion and Future Directions

Leadership in healthcare and medical education has evolved from trait-based models of the past to competency-based and relational approaches that reflect the complexities of modern clinical environments. Frameworks such as CanMEDS and ACGME have successfully embedded leadership within professional practice, yet challenges remain in clearly defining, assessing, and sustaining leadership competencies across diverse contexts. The ongoing tension between viewing leadership as an individual skill set versus a collective, relational process highlights the need for a more integrative approach. This is the challenge which presents itself to health profession educators.

As health systems face rapid technological innovation, shifting pedagogical paradigms, and increasingly globalized challenges, leadership in medical education must adapt accordingly. Future leaders will require not only technical proficiency and clinical expertise but also digital literacy, emotional intelligence, cultural humility, and systems thinking with a profound knowledge of simulation, artificial intelligence, and virtual and augmented reality. All these elements are critical to fostering collaboration, equity, and resilience in a healthcare landscape that is more interconnected, dynamic, and ethically complex. The VITAL Leadership Competency Framework for Healthcare Education is a step to base future curricula on leadership.

Ultimately, preparing the next generation of health professionals demands leadership development that is evidence-informed, adaptable, and globally relevant. By rethinking leadership as both a shared responsibility and a personal commitment, health professions education can equip future practitioners to navigate uncertainty, inspire innovation, and shape healthcare systems that are safe, equitable, and sustainable.

References

1. Alluhaymid Y, Alalwan A, Alruwaitea A. Perspectives of family medicine residents in Riyadh on leadership training: a cross-sectional study. BMC Med Educ. 2023;23:183. https://doi.org/10.1186/s12909-023-04188-2.
2. Fennell KM. Conceptualizations of leadership and relevance to health and human service workforce development: a scoping review. J Multidiscip Healthc. 2021;14:3035–51.
3. Rodríguez-Feria P, Czabanowska K, Babich S, Rodríguez-Sánchez D, Carreño Hernández FL, Hernández Florez LJ. Defining leadership in undergraduate medical education, networks, and instructors: a scoping review. International Medical Education; 2023.
4. Murray S. Hidden in plain sight: finding a balance between assessment and learning in competency-based education in Canadian Health Care. 2023.
5. Boardman NK, Munro-Berry J, McKimm J. The leadership and followership challenges of doctors in training during the COVID-19 pandemic. Br J Hosp Med. 2021;82(2):1–9.
6. Mitchell M. Evaluation of nurses' knowledge related to early recognition of deteriorating patients; 2020. Doctoral dissertation, Grand Canyon University.
7. Bates JE. Graduate Medical education after implementation of the ACGME CLER program: perspectives of teaching hospital leaders, designated institutional officials, and GME program directors.
8. Dias JM, Halimi A, Ghorbani SS, Jarrahi AM, Al-Marzouqi A. The effectiveness of virtual simulation in knowledge of nurses: a protocol for systematic review and meta-analysis of randomized controlled trials.
9. Gustafson S, Poynter SE, Turner TL, Condus M, Waggoner-Fountain LA. Starting with the end in mind: transformative curriculum development in CBME. Curr Probl Pediatr Adolesc Health Care. 2024:101678.

10. Chan J, Man K, Dias JM. Strategies to incorporate generative artificial intelligence in simulation-based education among undergraduate students of health care professions. Clin Simul Nurs. 2025;16 https://doi.org/10.1016/j.ecns.2025.101795.
11. Genza GM. But what is leadership? A systematic review of the leadership concept in view of heightened educational leadership in Africa. J Educ Pract. 2021;
12. Huikko-Tarvainen S. Elements of perceived good physician leadership and their relation to leadership theory. Leadersh Health Serv (Bradford, England). 2021;35:14–29.
13. Botha AP, Coopasamy S. Leadership 4.0: leadership changes required in the South African petroleum industry to support the fourth industrial revolution. S Afr J Ind Eng. 2022;
14. Tolentino R, Baradaran A, Gore G, Pluye P, Abbasgholizadeh-Rahimi S. Curriculum frameworks and educational programs in AI for medical students, residents, and practicing physicians: scoping review. JMIR Med Educ. 2024;10(1):e54793.

23 The Future of Medical Education: A Medical Student Perspective

Hasan Zaidi, Hussain Zaidi, and Shane Zaidi

Key Points

- Medical education must balance digital innovation with authentic patient interaction.
- Microlearning improves retention by delivering knowledge in short bursts.
- Large language models enable interactive, personalized tutoring with rapid explanations.
- Artificial intelligence in learning supports research, assessment, and simulation but raises ethical issues.
- Flipped classroom promotes learning by shifting core content outside class, focusing on application during contact time.

23.1 Introduction

Medical education is evolving at an unprecedented pace. The traditional didactic lectures of the Flexnerian era are being reshaped by a post-COVID paradigm shift. Personalized learning is on the ascent, enabled by digital tools that harness algorithms to optimize retention and identify weaknesses in knowledge. These innovations widen access to medical education globally and may help standardize curricula, reducing dependence on local variation in teaching quality. Large language models

H. Zaidi
Imperial College, Medical and Bioengineering, London, UK

H. Zaidi
St Georges Hospital Medical School, Department of Bioengineering, Imperial College, London, UK

S. Zaidi (✉)
The Royal Marsden Hospial and ICR, London, UK

J. Sandars et al. (eds.), *Modern Medical Education*,
https://doi.org/10.1007/978-3-032-27958-3_23

(LLMs) make it possible to ask unlimited questions via Socratic-style digital dialogue, while smartphone apps support microlearning (curated knowledge in short, focused bursts available anytime, anywhere).

This chapter traces the trajectory of medical education from Flexner to COVID-19 and into the age of AI, from a students' perspective. It analyses advantages, limitations, and risks, and reflects on how technology might shape the identity and practice of the next generation of doctors.

23.2 From Flexner and Halsted to the GMC: Why the Foundations Still Matter

Abraham Flexner's 1910 report reset medical education toward lab-based science, with the introduction of rigorous standards to be upheld by university hospitals [1]. Prior to this, there were many medical schools of varying quality—Flexner decided that, to improve standards, the number of medical schools was to be decreased and the prerequisites to entry were enhanced. There was also a transition to a scientific curriculum, supported by research. Subsequent medical students embarked on an apprenticeship-based course. The Halsteadian ethos of graduated responsibility in defined residency periods, summarized as "see one, do one, teach one," became the norm [2]. These historical anchors explain the dominance of hospital placement-based learning.

Contemporary standards now broaden those foundations. The General Medical Council's Outcomes for Graduates convey the importance of nurturing patient safety, professional values, communication, health promotion and prevention, and having robust knowledge of the social determinants of health [3]. This reflects a shift from a narrow biomedical model to one that critical systematic thinking, teamwork, equity, and population health are all new competencies that digital tools can help to deliver.

Globally, variations in governance mirror this trend. The Accreditation Council for Graduate Medical Education (ACGME) in the USA has broadened competencies beyond medical knowledge into professionalism, communication, and systems-based practice [4]. Similarly, European frameworks such as the Bologna Process have sought to harmonize standards across borders. Thus, while Flexner's spirit of scientific rigour remains the bedrock, modern frameworks place equal weight on softer skills and holistic understanding.

The COVID-19 pandemic marked a transition point. As campuses closed, medical schools pivoted to virtual platforms at speed. What began as a contingency measure became the usual infrastructure: online lectures, remote assessments, virtual case discussions, and cloud-based resource banks. This has been evidenced by surveys; Dost et al. [5] reached out to 2721 UK medical students across 39 schools and found a marked rise in time spent on online platforms during the first pandemic wave. Students highlighted flexibility, self-paced study, and access as key benefits; common barriers included family distractions (26.8%) and connectivity (21.5%). Crucially, the student consensus varied in its view of online practical skills. Eighty-two percent felt online teaching could not adequately replace clinical skill development, reaffirming the centrality of direct patient contact for competence and confidence.

The broader literature similarly notes that online learning can achieve comparable knowledge outcomes to face-to-face teaching in some contexts [6]. It is also found that students appreciate online teaching as successfully implemented when educators prioritize design quality, interaction, and student support [7, 8]. The latter can be in the form of online drop-in question-and-answer calls. Details that might seem minor can actually matter more than the content itself-because when resources are not engaging, students quickly lose the motivation to learn. From a medical student perspective, we note that the most powerful advantage to asynchronous learning is the time made free to pursue co-curricular activities. The pandemic clarified two important aspects about medical education: first, medical education is no longer location-bound, second, authentic clinical exposure remains irreplaceable.

That is not to say that virtual classrooms and online resources are without their clinical advantages—flipped classrooms allow us to use physical space for thinking, not transmitting. In flipped learning, students cover foundational content asynchronously (book chapters, short videos, quizzes), prior to using Team Based Learning (TBL) live sessions for discussion, application, and feedback [9, 10]. Students come to sessions with a firm grasp of key concepts and are not disadvantaged if they miss a few seconds of a lecture. This suits what students want from their education: the "information layer" is scalable and rewindable, and limited synchronous time is reserved for clinical reasoning, problem-solving, and personalized one-to-one feedback. This is consistent with Dost et al. [5], which reports that clinical students often value synchronous tutorials for case discussion, whereas preclinical students prefer curated, concise videos to clarify concepts.

International studies reflect similar findings. A Canadian survey of 1158 medical students found that while 90% valued recorded lectures for flexibility, only 28% believed clinical competence could be adequately achieved through online methods alone [11]. In India, where bandwidth issues are common, 37% of students cited technological barriers as their primary obstacle [12]. Thus, the pandemic accelerated global experimentation but reinforced the universal indispensability of bedside learning.

The standard curriculum has also been reframed. Early clinical exposure is common in modern medical schools, with many having dedicated Early Years Clinical Experience (EYCE) modules. Exposing students to clinical environments at an early stage in their careers helps them to link their "classroom" learning with real-world practice and develop a professional identity early on, fostering a deeper understanding of patient care. Students subsequently can better understand what is expected of them professionally and are motivated when they better appreciate how their esoteric knowledge can be applied in healthcare settings. These experiences are vital to develop the interpersonal skills required to be a doctor. There is also a greater focus upon modules relating to professional values and behaviors—especially with an increase in asynchronous learning, communication skills sessions are a vital aspect of modern medical education. Supervised teaching now involves both peer-to-peer role play situations and simulated patients portrayed by dedicated actors. IQ (Intelligence Quotient) is not all that matters—we nurture our EQ (Emotional Quotient) through practising empathy and by assuming patient perspectives. These help to promote and ensure future doctors have appropriate emotional intelligence and are effective at communicating clearly and concisely to patients. These skills are examined within traditional OSCEs (Objective Structured Clinical Examinations)—one common standardized examination station concerns breaking bad news, allowing students to prepare themselves in safe, supervised settings before preparing them for the wards. Contemporary curricula reach beyond pathophysiology to include lifestyle medicine, prevention, public health, health inequalities, and systems-based practice, following GMC guidance. As the country, and its health system, face ageing populations and multimorbidity, doctors must counsel on behavior change, understand community context, and navigate multidisciplinary pathways.

Medical ethics has become an essential component of modern medical curricula, reflecting the increasingly complex moral landscape in which doctors practice. From an early stage in their medical careers, students are taught to navigate issues such as patient autonomy, consent, confidentiality, equity of access, and end-of-life care. Ethical dilemmas may be integrated into Case-Based Learning tutorials, illustrating to students that ethical reasoning is inseparable from clinical reasoning. The 2010 Marmot review [13] highlighted the social determinants of health—how the conditions in which people are born, grow, live and work can lead to health inequalities. The findings of this report are now taught in specialized public health focused modules, helping students recognize that effective healthcare requires tackling upstream social factors, and not just treating disease at the bedside. In doing so, future doctors will be more aware of the need to advocate for healthier living conditions, early intervention and public health strategies to prevent disease before it arises.

Moreover, previously ignored voices are being heard. Webinars and remote guest lectures allow world-leading public health, primary care, and global health expertise to reach students, thus giving international views a platform, irrespective of geography, increasing accessibility. Similarly, we now see lectures from people termed "human libraries" (those with lived experiences), helping future clinicians understand what patients go through.

23.3 What Is a Spiral Curriculum?

The rigid "two preclinical years followed by three clinical" split is no longer the only option. Many holistic programmes now introduce patient contact from year one, with basic and clinical sciences learned in parallel. A spiral curriculum repeatedly revisits core concepts with increasing complexity and clinical relevance, supporting cumulative learning and transfer to practice [14]. Digital platforms, especially those with adaptive quizzing tools, map well onto spirals, surfacing individual gaps and timing revisits to optimize long-term retention. Many medical schools are ensuring key concepts are revisited repeatedly throughout a course, but each time at a deeper and more complex level. Instead of covering a topic once and moving on, students build on their prior knowledge, thus linking new information to what they already know to form a mental map. In medical education, this might mean learning the basics of anatomy in early years, then revisiting the same systems later in clinical years, reinforcing knowledge into long-term memory.

Case and Problem based learning (CBL and PBL) are well-established approaches within medical education that use specific real-world patient-centred scenarios to promote active learning and the development of clinical reasoning.

Students are guided to integrate prior knowledge with new information through collaborative discussion. In PBL, students are typically presented with a case for open inquiry without pre-reading; requiring students to identify their own knowledge gaps and self-direct subsequent learning. In PBL, the facilitator acts primarily as a guide, encouraging exploration of the topic rather than directly leading the session. In contrast, CBL is often more structured with defined learning objectives, pre-reading materials and greater input from the facilitator to ensure learning objectives are covered.

Formative assessment is foundational for these models. Frequent, low-stakes opportunities known as individual or team readiness assurance tests (iRAT/tRAT) are used to reduce anxiety towards formal assessments, helping students develop their examination technique. Clinical workplace-based assessment is adjudicated through the direct observation of practical skills (DOPS), a modern rendition of the "see-one, do-one" attitude where medical students can practice on real patients, in controlled settings (after having practiced on simulated models, whether these be latex or virtual reality).

Systematic reviews confirm benefits: Strobel and van Barneveld found PBL graduates demonstrate superior long-term knowledge retention and interpersonal skills, even if short-term test scores are sometimes lower. For students, this means emerging better prepared for uncertain, multidisciplinary real-world practice.

23.4 Microlearning and the Science of Memory

Microlearning (short, focused bursts of content learning) aligns with the unpredictable rhythms of clinical training, further into our medical careers, we have less dedicated time for studying. On top of their undergraduate degrees, students must also learn how to learn efficiently—after all, medicine is a profession that requires life long learning. When we pair microlearning with spaced repetition and retrieval practice, we leverage robust cognitive psychology: spacing boosts durable learning, and testing oneself enhances retention more than re-reading. Open-source platforms like Anki make this practical and equitable, enabling community-shared decks across topics. YouTube resources have become an important supplement to formal medical education. Many students use these videos for concise, visual expectations of complex topics like anatomy, physiology, or pharmacology. Channels run by clinicians, educators, and universities provide accessible tutorials in different languages, and their rewindable, on-demand nature makes these lectures well suited to microlearning and flipped classrooms. Without universities directing them, most students have adopted active learning strategies;

spaced-repetition flashcards (Anki) and single best answer (SBA) question banks with detailed answer explanations being the two most prevalent, as these styles are recognized as evidence-based approaches to long-term knowledge retention. Anki allows students to either create their own flashcard question sets (known as decks) or download decks from older students or the internet. One commonly downloaded deck is called Anking, which is tailored towards the USMLE exam. The dissemination of knowledge has been freed from the printing press, globalized by the internet. Question banks create a learning environment that replicates common multiple-choice exams. These provide students with opportunities to apply knowledge to clinical scenarios, with detailed explanations providing immediate feedback. These methods, frequently used in conjunction with each other, are often perceived as more efficient and engaging than passive reading of textbooks. Iterative, daily retrieval combats forgetfulness and builds a strong scaffold for clinical decision making under pressure.

23.5 The Birth of Large Language Models (LLMs)

Medical students can use AI tools such as ChatGPT as a highly adaptable tutor (Indeed, one that is available 24/7, never fatigues, and adjusts explanations to the student's level of understanding, unlike textbooks, students can engage with AI tools in a Socratic dialogue, asking unlimited follow-up questions to clarify complex physiological pathways, pharmacological mechanisms or ethical dilemmas. This interactivity with a LLM transforms passive reading into an active learning process. AI can break down abstract concepts into manageable steps and even generate practice questions on demand. From a medical student perspective, this is valued during revision periods—for it is difficult to arrange personal discussions with experts outside tutorial settings. When struggling to understand a concept, one can ask an LLM to explain the idea at different spiralling levels.

23.6 Commercialization of AI in Medical Training

Private companies have picked up on what students desire. Artificial intelligence is being incorporated into new revision tools for Objective Structured Clinical Examinations (OSCEs). One novel application available in the United Kingdom is an online platform allowing students to practice information-giving stations and taking histories from a virtual interactive AI patient. These patients simulate real-life clinical encounters, providing immediate, tailored feedback on communication skills. Furthermore, students can track their progress and target specific areas for further practice. With the advent of artificial intelligence, learning is more personalized than ever.

23.7 Emerging Applications of AI for Learning and Research

Another emerging usage of AI is to summarize literature. Tools underpinned by large language models (LLMs) are capable of rapidly processing and condensing research articles, such as those indexed in online libraries such as PubMed. By generating such concise summaries, AI is making research more accessible. With such tools, literature reviews become easier to conduct, supporting evidence-based learning. These devices also allow students to expand the scope of their projects by reducing cognitive load. However, caution must be taken. Concerns remain regarding the accuracy and reliability of AI-generated summaries. Whilst AI-driven summarization has the potential to simplify the process of conducting a literature review, students must remember LLMs may fabricate information. This is often referred to as "hallucination," when AI generates plausible but false or nonsensical information. The term "hallucination" in relation to Large Language Models (LLMs) arises from the way these systems generate text. An LLM is a program that mimics the way humans produce natural language. These are trained on a large dataset to predict the most likely next word in a sequence, based on patterns they have previously encountered during their "training." They do not possess an intrinsic understanding of factual accuracy, instead relying on probabilistic associations between words and phrases. As a result, when asked to provide information, these models may produce outputs that are linguistically coherent and plausible but fabricated, factually incorrect or linked to fictional sources. Despite this, medical students increasingly turn their backs on textbooks and towards AI tools, like ChatGPT, to fulfil learning objectives. These are perceived to be less time consuming and allow students to ask follow-up questions to further clarify concepts. AI platforms offer immediate answers and explanations tailored to a student's level of understanding. There is also a risk of superficial learning with reduced long-term knowledge retention, and the potential erosion of evaluating primary sources may damage the development of key critical thinking skills. Textbooks, though less interactive, are curated by subject experts and undergo rigorous peer review, ensuring accuracy and reliability. Therefore, the common view is that medical students must not become overly reliant on AI tools. If medical students become accustomed to on-demand answers, they may struggle to tolerate uncertainty in clinical practice. AI systems are only as unbiased as the data they are trained on, meaning stereotypes or inequalities present in datasets could filter into explanations—Western data generates Western ideas. Looking into the future, the convergence of AI, virtual reality, and wearable sensors may offer immersive training that blends cognitive knowledge with psychomotor skills. Medical students may one day learn about rare cases on virtual ward rounds of AI-generated patients, yet authentic patient interaction is irreplaceable. Many ethical questions surround the application of AI. What were models trained on? Was informed consent obtained? The problems of inductive reasoning -lesser seen diagnoses risk falling under the radar. Students must hold responsibility for their machines and keep these questions in mind as the digital healthcare landscape continues to transform.

23.8 Conclusion: Preserving Medical Education

Medical education has journeyed from the rigid structures of Flexner and Halsted to a modern ecosystem shaped by pandemics, digital innovation, and artificial intelligence. The trajectory illustrates a persistent truth: while tools and methods evolve, the fundamental goal of training competent, compassionate, and critically minded doctors remains unchanged. The rise of AI, microlearning, and virtual platforms offers unprecedented opportunities for personalization, accessibility, and efficiency, yet these benefits carry risks—superficial knowledge, over-reliance on algorithms, and erosion of critical thinking. At the same time, the irreplaceable elements of bedside learning, professional identity formation, and ethical reasoning must remain at the centre of medical training.

The doctor of tomorrow must therefore embody a unique synthesis: scientifically rigorous, technologically fluent, ethically grounded, and empathetically attuned to the lived realities of patients. By harnessing innovation while safeguarding humanity, medical education can prepare a generation of physicians equipped to meet the challenges of twenty-first-century healthcare.

References

1. Flexner A. Medical education in the United States and Canada. Boston: Updyke; 1910.
2. Halsted WS. The training of the surgeon. Bull Johns Hopkins Hosp. 1904;15:267–75.
3. General Medical Council. Outcomes for graduates. London: GMC; 2018.
4. Swing SR. The ACGME outcome project: retrospective and prospective. Acad Med. 2007;82(12):1200–10.
5. Dost S, Hossain A, Shehab M, Abdelwahed A, Al-Nusair L. Perceptions of medical students towards online teaching during the COVID-19 pandemic: a national cross-sectional survey of 2,721 UK medical students. BMJ Open. 2020;10:e042378.
6. Pei L, Wu H. Does online learning work better than offline learning in undergraduate medical education? A systematic review and meta-analysis. Med Educ Online. 2019;24(1):1666538.
7. O'Doherty D, Dromey M, Lougheed J, Hannigan A, Last J, McGrath D. Barriers and solutions to online learning in medical education: an integrative review. BMC Med Educ. 2018;18:130.
8. Kay D, Pasarica M. Using technology to increase student (and faculty) satisfaction with engagement in medical education. Adv Physiol Educ. 2019;43(4):408–13.
9. Prober CG, Heath C. Lecture halls without lectures—a proposal for medical education. N Engl J Med. 2012;366(18):1657–9.
10. Bishop JL, Verleger MA. The flipped classroom: a survey of the research. In: Proceedings of the ASEE Annual Conference & Exposition, June 23–26; Atlanta, GA. Washington, DC: ASEE; 2013. Paper ID 6219.
11. Tsang KK, Latchman A, Singhal N, et al. A survey on Canadian pediatric hospital clinical/medical teaching unit implementation during the first and second wave of the COVID-19 pandemic. BMC Med Educ. 2021;21:570.
12. Singh K, Bharatha A, Sa B, Adams OP, Majumder MAA. Online learning experiences of medical students in India during COVID-19. BMC Med Educ. 2021;21:181.
13. Marmot M, Bell R. Fair society, healthy lives. Public Health. 2012;126(Suppl 1):S4–10. https://doi.org/10.1016/j.puhe.2012.05.014.
14. Harden RM, Stamper N. What is a spiral curriculum? Med Teach. 1999;21(2):141–3.

Involving Students in Decision Making 24

Bahaa Aldeen Abdulrahman Hadi

Key Points

- Partnership turns student voice into shared responsibility and timely action, improving quality, clarity, and trust across the learning environment.
- Authentic decision rights, transparent processes, and inclusive representation distinguish meaningful partnership from tokenism.
- Psychological safety, assessment literacy, and continuous quality improvement skills are teachable capabilities that enable students and staff to co-create rigorous, fair decisions.
- Programmatic assessment is a natural home for partnership, from co-blueprinting and feedback design to equity audits.
- Light-touch evaluation that combines data with narrative sustains momentum and helps meet accreditation expectations.

24.1 Introduction: From Feedback to Shared Stewardship

Imagine a third-year student on a night shift who notices a recurring handover gap that leaves interns scrambling at dawn. In a traditional school, that observation might vanish into an end-of-rotation survey. In a partnership-oriented school, the same student has a seat—and a say—on a learning environment group with the authority and support to test a solution. Within weeks, a student–faculty team pilots a checklist, examines safety and workflow data, and decides together whether to spread the change. The scene captures the promise of partnership: it makes the system more responsive while teaching the habits of collaborative clinical practice that graduates will need.

B. A. A. Hadi (✉)
Medical Education, College of Medicine, University of Kerbala, Kerbala, Iraq
e-mail: bahaa.h@uokerbala.edu.iq

J. Sandars et al. (eds.), *Modern Medical Education*,
https://doi.org/10.1007/978-3-032-27958-3_24

Across regulatory traditions, accreditation and quality assurance frameworks now expect schools to involve students meaningfully in educational decisions. These expectations are explicit in global and national standards and link to quality management, learning environment oversight, and evidence-informed improvement [1–4]. Contemporary theory explains why partnership works. When students experience real agency and belonging, motivation and engagement grow [7]. When psychological safety is deliberately cultivated, people speak up, examine data, and improve complex systems together [8]. The result is both pragmatic and principled: decisions become clearer and fairer, cultures more candid and inclusive, and learners rehearse the co-production skills modern health systems require [5, 6, 13].

24.2 Conceptual Foundations That Make Partnership Work

Partnership reframes students as colleagues in educational work, not customers. It is a move from sporadic consultation to shared problem solving with reciprocal responsibilities and benefits. Three strands of evidence help leaders design partnerships that endure:

Motivation matters. For example, Self-Determination Theory identifies autonomy, relatedness, and competence as basic needs that sustain engagement; authentic roles with clear scope and responsibility support all three needs, turning participation into learning rather than service [7].

Climate matters: psychological safety—people's shared belief that they can ask questions, challenge assumptions, and admit mistakes without fear—predicts learning behaviors and performance across teams [8]. It rarely happens by accident; it is created through explicit norms, inclusive facilitation, and predictable processes.

Method matters: continuous quality improvement, often using Plan–Do–Study–Act (PDSA) cycles, gives partnership a disciplined rhythm—clarify the aim, test a change, study outcomes and equity impacts, and decide together what to adopt, adapt, or abandon. Used well, PDSA helps small teams make timely, data-informed decisions without bureaucratic drag [9].

Assessment is a particularly fertile domain for partnership. Programmatic approaches depend on transparency, multiple low-stakes data points, and routine sense-making. Students add value by co-designing blueprints and feedback, by serving as trained item writers and reviewers with psychometric oversight, and by co-interpreting equity audits—all without compromising rigor [10–12]. More broadly, co-production in education mirrors the movement to co-produce care with patients and communities, preparing students for the realities of modern health systems [13].

24.3 Where Students Can Shape Decisions in Practice

The issue is not whether to involve students everywhere, but where their perspective and energy can genuinely shape outcomes. At the institutional level, students can contribute to strategy, curriculum and assessment governance, equity policy, and accreditation self-study. Decision rights here can include voting seats on curriculum and assessment boards, co-chair roles on learning environment groups, and named responsibilities within quality assurance activities, supported by clear terms of reference, induction, and mentorship [1–4]. At the program level, partnership often centers on curriculum mapping and sequencing, assessment blueprints, feedback policies, and admissions design. Co-design workshops and partnership microgrants help teams redesign modules, audit inclusion, and prototype new feedback models. Structured roles in standard setting or multiple mini-interview development work well when training, calibration, and conflict-of-interest protections are in place [2, 10, 11]. At the course or clinical team level, students co-author cases, co-lead PDSA projects on safety and wellbeing, and steward always-on feedback channels that surface issues early and route them to action. To make scope and influence explicit from the start, a concise charter helps teams align quickly and act predictably (Table 24.1).

What distinguishes meaningful involvement across levels is clarity of scope and influence. Effective charters specify what is on and off the table, how decisions will

Table 24.1 Student–Faculty Partnership Charter (template)

Section	Required content	Example phrasing
Purpose	Why the partnership exists	"To enable students and staff to co-produce decisions that improve educational quality, equity, and safety" [1–6, 14]
Scope of decisions	What is in and out of scope	"In scope: Assessment blueprints, feedback policy, learning environment priorities. Out of scope: Individual HR matters" [1–4, 10]
Decision rights	Authority levels	"Student members hold full voting rights; co-chairs rotate annually (one student, one faculty)" [1–6, 14]
Membership and representation	Composition, terms, inclusion	"Two students per year group; 12-month terms; stipend available; accessible meeting times" [4–7, 14]
Roles and responsibilities	Expectations for all members	"Prepare by reviewing pre-reads; declare conflicts; uphold confidentiality; model respectful dialogue" [2–4, 8]
Psychological safety norms	Ground rules	"One mic, many voices; disagree with ideas, not people; clarify next steps" [8, 14]
Data use and stewardship	Access and ethics	"Role-based access; anonymize datasets; student co-analysts trained in data ethics" [2–4]
Meeting cadence and quorum	Timing and quorum	"Monthly meetings (90 min). Quorum: ≥60% members including ≥1 student co-chair" [1–4]
Escalation and appeals	How items escalate	"Unresolved items escalate to the Education Board within two weeks; written rationale provided" [1–4]
Feedback loops	Transparency mechanisms	"'You said, we did' log updated monthly; public decision diary with reasons and data" [4, 9, 14]
Recognition and compensation	Pay/credit	"Student co-chairs: stipend; members: micro-credential and authorship where appropriate" [5–7, 14]
Review cycle	How the charter evolves	"Biannual review in a joint workshop; revisions by simple majority" [4, 9, 14]

be reached, what data will inform deliberation, and how rationales will be communicated. Transparency is not a courtesy; it is the antidote to tokenism. Publishing decision diaries, maintaining "you said, we did" logs, and closing feedback loops consistently help people see the pathway from input to change [1–4, 14]. Without such clarity, even well-meaning structures drift toward symbolism.

24.4 Making Decisions That Are Fair, Timely, and Data-Informed

Fairness and timeliness come from design, not good intentions. Committees that work well have explicit mandates, balanced membership with real student decision rights, quorum rules that protect representation, and clear approaches to consensus with timeboxed fallbacks to a vote when needed. They put data on the table early and often: outcomes and psychometrics for assessment, learning environment indicators and climate scores for wellbeing, and equity audits that examine differential attainment and access. They also record why decisions were made, not just what was decided, so that future members can learn from trade-offs rather than relitigate them [1–4, 8, 10–12, 14]. A brief Terms of Reference checklist keeps these basics visible and repeatable in daily work (Table 24.2).

The PDSA method helps teams match their pace to the stakes of the decision. Small, low-risk changes can be tested quickly and adjusted, while larger, more

Table 24.2 Committee Terms of Reference checklist for student decision rights

Domain	Questions to specify	Example text
Mandate	What outcomes is the committee accountable for?	"Accountable for ensuring fair, coherent, and transparent assessment across the program" [1–4, 10]
Authority	Which decisions are final here?	"May approve exam blueprints, rubrics, and feedback timelines" [1–4, 10]
Membership	Who sits on the committee and why?	"Four faculty, four students (voting), one psychometrician, one administrator" [1–6, 10, 14]
Selection	How are student members recruited and supported?	"Open call; brief statement of interest; orientation and mentorship provided" [5–7, 14]
Decision-making	How are decisions reached?	"Modified consensus with fallback to majority vote; co-chairs announce rationale" [1–4, 14]
Quorum	What constitutes quorum?	"≥60% members present, including at least two students" [1–4]
Conflict of interest	How are COIs managed?	"Declare COIs at item start; recusal recorded in minutes" [2–4]
Data for deliberation	What data inform decisions?	"Item stats, equity audits, climate surveys; data pack distributed one week prior" [4, 8, 10, 14]
Timelines	How are timelines safeguarded?	"Time-boxed decisions; fast lane with retrospective review in 30 days" [4, 9, 14]
Transparency	How is rationale shared?	"Decision diary published with options considered and reasons chosen" [4, 14]

Table 24.3 Capability-building map for student and staff partners

Area	Minimum transparency standard	Evidence/artifacts	Owner	Review cycle
Blueprint access	Students can view scope and weighting	Posted blueprint; briefing slides	Assessment office	Each term [10]
Standards	How passing standards are set and reviewed	Standard-setting report; student brief	Psychometrician	Each major assessment [10, 11]
Feedback	What feedback is given and when	Rubrics; turnaround SLA; exemplars	Course lead	Each assessment [10–12]
Appeals	Clear, timely, fair process	Appeals flowchart; timelines	Registrar	Annual [1–4]
Data use	What data are collected and how used	Data inventory; consent statement	QA lead	Annual [2–4]
Equity	Routine equity audit and mitigations	Audit summary; action log	EDI lead	Biannual [4, 14]

consequential changes receive more careful study before being scaled. Small tests of change allow student–faculty teams to learn quickly and adjust before scaling. The Study step examines not only whether a change worked but for whom it worked, checking for unintended inequities before spread. Many schools also predefine fast lanes for urgent issues with retrospective review, a practical compromise that preserves momentum without sacrificing oversight [9]. Where assessment decisions are involved, predictable transparency standards help students and staff orient to processes and timelines before tensions rise, which strengthens both trust and performance (Table 24.3).

24.5 Preparing Students and Staff for Partnership

Partnership rises or falls on preparation. Students benefit from orientation to governance basics, including how to read a terms of reference, how agendas and quorum rules shape influence, and what voting and escalation mean in practice. Assessment literacy matters: understanding blueprints, standard setting, and item statistics equips students to contribute substantively rather than symbolically. Continuous Quality Improvement (CQI) skills make contribution practical—writing a clear aim statement, choosing measures that matter, and analyzing simple run charts. A foundation in equity and bias is essential for effective student participation, especially when students gain access to sensitive institutional information [2, 4, 7]. Implementing clear boundaries is crucial for having access to sensitive information, such as, anonymization of data sets and statements of conflict of interests. Targeted preparation on governance, assessment, CQI, equity, and facilitation can be mapped and delivered efficiently to students and staff together so they grow a shared language and toolkit (Table 24.4).

The active inclusion of a diverse student population is usually made compulsory through diversity, equity and inclusion (DEI) guidance, but needs to be carefully implemented to ensure it does not inadvertently favor already privileged groups [4, 10, 14]. Another foundation is data ethics and stewardship, especially when students participate in management since they may have access to confidential data related to entry and progression but also decisions on personnel. As programs adopt learning analytics, the difference between helpful illumination and harmful surveillance often lies in how decisions are made. Co designing analytics policies with students keeps consent, purpose limitation, and proportionality in view. Students can advise on which metrics are meaningful, which are likely to be misinterpreted, and how to present progress without labeling or ranking individuals. Publishing a data inventory, access rules, and a plain language statement of purposes builds trust. Shared interpretation sessions—brief, scheduled, and psychologically safe—can turn dashboards into learning tools rather than compliance screens [4, 14]. The same partnership habits that improve curricula and assessment can make analytics ethical and useful.

Faculty and professional staff need development, too. Moving from representation to co-production is a pedagogical shift. It requires inclusive facilitation that invites divergent views while protecting people, comfort with transparency in programmatic assessment, and habits of sharing data early and interpreting it with students, not for them. Mentorship pairings and communities of practice help both groups learn alongside one another, and stipends or workload credit signal that the work is valued, integral contribution, not an extracurricular activity [5, 6, 8, 10–12, 14]. A practical way to start is to pair each student partner with an experienced faculty mentor and a concrete role. For example, a student on the assessment board might present a short analysis of item performance and alignment at each meeting, coached by a psychometrician [10, 11]. A student co-chair on the learning environment group might lead the monthly review of speaking-up data, supported by a faculty wellbeing lead who can act on patterns [3, 8]. Such anchoring tasks turn enthusiasm into repeatable contributions.

Table 24.4 Programmatic assessment transparency policy checklist

Audience	Competency	Learning objectives	Delivery	Duration	Evidence of completion
Students	Governance literacy	Explain TORs, quorums, voting, escalation	Interactive workshop + primer	2 h	Short quiz; participation [1–4, 14]
Students	Assessment literacy	Interpret blueprints, standard setting, item stats	Case-based session + sandbox	3 h	Reviewed sample items [10–12]
Students	CQI/PDSA	Draft aims and measures; read run charts	Hands-on lab	2 h	PDSA plan submission [9]
Students	Equity and bias	Apply an Equity Impact Assessment	Scenario + rubric	2 h	EIA worksheet [4, 14]
Faculty	Partnership pedagogy	Move from representation to co-production	Seminar + reflection	2 h	Reflective memo [5, 6, 14]
Faculty	Inclusive facilitation	Run meetings that support psychological safety	Practice with feedback	2 h	Observed facilitation [8, 14]
Both	Data ethics/ stewardship	Use anonymization and role-based access	Microlearning + checklist	1 h	Signed checklist [2–4]
Both	Consensus skills	Use NGT/Delphi appropriately	Simulation	1.5 h	Facilitator sign-off [1–4, 14]

24.6 Common Concerns and How to Respond

Colleagues sometimes ask whether student participation will dilute academic standards. Experience from programmatic assessment suggests the opposite. When students help blueprint assessments and co-create feedback processes, perceived alignment and fairness improve, appeals decline, and item performance can strengthen because relevance is checked in real time [10–12]. There are also concerns about confidentiality, especially around admissions or personnel decisions. These concerns can be addressed by defining clear boundaries and training rather than exclude students. Role-based access, anonymized data, conflict-of-interest declarations, and clear withdrawal procedures protect individuals while preserving the benefits of broader scrutiny [2–4]. Speed is another concern. Groups can be slow, but a small, well-focused team with a PDSA approach is often faster than traditional top-down cycles because solutions are more feasible and buy-in is built along the way [9]. Finally, there is a lot of concern that the partnership strains professional boundaries. For example, a student partner is not to make decisions about the professional character of a classmate, but as partner in reviewing and ensuring that there is justice in the assessment of the classmate. This distinction can be maintained by defining clear boundaries from the beginning. The effective partnership depends on clear charters specifying what is "on the table and closed" and strong conflict of interest declarations [2–4]. Joint training on the basics of governance supports both students and staff to navigate these challenges. Finally, it is important to remember that the partnership is about making the education system fair, explicit and more responsible for all [5, 6, 14].

A related challenge is to navigate the socio-cultural hierarchies found in traditional educational medicine, which can suppress the student's voice. Intentional design is required to overcome the dynamics of this challenge. The most important element is the cultivation of psychological safety—which is a shared belief that it is safe to speak without fear [8]. It can be achieved through several basic rules and inclusive actions, such as when the chair deliberately "invites quiet voices" to ensure all views are heard and considered. This work should be supported by structural changes, transparent recruitment of students and flexible planning and compensation levels, to ensure that participation is not limited to the most privileged [4, 10, 14].

24.7 Building a Culture That Sustains Partnership

Structures matter, but culture carries partnership forward. Culture is modeled in how chairs run meetings, how dissent is treated, and whether justification for decisions is shared publicly. A chair who starts by stating the purpose, invites quieter voices first, asks for data before opinions, and ends with a clear decision and a plan to revisit the decision is essential for teaching partnerships [8]. Recognition systems reinforce the message. For example, faculty promotion criteria can reward educational leadership and partnership expertise, and student transcripts or portfolios can record meaningful governance roles and CQI projects. These signals are integral to the hidden curriculum [5, 6, 14]. Language is another lever. Saying "our assessment system," asking "what would make this safer to try next month?," and closing with "what will we learn if we do this?" nudges teams toward shared ownership and learning.

24.8 Equity-First Design in Everyday Decisions

Equity should be designed from the outset. A wider range of students can be invited into roles through transparent recruitment, flexible scheduling, and compensation for substantial contributions. Equity questions can be asked of every major decision: Who benefits? Who bears the cost? What patterns in attainment or access might shift? What mitigations can we add now to avoid predictable harms? A brief Equity Impact Assessment worksheet can become routine and co-completed by student and faculty partners, and helps normalize this habit (Table 24.5). Over time, as equity audits are repeated, the conversation shifts from one-off accommodations to systemic design [4, 10, 14]. Admissions is a sensitive domain where careful partnership can align values and practice. Students can co-author multiple mini-interview prompts that probe teamwork, integrity, and openness to feedback and can serve as trained assessors in defined stations with calibration and explicit rejection procedures. Some schools report improved inter-rater reliability and stronger early professionalism ratings after such changes, coupled with routine equity and bias audits co-led by students [2]. Equity audits for assessment should be based on psychometric discussions and shared evidence, not seniority [1–4, 8, 10–12, 14].

Table 24.5 Equity Impact Assessment worksheet

Barrier to equity	Equity-centered strategy	Measured outcomes
Socioeconomic disparity	Financial stipends for student representatives, flexible scheduling, remote participation options	Participation rates from low-income backgrounds
Cultural and linguistic barriers	Translation services, cultural liaison roles, inclusive meeting practices	Participation rates across cultural backgrounds
Academic performance bias	Competency-based rather than grade-based selection	Portfolio assessment, peer nomination, skills-based evaluation; academic diversity among representatives
Disability accommodation	Universal design principles	Accessible meeting formats, assistive technology, flexible participation modes; full participation across disability status

24.9 Measuring What Matters Without Creating Heavy Bureaucracy

Evaluation does not need to be elaborate to be useful. A light-touch dashboard that combines simple run charts for a few indicators with a short monthly narrative can keep partnership on track without reporting fatigue. Process indicators might include representation and retention on committees and a brief psychological safety check. Output indicators might track the adoption of co-created policies or feedback tools. Outcomes might look at speaking-up rates, feedback timeliness, or perceived assessment transparency. Equity is best tracked as a routine selection of major indicators by cohort or background, with attention to both gaps and improvement over time [1–4, 8, 10–12, 15]. Narrative has a place alongside numbers. Short, structured reflections from student and faculty partners—what we tried, what we learned, what we will do differently—help others see the work from the inside and spread practical wisdom.

24.10 Implementation, One Disciplined Step at a Time

Schools that sustain partnership tend to start small and build the partnership before they scale. Begin with listening and mapping to identify existing structures, where students already sit, what influence they have, and where bottlenecks exist. Co-create a short partnership charter that clarifies purpose, scope, and decision rights (Table 24.1), and publish a visible "you said, we are doing" log to build trust through small wins. Next, build capability and run one or two pilots in high-yield areas such as a co-blueprinting cycle for a major assessment, a co-design workshop to improve a module or placement, or a learning environment huddle that pairs rapid-response commitments with a public decision diary. Provide induction for all partners and pair students with mentors who can open doors and debrief after challenging interactions. Finally, evaluate, refine, and spread. Review indicators together, adjust terms and supports, extend student decision rights to additional committees, and embed partnership metrics into existing quality dashboards and annual reports. Keep the momentum modest and predictable; reliability builds culture [1–4, 9–12, 15].

24.11 Conclusion

When students help shape the systems that shape them, everyone benefits. Partnership makes education clearer, fairer, safer, and quicker to improve. It also grows the kind of professionals our health systems need: collaborative, reflective, ethical, and ready to co-produce solutions with others. Start where you are, be transparent about constraints, invest in capability and trust, and make partnership a habit rather than an event.

References

1. World Federation for Medical Education. WFME global standards for quality improvement: basic medical education. Copenhagen: WFME; 2020.
2. Liaison Committee on Medical Education. Functions and structure of a medical school: standards for accreditation of medical education programs leading to the MD degree. Washington, DC: AAMC and AMA; 2023.
3. General Medical Council. Promoting excellence: standards for medical education and training. London: GMC; 2015.
4. European Association for Quality Assurance in Higher Education. Standards and guidelines for quality assurance in the European Higher Education Area (ESG). Brussels: ENQA; 2015.
5. Matthews KE. Five propositions for genuine students as partners practice. Int J Stud Partners. 2017;1(2):1–9.
6. Bovill C. Co-creating learning and teaching: towards relational pedagogy in higher education. London: UCL Press; 2020.
7. Ryan RM, Deci EL. Self-determination theory: basic psychological needs in motivation, development, and wellness. New York: Guilford Press; 2017.
8. Frazier ML, Fainshmidt S, Klinger RL, Pezeshkan A, Vracheva V. Psychological safety: a meta-analytic review and extension. Pers Psychol. 2017;70(1):113–65.
9. Reed JE, Card AJ. The problem with plan-do-study-act cycles. BMJ Qual Saf. 2016;25(3):147–52.
10. Heeneman S, Oudkerk Pool A, Schuwirth LWT, van der Vleuten CPM, Driessen EW. The impact of programmatic assessment on student learning: theory, practice and implications for medical education. Med Teach. 2015;37(7):695–702.
11. Norcini J, Anderson MB, Bollela V, Burch V, Costa MJ, Duvivier R, et al. 2018 consensus framework for good assessment. Med Teach. 2018;40(11):1102–9.
12. Double KS, McGrane JA, Hopfenbeck TN. The impact of peer assessment on academic performance: a meta-analysis of controlled studies. Educ Psychol Rev. 2020;32(2):481–509.
13. Batalden M, Batalden P, Margolis P, Seid M, Armstrong G, Opipari-Arrigan L, et al. Coproduction of healthcare service. BMJ Qual Saf. 2016;25(7):509–17.
14. Sclater N. Learning analytics explained. New York: Routledge; 2017.
15. Kirkpatrick JD, Kirkpatrick WK. Kirkpatrick's four levels of training evaluation. Alexandria: ATD Press; 2016.

Entrepreneurial Mindsets in Medical Education: Empowering Future Physicians

25

Rafia Minhas and Noor-i-Kiran Naeem

Key Points

- Physicians with entrepreneurial mindset are prepared to innovate and lead in uncertain healthcare contexts.
- Core traits of this mindset include; opportunity recognition, creativity, resilience, and adaptability.
- Global models emphasize context-specific innovations.
- Strategies of experiential learning, interdisciplinary collaboration, design thinking, mentorship and reflection are effective in nurturing this mindset.
- Barriers in implementation of the mindset should be overcome to ensure sustainable and equitable healthcare innovation.

25.1 Introduction

As healthcare evolves, the roles of physicians have diversified tremendously. In addition to patient care, the physician of today needs to be innovative, adaptive and lead in the face of uncertainty. Entrepreneurship is redefining healthcare rapidly. It provides an opportunity to innovate, create value and solve problems. A physician with an entrepreneurial mindset identifies opportunities in systems and creatively solve problems, thereby improving patient care and health outcomes. This mindset is essential to keep the healthcare system sustainable and adaptive. Entrepreneurship in the health industry focuses on improving the care-delivery, health services and healthcare-products. The vulnerabilities of healthcare systems can be addressed by

R. Minhas (✉)
Department of Medical Education, Central Park Medical College, Lahore, Pakistan

N.i.K. Naeem (✉)
Department of Medical Education, ABWA Medical College, Faisalabad, Pakistan

J. Sanders et al. (eds.), *Modern Medical Education*,
https://doi.org/10.1007/978-3-032-27958-3_25

entrepreneurial initiatives [1]. Bridging entrepreneurship in medical education aims to help solve the challenges faced by the healthcare and facilitate its evolution.

25.2 Defining Entrepreneurial Mindset in Medicine

Entrepreneurship is the capability to recognize an opportunity, be innovative, and proactively take actions for improvement. It is embedded in the concept of thinking out of the box to create value. Its success is directly proportional to the mindset of the individual. An entrepreneurial mindset manifests itself through risk taking, innovation and creativity. It is not the pursuit of commercial benefits, rather, it is the cognitive ability to reframe the situations so that challenges become opportunities for growth, innovation and problem solving [2]. Decision making improves, when failures and problems are seen as learning opportunities instead of an end point [3]. An entrepreneurial mindset is a growth oriented outlook. It enables an individual to respond to uncertainty. It is depicted by the internal locus of control and tolerance for ambiguity. It influences not only the way of thinking, but also shapes the behavior of an individual to become resilient proactive and confident [4].

In healthcare, entrepreneurship responds to the call to create cost effective and sustainable solutions in resource limited and ambiguous situations. Entrepreneurial skills can be developed through experiential learning. A systematic approach is effective in cultivating this mindset in healthcare professionals [5]. Individuals who push boundaries, deviate from the traditional norms, and challenge the orthodox thinking, are the ones who can solve the healthcare problems in future. This process of creative destruction, is a key element in taking the healthcare industry forward. It paves new pathways for physicians to lead and innovate the healthcare profession [6].

If physicians fail to develop an entrepreneurial mindset, patient care will be compromised. Rather than leading the healthcare system, they will fall prey to it and rely on external factors to innovate and solve their problems. Cultivating an entrepreneurial mindset in medical professionals, gives them the power to identify the weaknesses and capitalize upon the opportunities within their systems. During this entire process, professional ethics and patient needs remain the core elements; never to be compromised.

Entrepreneurial mindset in medicine, therefore, is not an elective, but a core professional competency. It equips our future generations to be the catalysts of change and innovation for better health outcomes.

25.3 Traits and Competencies of the Entrepreneurial Mindset

Entrepreneurial mindset is a set of qualities that are diverse in nature. It ranges from optimism, internal locus of control and resilience to tolerance for ambiguity and sense of humor regarding oneself. It is the adaptive thinking, how one perceives success, difficulty, and failure [4]. It urges healthcare professional to bring a change in the system for its betterment.

The European Commission has developed an Entrepreneurship Competence Framework, which identifies the domains representing the entrepreneurial mindset [7] These include communication, collaboration, critical thinking, opportunity recognition, adaptability, problem-solving, taking initiatives, self-reliance, innovation and creativity, risk management, and future orientation, to name a few. For medical students, these domains translate into professional behaviors such as leading multidisciplinary teams, anticipating health care needs, and applying innovative approaches to clinical practice.

Among the above-mentioned traits, the most central trait is opportunity recognition, which involves the ability to detect unmet health care needs and envision new ways of addressing them. Research shows that this skill is directly linked to prior knowledge, information processing, pattern recognition, and alertness. It has been postulated that these cognitive and soft skills can be acquired and polished through education [8].

Creativity is one of the important traits of an entrepreneurial mindset, as it helps the individual develop new ideas and recombine existing resources in new ways. In medicine, creativity drives advances in diagnostic technologies, digital health tools, and patient centered care models. By encouraging students to "think outside the box." Medical teachers can nurture this innovative problem-solving in their students in research and educational contexts alike.

Cognitive adaptability is a skill that enables a physician to adjust in uncertain clinical environments. It is demonstrated in the students by being flexible, proactive, and self-regulating in their thought processes in a given uncertain environment. This lays the foundation of an entrepreneurial mindset and enables the physicians to tolerate ambiguity without compromising their decision-making process.

It is interesting to note that the traits of entrepreneurial mindset are not alien to the medical profession. They are related to the international guidelines of healthcare. The CanMEDS framework advocates the physician to act as a "Leader." This role requires the doctor to address the complexity of systems, lead change, and demonstrate systems thinking. These skills are also an integral part of entrepreneurial mindset. In the USA, the Accreditation Council for Graduate Medical Education (ACGME) defines the core competencies for its physicians. The ACGME competencies of communication skills, leadership, problem-based learning, and improvement align with entrepreneurial mindset.

25.4 Global Trends in Innovation and Entrepreneurship Education

Healthcare entrepreneurship is an interdisciplinary area, where medicine, innovation, economics, entrepreneurship, and even management come into play. This creates opportunities for knowledge transfer and synergies. The Bio design program, of Stanford University, in USA, has a multidisciplinary curriculum that aims to train leaders in healthcare innovation. [9]. It focuses on teamwork, networking, and critical thinking. Learning from each other is a key element of this project. Stanford University, also provides training to global audience through its "Global Faculty in Training" program. This enables the learners to apply their skills in local contexts and be the catalysts of change.

In Europe, the European Institute of Innovation and Technology (EIT) has established itself as a significant innovation community. Its sub-community EIT Health, focuses on healthcare delivery, public awareness and disease prevention. It aims to harness the entrepreneurial capacity of the region to benefit local healthcare. This platform provides boot camps and short courses in addition to a structured master's program [10].

Low- and middle-income countries (LMICs), including low-income regions, like Africa and Latin America, are also benefiting from health entrepreneurship education. The primary focus in these contexts is to design sustainable and affordable solutions that are workable in the local contexts. This approach integrates with the concepts of social entrepreneurship, a basic model of healthcare industry. Within LMICs, an entrepreneurial mindset enables students and professionals to solve their healthcare problems creatively. An example is the innovation hubs in Makerere University, Uganda where medical students are encouraged to co-create low-cost health solutions for local communities. A similar program in Latin America facilitates the development of frugal innovation—solutions which are not only contextually relevant, but are also affordable for the resource constrained nations. Such initiatives highlight the adaptable nature of entrepreneurial education that can be contextualized across the diverse socio-economic landscape.

Various significant themes emerge from these global initiatives. First, interdisciplinary and project-based learning activities creates a learning environment where entrepreneurship education in medicine thrives. Secondly, collaborations with external stakeholders (investors, policymakers, and communities) are crucial for transforming the innovative ideas into practice. Providing authentic and supportive learning opportunities, like, hackathons, simulations, and, incubators bridge the gap between theory and its application. Role models shape the entrepreneurial confidence and resilience of their mentees. Therefore, numerous mentorship opportunities are provided to the learners throughout their learning process.

25.5 Impact on Medical Practice and Education

When healthcare students are exposed to entrepreneurship during their medical curriculum, an unexpected outcome is observed. These physicians embrace creativity as part of their professional identity. They tolerate ambiguity and think systematically. This integration transforms their medical practice. It changes their way of thinking, methods of leading their organizations and decision making. They become critical thinkers: adaptive and resilient. They can now create cost effective solutions for their local issues. An example of this is Dr. Devi Shetty, a cardiac surgeon in India who designed low-budget cardiac care model. This model provides easy access to surgery in under-resourced regions. It underpins the role of creativity and innovation in face of challenge.

Entrepreneurial mindsets empower the physicians to improve the healthcare systems. They can identify gaps and rise up to solve the challenge. They are resilient, confident, and creative to design sustainable solutions. They learn from cross-disciplinary interactions to solve their own issues. A relevant example is of Dr. Atul Gawande, who developed surgical safety checklists on the concepts of aviation industry. This initiative has reformed healthcare delivery. This mindset in medical students enables them to become leaders of change and competent physicians, both at the same time.

Digital innovation, telemedicine, and artificial intelligence is a domain that is rapidly revolutionizing the healthcare. Entrepreneurial mindset can make the best of the opportunities these platforms provide. This can not only revolutionize the practice model of clinical medicine but also create new opportunities for growth. An example of this is Dr. Eric Topol, a cardiologist and digital health expert, who has integrated AI, genomics, and wearable technologies for improved healthcare.

Finally, an entrepreneurial mindset enhances the research and innovation capacity of physicians. Clinicians who approach problems with this mindset are more likely to translate research into practice, develop medical devices, and collaborate with industry to scale their innovations. A Malaysian study reports that medical students demonstrate the same entrepreneurial motivation as shown by their peers from other non-medical fields [11]. One may feel that medicine is very different from entrepreneurship, but a detailed analysis demonstrates that both share many common themes like communication skills, critical thinking, resilience, and problem solving.

The entrepreneurial mindset, therefore, augments the medical profession. It does not steer the learners away from patient care. Instead, it empowers them to bring change and cater to the evolving demands of the healthcare industry.

25.6 Role of Institutions in Nurturing Entrepreneurial Thinking

Higher education institutions (HEIs) are the essential ecosystems where medical students can nurture their entrepreneurial mindsets. These centers of knowledge, provide their students, safe platforms for experimenting with creativity and innovation. The students, develop leadership skills, and translate their ideas into action. An institutional culture, that allows creativity, flexibility, and problem-solving, fosters entrepreneurial thinking among its learners [12].

Institutes can act as "entrepreneurial ecosystems" by providing a conducive environment that delivers entrepreneurship education to their learners. A successful entrepreneur inspires, guides and mentors these students; the institutional policies provide support, and designated departments ensure collaboration between external funders and real-world stakeholders.

Cross-disciplinary culture provides diverse learning opportunities, in the form of simulations, clubs, hackathons and business plan competitions. These events promote creativity and collaboration, essential for an entrepreneurial mindset. As a result, the entrepreneurial awareness increases and the students are able to transition an idea from its conception to the final stages of its practical implementation. These clubs, simulations and hackathons, improve the students' opportunity recognition ability and self-confidence in pursuing innovation.

Faculty development has a crucial role in cultivating entrepreneurial mindset. They need to be trained in reflective practices, design thinking and innovative pedagogy, to efficiently train students. Without a well-trained faculty, entrepreneurial education will be a superficial and elective component of the curriculum instead of being integrated into the main program. Therefore, lack of faculty training and rigid curricula are the major barriers to cultivating entrepreneurial mindset.

There are many challenges in aligning the institutional priorities with entrepreneurial goals. Medical schools normally prioritize traditional academic outcomes (publications, board exam performance) over innovation. Resource constraints (especially in LMICs) can limit access to mentorship, funding, and infrastructure. Cultural resistance is another major issue, where faculty perceives entrepreneurship as a business model instead of an innovation opportunity.

HEIs, however, can purposely embed entrepreneurial education into their curricula through leadership commitment, policy support, and by providing dedicated centers. Thus, they equip their students with entrepreneurial competencies and strengthen their own significance in addressing both local and global healthcare challenges.

25.7 Evidence-Based Educational Strategies

Fostering an entrepreneurial mindset in medical education calls for intentional strategies that blend theory with practice [13]. Contrary to the traditional didactic methods, entrepreneurial learning is inherently experiential. It requires the students to experiment different ideas, navigate ambiguity, and reflect on the outcomes. Evidence advocates that active, integrated, and contextually relevant pedagogical methods are essential for cultivating entrepreneurial competencies.

One widely applied approach is project-based learning, where students work on real-world problems in teams. Such projects enable learners to apply theoretical knowledge to practical challenges, enhancing creativity, problem solving, and resilience. For example, medical students in innovation tracks in U.S. Universities have designed low-cost devices and community health interventions as a part of their capstone projects.

Interdisciplinary collaboration is another proven strategy. By working alongside engineers, business students, and data scientists, medical learners gain exposure to diverse perspectives and skillsets. Studies show that interdisciplinary teamwork significantly improve opportunity recognition, systems thinking, and leadership skills.

Design thinking (human centered approach to innovation) is increasingly integrated into medical curricula. It emphasizes empathy, interactive prototyping, and co-creation with patients and communities. Research in medical education demonstrates that design thinking enhances students' tolerance for ambiguity and their ability to generate novel solutions to clinical problems.

Mentorship and role modeling are equally critical. Bandura's social cognitive theory explains how observing entrepreneurial role models builds learners' self-efficacy, shaping their beliefs about what they can achieve [14]. Mentorship programs that pair students with physician-innovators or healthcare programs that pair students with physician innovators or healthcare entrepreneurs have been shown to increase persistence, risk tolerance, and career aspiration in innovation pathways [15].

Reflective practice ensures that students frame failures not as setbacks but as learning opportunities. By incorporating structured reflection into innovation projects (through journaling, peer feedback, or debrief sessions), learners can develop metacognition, resilience, and adaptability. Reflection thus consolidates both the cognitive and emotional aspects of entrepreneurial growth.

Finally, extracurricular opportunities such as entrepreneurship clubs, hackathons, and innovation competitions provide informal yet powerful contexts for learning. A Chinese study showed that students who participated in entrepreneurship clubs, and pitch competitions report significant entrepreneurial awareness and intention compared to peers who only engaged in classroom-based training [8].

Together, these strategies underscore the importance of pedagogical alignment (aligning learners' needs, entrepreneurial outcomes, and instructional methods) which can be seen as a summary in Table 25.1 below. The Kolb's experiential learning cycle can provide a useful model for designing such aligned learning experiences in medical entrepreneurship education.

Table 25.1 Strategies for cultivating entrepreneurial mindsets in medical education

Strategy	Description	Key outcomes
Project-based learning	Students address real-world health challenges in teams	Creativity, problem-solving, resilience
Interdisciplinary collaboration	Teams of med students + engineers + business graduates	Systems thinking, leadership, opportunity recognition
Design thinking	Human-centered innovation, prototyping, empathy mapping	Tolerance for ambiguity, innovative solutions
Mentorship and role modeling	Pairing students with physician-innovators	Self-efficacy, persistence, risk tolerance
Reflective practice	Journals, peer feedback, structured debriefs	Resilience, metacognition, adaptability
Extracurricular activities	Clubs, hackathons, competitions, and incubators	Entrepreneurial awareness, initiative, networks

25.8 Barriers, Ethical Concerns, and Future Challenges

Integrating entrepreneurial mindsets in medical education appears very promising. However, its implementation is very difficult. Curricular rigidity is a major challenge. The medical curricula are so densely packed that it hardly has any space for the innovation skillsets. The second hurdle is faculty resistance. Most educators consider it futile for medical students. Lack of funds and resources also makes the implementation challenging. The implementation process also presents many ethical threats. If the entrepreneurship education is not well crafted, it will remain fragmented from the main curriculum. This will disrupt the delicate balance healthcare entrepreneurship intends to maintain. As a result, the learners will lean towards commercialization. They shall be prioritizing profit margin over the healthcare outcomes. Therefore, it is very important that the entrepreneurial training is well designed, and contextual to serve the local communities.

As technology evolves, new challenges shall arise in future. Data privacy, digital biases, and cyber-security breach are issues that are being countered. It is therefore important to train faculty to discuss these concerns with the students. This ensures that innovation is reinforcing trust and fairness in the society.

25.9 Conclusion

The authors argue that healthcare professionals need to transcend from their role of clinician to become innovators. This can be done by integrating entrepreneurial mindset in the medical curriculum. We have elaborated how this mindset impacts the learner and discussed the impact it may have on the healthcare industry. By recognizing the obstacles beforehand, the curriculum developers can ensure a great synergy between the two domains. As AI continues to advance, entrepreneurial education must address the demand for social accountability and ethical innovation.

The action plan is clear: faculty members, curriculum designers, and policymakers need to embrace entrepreneurship not as a peripheral skill but as a core central mindset. This way, they facilitate empowering future physicians to navigate uncertainty, lead with creativity, and create sustainable solutions for complex health challenges. Entrepreneurial mindset not only prepares learners to be future-ready professionals but compels them to become transformative leaders who create responsive and equitable healthcare ecosystems.

References

1. Lim WM, Ciasullo MV, Escobar O, Kumar S. Healthcare entrepreneurship: current trends and future directions. Int J Entrep Behav Res. 2024;30(8):2130–57. https://doi.org/10.1108/IJEBR-02-2023-0197.
2. Asenge EL, Diaka HS, Soom AT. Entrepreneurial mindset and performance of small and medium scale enterprises in Makurdi Metropolis, Benue State-Nigeria. Int J Innov. 2018;6(2):124–46. Available from: https://periodicos.uninove.br/innovation/article/view/16517.

3. Zhang Z, Chun D. Becoming entrepreneurs: how immigrants developed entrepreneurial identities. Int J Entrep Behav Res. 2018;24(5):947–70. https://doi.org/10.1108/IJEBR-07-2016-0214.
4. Daspit JJ, Fox CJ, Findley SK. Entrepreneurial mindset: an integrated definition, a review of current insights, and directions for future research. J Small Bus Manag. 2023;61(1):12–44. Available from: https://www.tandfonline.com/doi/abs/10.1080/00472778.2021.1907583.
5. Suryavanshi T, Lambert S, Lal S, Chin A, Chan TM. Entrepreneurship and innovation in health sciences education: a scoping review. Med Sci Educ. 2020;30(4):1797–809. Available from: https://link.springer.com/article/10.1007/s40670-020-01050-8
6. Zhang PC, Austin Z. To succeed as health care innovators, pharmacists need to cultivate an entrepreneurial mindset. Can Pharm J/Rev des Pharm du Canada. 2023;156(3):110–1. Available from: https://scholar.google.com/scholar_url?url=https://journals.sagepub.com/doi/pdf/10.1177/17151635231164622&hl=en&sa=T&oi=ucasa&ct=ufr&ei=hlSzaNyPGvnSieoPxKLpgQ0&scisig=AAZF9b-5W7mqMSxEliW-4ooz2G2.
7. You X, Wu W. Assessing the impact of Medical Education's Innovation & Entrepreneurship Program in China. BMC Med Educ. 2024;24(1):1–19. Available from: https://bmcmededuc.biomedcentral.com/articles/10.1186/s12909-024-05467-2.
8. Cui J, Sun J, Bell R. The impact of entrepreneurship education on the entrepreneurial mindset of college students in China: the mediating role of inspiration and the role of educational attributes. Int J Manag Educ. 2021;19(1):100296. Available from: https://www.sciencedirect.com/science/article/abs/pii/S147281171830394X.
9. Chua JYX, Kan EM, Lee PP, Shorey S. Application of the Stanford Biodesign framework in healthcare innovation training and commercialization of market appropriate products: a scoping review. J Med Syst. 2024;48(1) Available from: https://pubmed.ncbi.nlm.nih.gov/38647719/.
10. Prado AM, Sánchez-Gómez JI, Casamitjana N, Espriu M, Kumar P, Ngoye B, et al. Building management and innovation capabilities for global health: a senior executive program. Front Public Health. 2023;11:1053745. Available from: https://troped.org/.
11. Kumar KA, Ferdous Azam SM, Jayaram J, Arunasalam AP, Jeppu AK, Alwi MNBM, et al. Impact of entrepreneurial personality traits on nascent entrepreneurial behaviour of medical students: implications for medical education. Eurasian J Educ Res. 2023;2023(103):1–17.
12. Jiatong W, Murad M, Bajun F, Tufail MS, Mirza F, Rafiq M. Impact of entrepreneurial education, mindset, and creativity on entrepreneurial intention: mediating role of entrepreneurial self-efficacy. Front Psychol. 2021;12:724440. Available from: www.frontiersin.org.
13. Nor AI, Mohamed FS, Barre MM, Hussein MA. The role of higher education institutions in promoting entrepreneurship development. Cogent Bus Manag. 2025;12(1):2523417. Available from: https://www.tandfonline.com/doi/pdf/10.1080/23311975.2025.2523417.
14. DeCoito I, Briona LK. Fostering an entrepreneurial mindset through project-based learning and digital technologies in STEM teacher education. In: Integrated science. Cham: Springer; 2023. p. 195–222. Available from: https://link.springer.com/chapter/10.1007/978-3-031-17816-0_9.
15. Olawale D, Spicklemire S, Sanchez J, Ricco G, Talaga P, Herzog J. Developing the entrepreneurial mindset in STEM students: integrating experiential entrepreneurship into engineering design. Int J Process Educ. 2020;11(1):41–7. Available from: https://www.ijpe.online/2020/entrepreneurial.pdf.

26 Understanding the Action Research Journey

Nirmala Rege, Sucheta Dandekar, and Farzana Mahdi

No action without research, no research without action.

–Kurt Lewin

Key Points

- Action research is a method of progressive problem solving by analyzing day-to-day realities in an organization or in community, wherein practitioners usually serve as active participants rather than researchers.
- Action research takes place in a setting where conflicting values or hierarchy coexists but is capable of bringing positive change.
- Action research is always situational, collaborative, participatory, self-evaluative, reflexive, and significant.
- There are challenges and multiple ethical issues but they can be overcome if transparency and honesty is maintained throughout the research process.
- Successful action research depends on building trust among participants, empowering them to contribute to new knowledge and create transformative, lasting changes in their practice.

26.1 Introduction

Action research originated in 1946 from the social-psychology work of Kurt Lewin, the father of modern social psychology [1]. Interest in action research continues in diverse fields such as social studies, educational science, health, psychology, organizational development, etc. even after a period of almost 75 years. Through action research, Lewin provided a practically oriented research approach to solve social problems. It stems from social science research, which is primarily qualitative research but differs from the latter in the sense that it does not solely focus on

N. Rege · S. Dandekar · F. Mahdi (✉)
Era's Lucknow Medical College and Hospital, Era University, Lucknow, India

J. Sandars et al. (eds.), *Modern Medical Education*,
https://doi.org/10.1007/978-3-032-27958-3_26

understanding social arrangements or the practice but on the specific problem in a defined context, with an aim to attain a desired solution [1]. Thus, it involves both, problem solving process (doing research) and use of solution (taking action) together. This also means that the generated knowledge from the research is validated through its immediate application in the practice. During the process, action research relies on the collection and analysis of data by the stakeholders, who decide what action needs to be taken, by reflecting on the data and the process. Thus, action research empowers the stakeholders to use critical reflection [2, 3]. The stakeholders collaborate and cooperate with the researcher to participate in the action research. The end result is improvement in their current practices with a transformative change within them.

Action research also differs from the applied research, wherein the knowledge is generated first by the researcher and then offered for use. Professional consultants are sometimes appointed to identify the problem and provide solutions in an organization. Thus they work for the stakeholders. Action research goes beyond such consultancy. In action research stakeholders become partners in creation of knowledge. However, action research may overlap or begin with the consultancy [1].

26.2 Why Action Research in Health Professions Education?

Today's healthcare system is undergoing a rapid change due to the emerging health needs. Population and individual health depend on the environment where we live, which in turn is influenced by economy and demography. With an increase in the geriatric population worldwide, there is a significant change in demography. The rate of migration to other countries has increased due to the availability of travel facilities, better job opportunities as well as other adverse conditions. This gets reflected in the disease pattern of the country to which people have migrated, e.g., the prevalence of diabetes is highest among migrants from India compared with other migrant groups in the United States. There is a shift from communicable diseases in children to non-communicable diseases (NCDs) in adults. NCDs affect young population, thereby decreasing working force and consequently affect the economy of a country [4]. In addition, newer and severe infections are creeping in and the rate at which they become epidemic or pandemic is alarming. Technological inventions, including AI and machine learning, have dominated the diagnostic and therapeutic areas. Newer therapeutic approaches are becoming available due to continuous research in the field and improved technological backup. At the same time changes in healthcare delivery are also observed- having home visits, online consultations, telemedicine etc. Needless to say, that expectations of patients have changed over the years. They expect their physician not only to be clinically competent but also to possess professionalism. There is an increased element of consumerism rather than considering the doctor-patient relationship to be altruistic. This demands that health professionals must acquire appropriate competencies along with adaptive learning abilities [5].

Health professions education (HPE) is a dynamic process and it keeps evolving by introducing responsive curricula, contextualized educational strategies, robust accreditation standards and mechanisms of change management to align with the changing scenarios [5]. While navigating these complex changes in HPE and healthcare systems, various issues or situations may emerge in educational contexts, either in educational components or settings. It is in this context that researchers can embark on an action research journey and judicially address the problem with the help of stakeholders. Hence it is essential for the health professions educators as well as practitioners to understand the nuances of action research.

26.3 Action Research Process

Action research is a cyclical process of reflection and action. It involves identification of problem, planning remedial action, its implementation and subsequent monitoring for outcomes. The major steps viz. (1) Problem identification, (2) Data collection, (3) Data analysis and (4) Action planning are undertaken by the stakeholders who participate in critical analysis of their own situation, followed by decision making.

A researcher for action research should have adequate training in action research as well as experience. The researcher plays a role in initiation of the enquiry, involves participants to take over the work and serves as a resource person throughout the process for data interpretation, offering advice or suggestions, identifying pitfalls etc. The researcher may be an external person or a group of teachers may work cooperatively without an external researcher [2]. In recent years, teachers commonly work together rather than relying on a professional researcher. All participants in the inquiry are considered as researchers [6].

Based on the willingness to invest time and efforts associated with research and change, mutual trust and motivation to improve practice, participants are included in action research. These are usually the stakeholders, e.g., faculty members, administrators, students, parents, patients or their combinations, who experience real-world problems. There may be others like administrators, university officials, sponsors, advisors, who may work at the periphery.

Researchers and participants together select problems within the educational setting or in health care systems, explore them systematically and contribute to generating new knowledge and its application to study its impact [7]. The participants contribute to selection of the problem and also help in exploring possible solutions. They collect both, quantitative and qualitative data. The qualitative element helps to address the complexity of the educational environment while quantitative element helps to observe the impact of the intervention undertaken [3].

Let us focus first on the model described by Kurt Lewin to understand the process. According to Kurt Lewin, action research has a two phase process:

1. *Diagnostic*, which stems from real world observations. The problems are investigated, analysed and hypothesis is developed and

2. *Therapeutic*, wherein a hypothesis is tested by conducting adaptive interventional studies in a real-life situation

This research involves cycles of planning, acting, observing, and reflecting. Lewin's model describes seven stages of action research [2].

- *Stage 1. Identification, evaluation and formulation of the problem*
  The problem may be an idea bothering stakeholders or something they wish to change, e.g., non-attendance by students or dissatisfaction with current T-L methods or assessment methods. The problem may be presented as perceived by the stakeholders but the real challenge may be deeper and could be uncovered later.
- *Stage 2. Fact finding*
  This requires gathering of data to get a complete description of the situation which helps to identify the real problem.
- *Stage 3. Review of literature*
  One needs to review the existing literature to gauge whether there is an already existing solution researched by someone else. Even if such a solution exists, its applicability to the current context and any existing gaps must be carefully evaluated. This process generates new insights that can guide subsequent actions to address the problem. The most tenable idea is the hypothesis.
- *Stage 4. Gather information which can serve as evidence*
  This helps in developing sufficient confidence in the hypothesis so that further action can be planned. No statistical testing is needed at this stage but it is essential to see whether the gathered information supports it. The research problem statement could undergo a revision at this stage. For example, absenteeism in class may not be due to their apathy towards a subject. The students may be prioritizing skill-lab training which they perceive as more important.
- *Stage 5. Preparation of action plan*
  This involves selection of research procedures viz. intervention planning, resources needed, data collection methods, and allocation of various tasks of the action plan. It requires discussions and negotiations with participants.
- *Stage 6. Implementation of action plan*
  Pertinent data is collected, classified, and analyzed. During this stage the tasks are monitored and feedback is given to the research team.
- *Stage 7. Interpretation of data and decision making*
  A detailed report is prepared backed by self-reflection. The project is evaluated and a decision is made to amend the action plan if the goals are not met with. So, a next cycle gets initiated with another action plan (Fig. 26.1).

Thus, action research is a step-by-step process, which is continuously evaluated over varying periods of time by a variety of mechanisms. This enables feedback to the researchers who can take decisions to modify the action plan to pursue different directions. Critical reflection on the content and process is a must but both action and reflection go together. In action research, one cannot have a stage of reflection

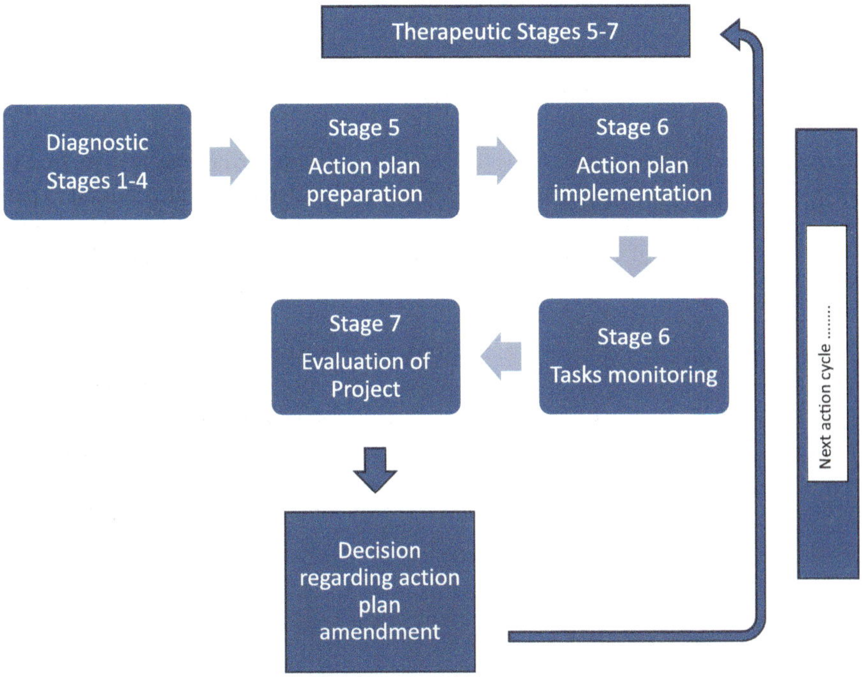

Fig. 26.1 Cyclical process of action research

followed by a stage of action. When both occur simultaneously, critical consciousness emerges, leading to further action [3].

Through these cycles, small scale, contextual initiatives get transformed into sustainable practices. They in turn trigger new cycles with different sets of questions and/or ideas for further inquiry.

26.4 Action Research Practices/Models

Diverse practices are observed under action research. In fact, action research serves as an umbrella term that represents a "family" of practices [1]. For example, three main forms of action research have been described viz. positivist, interpretive, or critical action research. The latter combines action research with critical social theory and is used in educational field. One more type is termed as participatory action research wherein the practitioners (e.g., faculty members) serve as participants and research partners. This is widely used in education. Other variants include action science, community-based participatory research, cooperative inquiry, action learning, appreciative inquiry, developmental action inquiry, and living theory approach [1, 7, 8].

There are three models of action research related to educational areas [9] which are described as follows:

- *Technical action research*: Its main purpose is to improve educational practice to achieve desired outcomes. For instance, when an educational institute collaborates with a university to test an idea, the resulting action research may be guided primarily by the university as the researcher, rather than by the practitioners themselves. Thus, a one-way relationship exists between the two.
- *Practical action research*: It is initiated by the teachers or the educational institution where the line between researcher and practitioner blurs, thus establishing a mutual relationship. This is participatory action research. Generally, the scope of such projects is small.
- *Critical action research*: This is also termed as emancipatory research. It is driven by the goal of liberating individuals or groups from irrationality, injustice, and inequity. At its core, it seeks to empower the underprivileged. These three models are also termed as collaborative action research (CAR).

It is beyond the scope of this chapter to provide details of the action research variants. It suffices to say that growing interest and work in action research has led to the birth of a peer reviewed journal "Action Research," published by SAGE [1]. This journal has an impact factor of 2.1 and it serves as a platform for the development of the theory and practice of action research.

26.5 Core Features of Action Research [1–3]

Whatever may be the practice or model of action research that is followed, to call it as action research it should have the following features:

- *Situational*: Action research is always contextual. Diagnosis of a problem takes place in a specific context and attempts to solve it also occurs in that context. Thus, creation of new knowledge through action research is always in the context of existing practice. It never aims at generalization of new knowledge.
- *Collaborative*: The teams of researchers and participants work in partnership. The features of the relationship the research team has with stakeholders determines the quality of the research.
- *Participatory*: Researchers involve the stakeholders appropriately in discussing and framing research questions, designing action plans, evaluating the process and decision making for change. The stakeholders also get engaged in the process. Thus, the line between researchers and participants merges and the participants become true partners over the period.
- *Self-evaluative*: Each and every stage of action research is continuously evaluated to provide feedback to the researcher and participants.
- *Reflexive*: It is the extent to which the action researchers explicitly locate themselves as change agents. Action researchers must acknowledge influence of context and researcher's perspective about the research process. They should examine how their own judgements, thoughts and feelings, and biases may affect a situation or may have led to a particular conclusion. Hence a self-conscious critique is

important in action research. Critical reflections constitute both, appraisal and evaluation of efforts to bring in change and impact of self on the research process.
- *Significant*: This is defined according to the impact of action research. Though solutions identified and tested through action research are meant to be applied for an immediate context, its significance should extend beyond this context. The insights from such action research should benefit similar settings elsewhere with similar problems or even bigger settings. In other words, it should be capable of benefitting other persons, communities, and the wider ecology.

26.6 Benefits of Action Research in HPE

Action research addresses problematic situations in settings that they range from classrooms to communities. This makes it possible to introduce innovations into ongoing practice, which is normally not conducive for change. It also improves communication between researchers and the stakeholders so that the stakeholders find their voice and representation in decision making. Apart from this, it also empowers the stakeholders [2].

It has been shown that action research fosters professional development. The reflexive practice of action research helps focusing on self-awareness, which itself is a prerequisite for professional development [6]. Working together on a common problem imparts a source of security, status and recognition and brings in a collective culture. During the process faculty members acquire new skills, find opportunities to sharpen their critical thinking/reasoning, and enhance the analytical power. Their reflective ability also increases and they nurture both, reflective teachers and researchers. Studies have shown that development of reflective teaching practices increases teacher's efficiency [2, 6]. In short, this research serves as a tool for in-service training of faculty, wherein the faculty members take charge of their own growth [10].

Action research bridges a gap between theory and practice. Many a times what is considered as best practice in teaching-learning or assessment or innovations in educational field may not be suitable to put into practice in a classroom. It may not match the daily schedule or daily needs of the classroom or institution. The teachers while using the innovation researched by someone else assumes a role of passive receiver. Values and concerns of the teachers or the problems in the given setting are not considered. This is termed as "Moses Effect." All these factors get mitigated if teachers conduct action research to make these innovations acceptable [11, 12].

Action research provides a ground for research-based education. It offers teachers ownership of effective practices [11]. A shift can occur in the behavior of participants as they start opting for evidence -based teaching rather than earlier opinion-based teaching. It helps in developing openness to the newer ideas.

Action research helps job analysis. It unfolds human relations and interpersonal communication in the organization [2]. This helps in the building of a community of practice [10].

26.7 Applications

Use of action research in health care was limited before 1980s. Its use has increased during 1990s resulting in more publications in health journals and as textbooks. It has been used for needs assessment studies as well as evaluating and changing health services in low-income countries, e.g., in Bolivia it was used to overcome maternal and neonatal health problems in rural areas through a community plan. Even in high-income countries, action research finds place in mental health research and indigenous health research, e.g., in Australia it has been used for the aboriginal Australian community to support its self-help group to design, implement and evaluate their activities [3].

Considering its practical utility, Stephen Corey, an educational researcher introduced action research for the first time in education in the 1950s [10]. The objective was to provide tools to the teachers for continuous improvement of classroom teaching-learning and its environment. Later on, there was some critique related to this and it resulted in decline of action research. In the 1970s it regained its place and value especially for continuous improvement in quality of education and teacher professional development programs. With technological advances, the sphere of action research has expanded due to effective professional networking. It is being used to assess institutional initiatives, refine educational policies and educational quality enhancement by the principals and administrators in partnership along with the teachers [10].

In HPE participatory action research is widely used now-a -days, which is primarily initiated by the faculty members who serve as action researchers [12]. The main goals of participatory action research in HPE are to improve existing practice, understand various factors responsible for the current practice and improve the environment in which the practice is ongoing. Faculty members usually show dedication towards these goals. Moreover, their ability to reflect, which they develop as teachers, plays a crucial role. The other helpful qualities are their pedagogical and research knowledge and skills, understanding of the self, capability to start change movement and sustain the desired changes in the education [6]. When they actively participate and self-experience, acceptability of innovations increases and they have a likelihood to get implemented [12].

Table 26.1 illustrates use of action research in some of the important domains of HPE. Few examples given below may motivate interested readers to read these publications and draw insights from them regarding how to use action research in HPE. Brown CT (2019) has highlighted how action research offers a learning opportunity for a student-researcher in the health education classroom and has expressed that student-teacher partnership in action research projects may lead to creation of better learning communities [13].

Table 26.1 Examples of studies using action research in various domains of HPE with the resultant impact and their retrieval information

Domain	Authors	Retrieval information	Impact
Curriculum development	Casey D.	Nurs Health Sci. 2007 Mar;9(1):5–13	Development of skills training program focusing on the health-promoting role of nurses
Curriculum reform	von Pressentin KB, Waggie F, Conradie H.	BMC Med Educ 2016; 16: 82 Doi: 10.1186/s12909-016-0607-3	Improvement of learning experience of students undergoing longitudinal integrated clerkship in the rural district health services.
Problems in educational setting	Findyartini A, Syah NA, Susilo AP, Nurokhmanti H, Qomariyah N, Greviana N, et al.	Medical Education Online, 28(1). Doi: 10.1080/10872981.2023.2185122	Challenges and opportunities for instituting student-centred learning in medical schools in a hierarchical cultural setting were identified with possible step forward in the form of mentorship model
Inter-professional education	Başer A, Şahin H.	BMC Med Educ 2025;25: 532 Doi: 10.1186/s12909-025-07085-y	IPE program on "Chronic Disease Management and Patient Safety" for students of medicine, dentistry, and health sciences
Assessment strategies	Terrón-Pérez M, Marcarell C, Corchón S.	Nurse Educ Pract. 2024 Oct;80:104095. Doi: 10.1016/j.nepr.2024.104095	Development of competency-based assessment template for oncology nurses for assessing knowledge, skills and attitudes
Simulation	Erlam G, Smythe L, Wright-St Clair V.	Nurse Educ Today; 2018; 61: 140–145	Identification of needs of undergraduate millennial nursing students learning in simulation environment
Digital learning tools	Keugoung B, Bello KOA, Millimouno TM, Sidibé S, Dossou JP, Delamou A, et al.	Learn Health Syst. 2020 Aug 28;5(4):e10244. Doi: 10.1002/lrh2.10244	Designing and implementing e-Health innovation, for mobilizing health district management teams in low-income countries

(continued)

Table 26.1 (continued)

Domain	Authors	Retrieval information	Impact
Student motivation	Dehnad A, Nasser H.	Acta Med Iran. 2014;52(6):473–80	Enhanced motivation of medical students to learn in an 'English for Specific Purposes' class and change in their classroom behaviour
Inclusive education	Foreshew A, Al-Jawad M.	Med Educ. 2022 Nov;56(11):1076–1085	Space created to build community for 'marginalised' students in medical college with creation of Inclusive Practice Partnership group for sharing experiences and advocating curriculum change. Development of anonymous system to report marginalising Behaviour. A series of recommended actions to decolonise and diversify medical curriculum movement.
Educational leadership	Cardiff S, McCormack B, McCance T.	J Clin Nurs. 2018 Aug;27(15–16):3056–3069	Development of person-centred leadership conceptual framework with explicit interplay between leadership relationships and context for nurse leadership
Leadership programmes	Spowart L, Inman AC, Hardy LJ, Dillon MJ.	BMJ Open. 2024 Mar 15;14(3): e079160. Doi:10.1136/ bmjopen-2023–079160	Development of online leadership workshops and their implementation for NHS health professionals to enhance the transferability of leadership skills gained during global health engagement in low- and middle-income countries

(continued)

Table 26.1 (continued)

Domain	Authors	Retrieval information	Impact
HPE training	Van Schalkwyk SC, Couper ID, Blitz J, De Villiers MR.	BMC Med Educ. 2020 May 14;20(1):154. Doi: 10.1186/s12909-020-02046-z	Development of framework for effective distributed health professions training and its subsequent implementation
Development of HPE research course	Scott KM, Hughes M, Davids J.	J. Clin Teach. 2021 Dec;18(6):614–20	Creation of a health professional education research course and development of capacity as teacher educators

26.8 Challenges and Ethical Issues

One of the challenges in action research is that it is time consuming. Duration of individual cycle and number of action cycles remain uncertain. Being a real-world project, delays are experienced [3, 7].

As mentioned earlier, the process of action research involves critical reflection and discussion within groups. Participants may consider these as face-threatening situations especially if their ideas or actions are critiqued [9].

The research findings may not get published as public health journals may find they are contextual and cannot be applied to other settings. There also may be no appreciation for the efforts of a researcher who engages the stakeholders to bring in change [3].

It lacks rigor of the other scientific research methods and there are concerns about its validity, [14] but it is a preferred alternative [2]. Compared to other interventional scientific studies [2], in most of the cases, it is difficult to get financial support for action research as the protocol is not very well defined. The researchers and participants usually remain unpaid. Working together and managing different or competing motivations of involved partners is difficult.

In addition, there are multiple ethical issues. As mentioned earlier, action research is collaborative but this collaboration needs to be voluntary. Sometimes administrators are interested in action research and may co-opt or coerce participants in the research merely due to hierarchical power. Power stems from assigned roles, hierarchical positions, academic background, and relational ties existing in an institution or between faculty members of an institution and external researcher from University or Ministry of Health or between researchers and communities [3]. More experienced researchers may impose on the colleagues their own plans during research, which affects the collaborative spirit. Anyone interested in conducting action research should be able to do so entirely by choice, without feeling pressured or compelled.

Students may get involved as participants or co-researchers. It is important to remember that students is a vulnerable population and all the care should be taken to protect their rights. No penalty, direct or indirect, should be imposed if they wish to leave the research even after signing informed consent.

Confidentiality of the participants should be maintained. Protecting anonymity is one way of ensuring confidentiality. However, both are linked with ethical issues of authorship and ownership. For example, participants may believe that they own the data of the action research and therefore wish that the report or the publication should bear their real name. They may demand co-authorship instead of their inclusion in acknowledgement. Action research is always participatory and cannot be conducted without discussions and involvement of participants. Hence it should be made clear to the participants at the time of informed consent and later on when findings are shared with the participants during the process of action research what role they will be playing and how that will be given due credit.

During action research participants do play a role in interpretation of data. Sometimes they may request to revisit the analyzed data especially when they perceive what they discussed is portrayed incorrectly or presented in a negative way. They have a right to do this but this request needs to be reported in the final report to observe transparency in the research. In such situation the participants may feel that their confidentiality is not protected.

The researchers should periodically disclose the benefits of action research project so that the participants recognize their varied motivations. These insights should be incorporated in the report as they determine whether the action research is technical, practical, or emancipatory, and highlight the personal motivations driving it. However, revelation of personal motivation may not be appreciated by the participants.

Although action research seeks to induce sustainable change, at times the changed practice may not continue, especially for externally initiated action research when funding stops or external researcher dissociates. Participants may be interested in continuing the change but may not be able to do so because they believe that they cannot pursue on their own. Therefore, participant empowerment is essential during the research process. The threat of abandoning the change is less in institutional faculty -initiated projects [9, 15].

26.9 Conclusion

Action research transforms education by empowering educators to become agents of change who systematically investigate and solve real-world challenges in their own practice. The cyclical process of action and reflection results in transformative changes which are long-lasting. It has promoted evidence-based educational practices and policies. Being a stakeholder-initiated inquiry, wherein stakeholders play a role of researchers, outcomes are better accepted. Most significantly, action research cultivates reflective practitioners who evolve from passive implementers into innovative problem-solvers, developing the critical thinking and adaptive capacity essential for life-long professional growth and educational excellence.

References

1. Bradbury-Huang H. What is good action research? Why the resurgent interest? Action Res. 2010;8(1):93–109.
2. Burns RB. Action-research. In: Introduction to research methods. 4th ed. London: SAGE; 2000. p. 443–58.
3. Baum F, MacDougall C, Smith D. Participatory action research. J Epidemiol Community Health. 2006;60(10):854–7.
4. Narayan KMV. Public health challenges for the 21st century: convergence of demography, economics, environment and biology: Nalanda distinguished lecture. Natl Med J India. 2017;30(4):219–23.
5. Frenk J, Chen L, Bhutta ZA, Cohen J, Crisp N, Evans T, et al. Health professionals for a new century: transforming education to strengthen health systems in an interdependent world. Lancet. 2010;376(9756):1923–58.
6. Zajic JO, Maksimovic J. Contemporary teachers' action research—basis for the development of reflective practice in education. Res Pedagogy. 2020;10(2):354–66.
7. Aulianda M, Djatmika ET, Handayati P. Critical review: action research. INOVASI. 2021;17(4):860–8.
8. Morales MPE. Participatory Action Research (PAR) cum Action Research (AR) in teacher professional development: a literature review. Int J Res Educ Sci. 2016;2(1):156–65.
9. Banegas DL, Villacañas de Castro LS. A look at ethical issues in action research in education. Argent J Appl Linguist. 2015;3(1):58–67.
10. Teachers Institute. The evolution of action research: From Kurt Lewin to modern education. Topic Wise Notes for Teaching & Education Courses. 27th Dec, 2023. (2025). Available on: https://teachers.institute/growth-and-development-of-educational-management/evolution-of-action-research/. Accessed 25 Aug 2025.
11. Lufungulo ES, Mambwe R, Kalinde B. The meaning and role of action research in education multidisciplinary. J Lang Soc Sci Educ. 2021;4:115–28.
12. Mubuuke AG, Leibowitz B. Participatory action research: the key to successful implementation of innovations in health professions education. Afr J Health Prof Educ. 2013;5(1):30–3.
13. Brown CT. The value of action research in health education. J Phys Educ Recreat Dance. 2019;90(5):52–5. https://doi.org/10.1080/07303084.2019.1583027.
14. Feldman A. Validity and quality in action research. Educ Action Res. 2007;15(1):21–32.
15. Nolen AL, Putten JV. Action research in education: addressing gaps in ethical principles and practices. Educ Res. 2007;36(7):401–7.

Training Medical Educators to Integrate Future Technologies Effectively

27

Suresh Narayanan and Vimala Ananthy

Key Points

- Insufficient faculty development leads to superficial technology use and resistance to pedagogical change.
- To effectively deliver a technology-based training program, identify the needs of the learner, frame the objectives of the session, develop resource materials, implement without any glitches, and evaluate using an appropriate assessment.
- Training sessions can be face-to-face, online, or hybrid, based on the availability of resources.
- The e-learning content must adhere to cognitive load theory and multimedia principles for better understanding.
- Comprehensive checklists or rubrics should be used to ensure consistency and quality in technology-enabled learning.

27.1 Introduction

Technology-enhanced learning (TEL) focuses on the use of digital tools to improve and support the learning experience. Educators have extensively used technology in student enrollment, resource sharing, subject content delivery, assessment, feedback, and analytics. The current generation of learners also prefers technology-based instruction over traditional learning, as it matches their learning style and improves accessibility [1]. The successful integration of technology depends not

S. Narayanan (✉)
Department of Anatomy, All India Institute of Medical Sciences—Madurai, Madurai, India

V. Ananthy
Department of Pharmacology, Mahatma Gandhi Medical College and Research Institute, Puducherry, India

J. Sandars et al. (eds.), *Modern Medical Education*,
https://doi.org/10.1007/978-3-032-27958-3_27

merely on its implementation but on the preparedness of educators to use it effectively. In this context, medical educators serve as agents of change as their knowledge, attitude, and technology practice will directly influence how students engage with these innovations [2]. This chapter explores the need for training medical educators on technology, training models/methods, designing technological content using multimedia principles, quality initiatives, and future trends. Thus, we aim to strengthen future medical education by empowering medical educators to utilize technology effectively.

27.2 Need for Training Medical Educators on Technology

Emerging technologies like virtual reality, artificial intelligence, massive open online courses, mobile apps, and gamification have transformed medical education by improving accessibility and promoting self-directed learning and student engagement [3]. However, many educators hesitate to incorporate these approaches into their routine teaching. Several factors contribute to their reluctance, including technological factors (such as perceived ease of use and accessibility), teacher-related factors (such as attitudes toward change, technological capabilities, pedagogical beliefs, and existing practices), and contextual factors (such as the level of institutional support). The lack of training is often considered the key barrier to effective technology integration. Insufficient faculty development leads to superficial technology use, missed opportunities for collaborative learning experiences, and resistance to pedagogical change. Implementing inappropriate technology can lead to poor student engagement and inadequate learning outcomes. Comprehensive training programs can address these challenges by equipping medical educators with the technical skills and pedagogical frameworks needed to integrate technology [2].

27.3 Framework for Technological Training

ADDIE (Analysis, Design, Development, Implementation, and Evaluation) is an instructional framework for delivering effective training programs.

Step 1: Analysis

To effectively design a training program, firstly, we need to identify the gap by assessing the current level of competency using surveys or standardized assessment tools. Gap identification helps clearly understand existing skills and areas that require improvement. Next, we need to define performance goals (i.e., what educators should be able to accomplish after the training program). Additionally, we need to identify available infrastructure, participant demographics, attitudes toward technology adoption, motivation levels, and current workload to improve the effectiveness of the training. The failure of implementing technology is not always related to a lack of training but rather to a lack of follow-up training, increased workload, and poor infrastructure [4]. For example, the educator may have demonstrated their ability to upload resource materials in a previous Learning Management System (LMS) workshop, but this may not be reflected in actual practice. In such a case, a simple infographic of the workflow can reduce the work burden and technical support can be improved to solve the problem rather than retraining the educators.

Step 2: Design

To effectively achieve the desired goal, it is important to frame learning objectives using SMART criteria (Specific, Measurable, Achievable, Relevant, and Time-bound) and Bloom's Taxonomy. An appropriate teaching strategy is selected among face-to-face sessions, online modules, and blended approaches. The common pitfalls in the design phase are (1) mismatch between training objectives and outcomes. For instance, the facilitators could have mentioned that "educators should enlist digital tools" as the objectives, but expect the "participants to independently create quizzes," and (2) choosing an inappropriate teaching method. For example, when the facilitators want to train the participants on a SCORM (Sharable Content Object Reference Model) compliant module that requires multiple steps for its designing, a hands-on practice for real-time support is preferred over video tutorials. Therefore, facilitators should always keep the training outcome in mind and design session objectives and teaching methods for its facilitation [4].

Step 3: Development

In this phase, the organizers identify digital tools and develop a detailed lesson plan, resource materials, communication strategy, and participant guides to align with the educators' routine workflow. Then, the training module should be tested through a pilot session with a small group of participants. This piloting checks whether the resource materials address the previously identified learners' needs. Based on feedback from this pilot, it is important to iterate and refine the materials [4]. The organizer's choice of technology should be based on educational goals, institutional capacity, and learner needs, and not for the sake of implementation. For instance, a recently established institution with students from diverse socioeconomic backgrounds wants to enhance the student's clinical skills training through digital tools. Choosing a virtual reality platform is not a feasible approach due to financial constraints. A feasible solution is to opt for a web-based virtual patient simulator that (1) focuses on improving diagnostic reasoning and patient management (matching the educational goal), (2) runs on standard devices (fitting the institution's capacity), and (3) allows students to use the web-based platform in their device (addressing the needs of the learner).

Step 4: Implementation

Here, the training is delivered using the chosen teaching method in the design phase, such as LMS, in-person, or hybrid. An effective training program begins with clearly communicating expectations, outlining the learning objectives, and informing participants about available support resources. Before the program, the organizers should ensure the physical space for the session, the technological setup, and the facilitator training. Some initiatives that enhance learning outcomes include managing technical glitches during the sessions, using case studies to make the content relevant, and asking questions to check for learner understanding. A common drawback during implementation is delivering too much theoretical content and a passive teaching process. Facilitators should incorporate hands-on activities and peer discussions to make the session interactive [4].

Step 5: Evaluation
The evaluation of the training program should align with the session objective using appropriate assessment methods. Educators should focus on the long-term impact by triangulating data from surveys, interviews, authentic work tasks, and reflective logs. The data gathered during the evaluation process can be used to refine training content, instructional strategies, and delivery methods for continuous improvement in future sessions. A common pitfall during training evaluation is relying heavily on self-reported data and focusing only on participant satisfaction. The participants may feel "confident" after the training sessions, but it is a subjective phenomenon and does not reflect the competence of the educator. Hence, the organizers should make sure that the participants are evaluated on the intended learning outcome [4].

27.4 Framework for Integrating Technology in Teaching Practice

The Technological Pedagogical Content Knowledge (TPACK) framework identifies the educator's current knowledge and skill in subject content, pedagogy, and technology. This framework also ensures that digital tools are selected and applied to enhance content delivery and pedagogical strategies rather than using technology for its own sake. This training model also emphasizes the alignment between learning objectives, pedagogy, and technology, creating an engaging and relevant teaching experience [5].

Here is an example of how the TPACK framework is used to select an appropriate technology and teaching method:

Content knowledge (CK): What subject content am I teaching? (e.g., cardiac anatomy).

Pedagogy knowledge (PK): Which teaching methods are suitable for learning this content? (e.g., case-based learning, team-based learning, draw-along techniques, 3-dimensional models).

Technology knowledge (TK): What digital tools can enhance this teaching experience? (e.g., LMS platforms, digital flashcards, gamified quizzes, clinical videos, 3-dimensional software).

Pedagogical Content Knowledge (PCK): Which pedagogical strategy effectively delivers the subject content? (Case-based learning aids in understanding clinical reasoning; team-based learning facilitates peer discussion and deepens conceptual understanding; and 3-dimensional models help visualize spatial relationships).

Technological Content Knowledge (TCK): Which technology delivers the subject content effectively? (LMS for resource sharing; digital flashcards for memorizing structures; videos for clinical reasoning; clinical videos to link anatomy with diagnostic imaging and patient cases; 3-dimensional software for spatial understanding).

Technological Pedagogical Knowledge (TPK): Which technology effectively delivers the pedagogical strategy? (Gamified quizzes with immediate feedback strengthen retention; LMS discussion forums facilitate collaborative learning and critical thinking abilities).

Technological Pedagogical Content Knowledge (TPACK): How can content, pedagogy, and technology be blended effectively in teaching? (Pre-class: Assign videos and digital flashcards via LMS for foundational knowledge (TK + CK). In-class: Use 3D software and draw-along techniques for visual and kinaesthetic engagement (PCK + TCK). During discussion: Apply case-based learning in small groups, supported by LMS forums for collaboration (TPK). Assessment: Use gamified quizzes with immediate feedback to reinforce knowledge and clinical reasoning (TPK + CK). Application: Employ simulation software or VR to link anatomy to clinical practice in immersive ways (TPACK fully integrated) [6].

The choosing of appropriate technology depends upon contextual factors (use of 3D apps in the classroom as compared to portable ultrasound machines in a clinical setting to teach cardiac anatomy), teacher's technology proficiency (tech-savvy teacher might prefer 3D apps over animated videos), students acceptability (students may choose a gamified quiz over interactive polls), and curricular demands (recorded videos or online quizzes for theoretical understanding and virtual patients for clinical skill application) [7]. Common issues with the TPACK framework include (1) difficulty in applying learned theoretical concepts in practice. For example, a lecturer understands the components of TPACK but fails to transfer them in routine teaching due to a lack of resources or unfamiliarity with the tool, and (2) even after technology is integrated, the learner might not see the relevance if assessment still focuses on rote knowledge. For example, a lecturer uses simulation-based software to teach surgical skills. However, the final exam is still a traditional multiple-choice paper, failing to reflect the hands-on or scenario-based learning that the technology supports.

27.5 Framework for Determining the Depth of Technological Integration

Another model is the SAMR framework that guides educators in the level of integrating technology into teaching and learning. The SAMR model includes:

Substitution (S): Technology is a direct substitute with no functional change. For example, uploading a pre-recorded video lecture in an LMS replaces the traditional lecture.

Augmentation (A): Technology still substitutes but adds some functional improvement. An example is administering digital quizzes in classrooms.

Modification (M): Technology enables significant redesign of tasks. For example, students collaborate on Google Docs to make diagnoses with real-time faculty feedback.

Redefinition (R): Technology facilitates the creation of new tasks previously inconceivable. For example, the LMS uses learning analytics to adapt content delivery based on individual student performance, providing targeted remediation, adaptive quizzes, and personal learning dashboards.

The SAMR model assists educators in evaluating their current use of technology and identifying ways to transition from basic substitution to transformative learning experiences. It promotes reflective teaching practices by assessing the impact of technology on learning outcomes. For example, an educator can reflect on whether the intended outcome of collaboration and clinical reasoning was achieved after implementing discussion forums in a digital platform. Ultimately, this model is a roadmap for guiding faculty development to enhance digital teaching skills [8].

27.6 Training Methods for Medical Educators to Integrate Technology

There are several training strategies, but the commonality is that the training should be based on a real-world, evidence-based approach that aligns with adult learning principles to integrate technology effectively. In face-to-face training programs, the facilitator first demonstrates how the digital tools work, followed by hands-on training for the participants. The major advantage of in-person training is that troubleshooting is addressed immediately through personalized feedback. Participants can ask questions in real-time, observe peer demonstrations, and engage in collaborative problem-solving. These workshops are most impactful when they include hands-on activities, small group collaboration, and immediate feedback [9]. In institutions where there are physical space constraints and logistical difficulties, online training is a suitable alternative. In online learning, the content is easily accessible, and the participants learn at their own pace [9]. A scaffolded approach where learners progress step by step without cognitive overload is ideal for online learning. For example, when training medical educators to use an LMS, the module sequence can include an introduction, uploading content, creating quizzes, and monitoring student performance. Incorporating drag-and-drop elements to check their understanding, discussion forums to clarify their queries, and downloadable tip sheets support real-world application and sustained use.

In peer mentoring, an experienced faculty member (the mentor) guides a less experienced colleague (the mentee) by demonstrating the skill, guiding the mentee, and allowing the mentee to take complete control. This guided approach enables the educator to ask questions directly and progressively attain competence. This method will be more effective when mentors and mentees share similar teaching backgrounds or challenges [10]. For example, a pathology teacher mentoring another pathology teacher makes the learning more relatable and directly applicable.

Lastly, project-based learning provides an immersive and outcome-oriented approach to integrating technology. For example, an educator designing an e-learning module will learn about student enrollment, sharing resources, creating assessments, providing feedback, and generating completion certificates. In this process, the educator has gained technological skills and innovative ways to address the problems. Practical issues in the e-learning module can be identified and rectified by incorporating peer review and piloting the project. This hands-on approach builds confidence in using technology and ensures its application is directly relevant and beneficial to student learning [11]. Together, these strategies provide a comprehensive and sustainable approach to building digital teaching capacity among medical educators.

27.7 Designing Technological Content Based on Cognitive and Multimedia Principles

Simply converting learning materials and PowerPoint presentations into videos and e-learning modules hampers learning because it creates information overload, lacks interactivity, ignores the learner's prior knowledge, and is often redundant. Therefore, educators must design technological content using established instructional designs, such as cognitive load theory and multimedia principles. Cognitive principles explain how information is processed in the brain. First, there are separate channels for processing visual and auditory information. Second, our working memory can process a limited amount of information. Finally, learning is an active process in which learners identify and select relevant materials, organize them into mental representations, and store them in long-term memory. Learning becomes inefficient if the information exceeds the learner's ability to comprehend and process it during learning. Understanding the three types of cognitive load (i.e., intrinsic, extraneous, and germane load) helps design effective instructional materials [12].

27.8 Minimize Extraneous Load (Unnecessary Mental Effort)

Coherence principle: Avoid material that hinders the learning process (In e-learning content, display only essential structures; avoid irrelevant images and music).

Signaling principle: Highlight essential material (In a video, use arrows to denote a particular part of an image or highlight text).

Redundancy principle: Graphics and narration should not be accompanied by on-screen text that repeats the narration (While narrating an anatomical image, do not add on-screen text).

Spatial contiguity: Place printed words near corresponding graphics (While explaining a pathogenesis of disease using an image, place the "label" close to the image, rather than listing it as a separate legend).

Temporal contiguity: Present corresponding narration and animation at the same time (When showing a suturing technique, the instructor's voice explains the step while it is being performed) [12].

27.9 Managing Intrinsic Load (Complexity of the Material Being Learned)

Segmenting principle: Break content into smaller chunks (e.g., in a surgical simulation video, split the procedure into preparation, incision, and closure).

Pre-training principle: Provide pre-training with basic terms and concepts (e.g., before an e-module on ECG interpretation, give an orientation of various waves in ECG and their causes).

Modality principle: Graphics are explained by spoken narration rather than on-screen text (An animation of how the heart pumps blood is explained through audio narration rather than on-screen text) [12].

27.10 Maximize Germane Load (Mental Effort Used for Knowledge Acquisition)

Multimedia principle: Present words and pictures rather than words alone (Show a diagram of receptor binding while narrating how beta-blockers work).

Personalization principle: Present words in conversational style rather than formal style (While explaining the histology of the thymus, state that this is the place where the student's immature T cells become competent T cells) [12].

27.11 Evaluating the Impact of Integrating Technology in Medical Education

The Technology-Enhanced Learning Evaluation Model (TELEM) guides medical educators in assessing the impact of educational technologies that have been implemented:

Level 0: Needs Analysis—Assess whether the implemented technology appropriately solves an identified problem statement. Example: Conduct surveys and faculty interviews to determine whether students struggle with self-paced learning and whether an LMS can improve content accessibility and engagement.

Level 1a: Learner Satisfaction—Assess the learner's usability and experience using post-session Likert scale surveys. Example: Administer a post-course questionnaire asking students to rate the LMS platform's ease of navigation, clarity of resources, and responsiveness.

Level 1b: Learning Gain—Assess the knowledge or skill improvement using pre-test-posttest or control group designs. Example: Compare pre- and post-course test scores in modules delivered via LMS to gauge knowledge retention.

Level 2: Curriculum Integration—Assess technology's impact when incorporated into the curriculum. Example: Track student performance across Phases 1 to 4 of the medical curriculum to determine if integrating LMS-based quizzes and discussions improves final exam outcomes.

Level 3: Institutional Impact—Examine sustainability, return on investment (ROI), and scalability. Example: Perform a cost-benefit analysis comparing LMS-based course delivery versus traditional face-to-face methods, factoring in faculty time, printing costs, and student outcomes [13].

27.12 Quality Initiatives in Technology-Enhanced Learning

Educators and learners are accustomed to traditional modes of instruction, and when they are exposed to a TEL environment, they expect improved usability and pedagogical effectiveness. Also, poorly designed digital content can lead to cognitive overload, learner disengagement, and poor learning outcomes. To address these shortcomings, quality assurance is needed for continuous improvement in TEL delivery. The Medical Education Unit (MEU) or Internal Quality Assurance Cell (IQAC) could take the initiative of collecting feedback from faculty members and students. The independent assessors can use comprehensive checklists or rubrics to assess key domains such as:

Learning Objectives (Specific, measurable, aligned with content and assessment)

Content Delivery (Use of multimedia, chunked information, clarity, cognitive load reduction)

Interactivity and Engagement (Opportunities for real-time interaction, collaboration, and application to clinical cases)

Assessment and Feedback (Formative and summative assessments with timely, constructive feedback)

Accessibility and Inclusivity (Universal design, mobile compatibility, support for low-bandwidth learners)

Support and Resources (Availability of LMS, trained IT staff, and learning aids)

Reflection and Collaboration (Promoting peer-to-peer and learner-instructor collaboration with space for self-reflection)

Ethics and Privacy (Adherence to data privacy laws and ethical handling of patient or clinical scenarios)

Monitoring and Improvement (Evaluation mechanisms using feedback, analytics, and external review)

These components are a foundation for structured self-assessment, peer review, and institutional evaluation, promoting excellence and accountability [14].

27.13 Future Trends in Technology-Enhanced Learning

Firstly, the growing affordability of technology will democratize access to high-quality learning materials and the expansion of open educational resources. Institutions will take initiatives to improve technological equality and inclusivity. Secondly, the ICT committee will prioritize the digital well-being of learners. The committee will emphasize professional and ethical behavior in digital spaces. It will take steps to maintain a mindful online presence, promote data ownership to avoid copyright issues, and upgrade infrastructure for improved data privacy and confidentiality [15]. Thirdly, faculty development initiatives such as just-in-time learning, microlearning modules, and virtual communities of practice are becoming core components of faculty development programs. Future workshops will focus on an integrated approach, where educators are trained to choose the right technology and teaching strategy [9]. Fourthly, regulatory bodies will develop technological competency for medical educators. Then, these statutory bodies will periodically assess their proficiency in creating and utilizing e-learning content.

References

1. Plch L. Perception of technology-enhanced learning by medical students: an integrative review. Med Sci Educ. 2020;30(4):1707–20. https://doi.org/10.1007/s40670-020-01040-w.
2. Grainger R, Liu Q, Geertshuis S. Learning technologies: a medium for the transformation of medical education? Med Educ. 2021;55(1):23–9. https://doi.org/10.1111/medu.14261.
3. Martin F, Dennen VP, Bonk CJ. A synthesis of systematic review research on emerging learning environments and technologies. Educ Technol Res Dev. 2020;68(4):1613–33. https://doi.org/10.1007/s11423-020-09812-2.
4. Chen P. Designing learning activities and instructional systems. In: Huang R, Spector JM, Yang J, editors. Educational technology: a primer for the 21st century. Singapore: Springer; 2019. p. 125–48.
5. Ait Ali D, El Meniari A, El Filali S, Morabite O, Senhaji F, Khabbache H. Empirical research on technological pedagogical content knowledge (TPACK) framework in health professions education: a literature review. Med Sci Educ. 2023;33(3):791–803. https://doi.org/10.1007/s40670-023-01786-z.
6. Jayatilleke A, Shah M. Examining the technological pedagogical content characteristics of games for medical education. Med Sci Educ. 2020;30(1):529–36. https://doi.org/10.1007/s40670-019-00891-2.
7. Boedeker PJ, Moreno NP, Newell AD, Maheshwari A, McMillin MA, Tippen SP, et al. Pedagogical content knowledge as a lens for transforming teaching in medical and health professions education. Med Sci Educ. 2025;35(3):1707–14. https://doi.org/10.1007/s40670-025-02325-8.
8. Grainger R, Liu Q, Gladman T. Learning technology in health professions education: realising an (un)imagined future. Med Educ. 2024;58(1):36–46. https://doi.org/10.1111/medu.15185.
9. Singleton R, Ruiz Cosignani D, Kam M, Clune M, Charlton A, Jowsey T. Faculty development for strengthening online teaching capability: a mixed-methods study of what staff want, evaluated with Kirkpatrick's model of teaching effectiveness. MedEdPublish. 2016;2023(13):127. https://doi.org/10.12688/mep.19692.2
10. Barr KP, Deluca K, Dicianno BE, Helkowski WM, Liu B. Group peer mentoring to improve faculty connections and enhance mentoring networks. Clin Teach. 2024;21(4):e13747. https://doi.org/10.1111/tct.13747.

11. Vyas R, Faith M, Selvakumar D, Pulimood A, Lee M. Project-based faculty development for e-learning. Clin Teach. 2016;13(6):405–10. https://doi.org/10.1111/tct.12486.
12. Mayer RE. Designing multimedia instruction in anatomy: an evidence-based approach. Clin Anat. 2020;33(1):2–11. https://doi.org/10.1002/ca.23265.
13. Pickering JD, Lazarus MD, Hallam JL. A practitioner's guide to performing a holistic evaluation of technology-enhanced learning in medical education. Med Sci Educ. 2019;29(4):1095–102. https://doi.org/10.1007/s40670-019-00781-7.
14. Dong C, Rajaratnam V. Evaluating synchronous online teaching in health professions education: a self-assessment rubric for educators. Med Sci Educ. 2025;35(3):1227–34. https://doi.org/10.1007/s40670-025-02353-4.
15. Naeem NI, Yusoff MSB, Hadie SNH, Ismail IM, Iqbal H. Understanding the functional components of technology-enhanced learning environment in medical education: a scoping review. Med Sci Educ. 2023;33(2):595–609. https://doi.org/10.1007/s40670-023-01747-6.

28 How to Integrate AI Education in the Health Sciences Curriculum

Rita Mojtahedzadeh and Aeen Mohammadi

Key Points

- AI is an important part of healthcare, influencing the quality of care.
- AI literacy is a core competency for medical sciences students.
- Integrating AI education into the curricula is a mandatory consideration today.
- Future physicians should understand AI and its responsible usage.
- Considering the overload of curricula, medical schools should take a suitable strategy for integrating AI education.

28.1 Introduction

Artificial Intelligence (AI) is rapidly changing the healthcare landscape and becoming part of everyday medical practice, from diagnostic imaging and clinical decision support to generative tools and virtual consultations. With this shift, it is increasingly important for medical science students to not only understand these technologies but also use them responsibly and effectively.

AI brings various potential benefits in clinical practice. Processing massive amounts of health data, improving diagnostic accuracy, and supporting more personalized care are examples of these benefits. However, alongside these benefits, new ethical dilemmas and practical concerns arise. Hence, as AI has become a crucial part of medical practice, future medical professionals need to be equipped with the right skills to navigate this evolving landscape [1].

R. Mojtahedzadeh · A. Mohammadi (✉)
Department of E-Learning in Medical Education, Center of Excellence for E-Learning in Medical Education, School of Medicine, Tehran University of Medical Sciences, Tehran, Iran
e-mail: r_mojtahedzadeh@tums.ac.ir; aeen_mohammadi@tums.ac.ir

J. Sandars et al. (eds.), *Modern Medical Education*,
https://doi.org/10.1007/978-3-032-27958-3_28

However, medical education has not fully adapted to these changes, and many undergraduate and postgraduate programs have not integrated AI education into their curricula. This has resulted in many trainees lacking even a basic understanding of how these systems function, which can potentially lead to misunderstandings or missed opportunities to use AI effectively in clinical care [2].

To address this gap, educators and administrators are calling for more systematically planned AI training. Key areas include understanding fundamental AI principles, developing data literacy, and applying these tools in real-world clinical settings. The Association of American Medical Colleges (AAMC) has reported that while many students already interact with AI tools, formal instruction remains limited [3].

If AI is here to stay in medicine, then preparing the next generation of physicians to use it wisely is no longer optional. Teaching AI in medical schools holds much promise. When appropriately integrated, AI can enrich how students learn and practice medicine. Adaptive learning systems and virtual patient simulations can offer tailored, hands-on experiences, allowing learners to work through diagnostic scenarios with real-time, AI-generated feedback. Tools like chatbots or smart quizzes can provide immediate, personalized responses to students' clinical decisions, helping them improve their reasoning and identify gaps in understanding. Exposure to AI not only has a positive impact on learning but also stimulates creativity in medical students, enabling them to create innovative solutions that improve care delivery [4].

To this extent, incorporating AI into the medical curriculum is more than just staying current with technology. Future clinicians should also be prepared to practice in a healthcare environment where digital tools play an increasingly central role. Equally, it can open new doors in research, innovation, and patient care, particularly when students are encouraged to engage critically and ethically with these technologies.

Despite the advantages, integrating AI into medical education has some challenges. Medical curricula are already densely packed, and adding new content often raises students' resistance, not because it is unimportant, but because faculty and institutions may lack the expertise or capacity to teach it effectively [3]. Technology also evolves rapidly, making it difficult for course content to keep pace. At the same time, many students use AI appropriately and effectively, sometimes finding themselves ahead of their institutions in expectations and readiness. Another concern is access to AI. Ideally, all students, regardless of where they study, should benefit from advances in AI education. Disparities in infrastructure, funding, and faculty development create significant differences in AI opportunities across schools. There are also important ethical dimensions to consider. AI tools can carry some biases, and their decision-making processes may not be clear. Students must understand these risks and learn how to apply AI in ways that are transparent, respectful of privacy, and aligned with values such as equity, fairness, and dignity [5].

Considering both the potential and the challenges involved, educators are now working to incorporate AI-related content into their teaching. There is a growing consensus that future medical professionals need more than just technical knowledge of AI; they must understand how AI functions, how to apply it responsibly, and when it is inappropriate to trust it. Medical education must ensure that graduates are confident in using AI to enhance care, without losing sight of the human judgment and ethical principles that remain at the heart of clinical practice.

This chapter discusses practical strategies, case studies, and curriculum development models that illustrate how AI can be thoughtfully embedded into medical education.

28.2 Core AI Competencies and Curriculum Frameworks

As medical schools begin to consider how to teach AI, a growing number of educators and organizations have developed competency frameworks to guide curriculum planning. These models offer structured approaches to help define what future physicians should understand about AI, machine learning (ML), and related fields. Despite differences in terminology or emphasis, many of these frameworks share common elements, such as the basics of AI and ML concepts, an introduction to data science and statistics, an understanding of how to evaluate AI tools, insight into clinical applications, and a focus on ethical and governance issues.

One well-known proposal by Schubert et al. (2025) outlines three levels of AI competence for clinicians: basic, proficient, and expert. These levels reflect the varying roles physicians might play concerning AI. In the *Basic level*, students should be able to use AI tools responsibly and understand their limitations. In the *Proficient level, the* clinician goes a step further, learning how to critically evaluate the outputs of algorithms, including performance measures and potential biases, and in the *Expert level*, physicians are expected to combine a strong technical background with clinical experience, allowing them to contribute to the design and implementation of new AI solutions [2].

Another model, developed in Singapore, classifies learners as consumers, translators, or developers [6]. *Consumers*: All physicians are considered consumers, meaning they need to use AI safely in practice. *Translators*: Some will become translators who help bridge the gap between data science and clinical care, and adapt existing tools for new contexts. *Developers*: A smaller group may take on the developer role, designing and building AI systems from the ground up.

These models highlight an important idea: not every medical student needs to become a programmer, but all should reach a level of fluency that allows them to assess and apply AI tools appropriately. Curriculum development should often address these levels of expertise.

Most of these frameworks begin by outlining the rationale for including AI in the medical curriculum, followed by clear learning objectives and suggested topics. They also recommend organizing content either chronologically (by year) or thematically (by domain), and offer guidance on instructional methods, from lectures and flipped classrooms to project-based learning and interdisciplinary workshops [7]. In a model proposed topics include:

Technical basics: fundamentals of data science, machine learning models, and statistical reasoning.
Clinical applications: examples where AI is used to show relevance.
Critical appraisal: interpreting AI performance and understanding how algorithms are trained and validated.
Ethics and policy: covering patient privacy, algorithmic fairness or bias, informed consent, accountability, and medico-legal responsibilities with AI use.
Hands-on skills: basic programming or data analysis tools, using AI software, or interacting with AI platforms in practical exercises.
Interdisciplinary collaboration: understanding the workflow between clinicians, data scientists, and engineers [7].

A study in 2024 aimed to define medical AI competencies for medical graduates in South Korea. They identified six core competency domains: "(1) understanding digital health and changes driven by AI; (2) fundamental knowledge and skills in medical AI; (3) ethics and legal aspects in the use of medical AI; (4) medical AI application in clinical practice; (5) processing, analyzing, and evaluating medical data; and (6) research and development of medical AI" [8]. The Medical Schools Council report emphasizes that data science and AI training should integrate health informatics, data governance, and digital professionalism, linking these digital health competencies into medical curricula [9].

In conclusion, curricula should treat AI both as a tool to be embedded in problem-solving exercises and as a topic to be taught theoretically and practically.

28.3 Educational Approach and Strategies

Medical schools are deploying multiple strategies to incorporate AI education into their curricula. This will occur both longitudinally, through the gradual introduction of AI concepts throughout the academic journey, and horizontally, via dedicated training modules. Strategies may include dedicated courses, integrated sessions, electives, dual-degree tracks, and interdisciplinary collaboration (projects).

28.3.1 Standalone Courses and Electives

One of the most common ways medical schools have begun integrating AI into their programs is through standalone courses and elective modules. Some institutions have taken the lead by embedding AI education into existing academic tracks. For instance, Harvard's Health Sciences & Technology program includes a one-month introductory course focused specifically on the role of AI in healthcare. Similarly, the Long School of Medicine in Texas has introduced electives on generative AI and the fundamental principles of machine learning, targeting first- and second-year students. At George Washington University, a two-week elective module entitled "AI Applications in Healthcare" is available to senior medical students. This course combines lectures with real-world case studies to explore how AI is used in diagnostics and medical research [3]. In Singapore, the Yong Loo Lin School of Medicine at the National University of Singapore offers a Minor in Biomedical Informatics, open to all undergraduate students. This program delivers education in data science, artificial intelligence, and digital tools specifically for healthcare, equipping students for both clinical and research roles [6]. Duke University has introduced a dedicated machine learning course for medical students, providing hands-on experience with algorithms and data interpretation. AI modules are increasingly delivered in radiology and pathology residency programs, where image analysis plays a central role and AI tools are rapidly becoming part of standard practice [7]. Likewise, at Tehran University of Medical Sciences, foundational principles of AI are taught within a broader course on health technology and informatics.

To sum up, most identified educational efforts in AI take the form of structured courses. A recent review showed that approximately half of all AI-related programs in medical education are delivered as formal courses, often supplemented with workshops, independent projects, or research opportunities [7].

28.3.2 Integration into the Existing Curriculum

In many cases, AI is integrated into standard coursework. Instead of introducing entirely new subjects, some programs are integrating AI-related content into existing clinical and scientific learning activities. For example, clinical reasoning sessions may now include scenarios where students interpret or evaluate AI-assisted diagnostic tools. In other settings, courses on genomics or epidemiology incorporate practical exercises that involve analyzing large datasets using AI methods. A class discussion on medical ethics might now include a session on the implications of AI in clinical decision-making, touching on topics such as algorithmic bias, data privacy, and accountability [3].

28.3.3 Dual-Degree and Tracks

A few institutions are developing integrated training pathways that combine medical education with AI. These programs are designed for students who want to go beyond basic literacy and develop a deeper, more technical understanding of AI and its role in healthcare.

One example is the dual MD/MSc program at UT Health San Antonio. In this model, medical students take a break after their third year to complete a one-year master's degree in AI, then return to finish their final year of clinical training. Harvard Medical School also supports students interested in pursuing research-focused careers through a PhD track in *AI in Medicine*. This program is designed for future physician-scientists who aim to develop AI tools that can advance biomedical research and clinical decision-making. These pathways prepare graduates to lead innovation in medicine, bridging the gap between front-line healthcare and cutting-edge technology [3].

28.3.4 Projects and Research

Another effective approach to AI education involves engaging students through hands-on projects and research. Rather than focusing solely on theory, these experiences encourage learners to apply AI concepts to real-world healthcare challenges.

At George Washington University's School of Medicine and Health Sciences, students enrolled in an AI elective complete the course by working on individual or group projects. The goal is not only to help students understand how AI can be used in clinical settings, but also to explore its limitations and ethical implications, especially regarding fairness and health equity.

Other schools have taken creative approaches by organizing AI-themed hackathons, where students collaborate to design digital tools that address specific problems in patient care. In some regions, such as Hong Kong and parts of Asia, student-led capstone projects have begun to focus on connecting AI applications with evidence-based medicine, offering a practical, research-oriented perspective on emerging technologies [6].

28.3.5 Interdisciplinary and Co-curricular Programs

Integrating AI into medical education often requires collaboration beyond the boundaries of traditional medical curricula. At many universities, medical students are encouraged to take courses in AI, data science, or machine learning through departments such as computer science, engineering, or public health. This cross-disciplinary approach not only broadens students' perspectives but also fosters essential skills for working in data-driven healthcare environments.

Duke University's "Machine Learning School" offers specialized training courses tailored for medical students, demonstrating an early commitment to interdisciplinary education in this area [7]. Similarly, some institutions promote joint seminars, collaborative projects, or shared research opportunities that bring together clinicians, AI scientists, and data engineers [6]. These collaborative experiences help bridge knowledge gaps, foster mutual understanding, and prepare future professionals to work effectively in multidisciplinary teams, a crucial skill in the evolving landscape of digital healthcare.

28.3.6 Continuing Medical Education (CME)

AI education doesn't stop at the undergraduate or postgraduate level. As technology continues to evolve, many institutions have begun offering CME opportunities to help practicing physicians stay up to date with developments in the field. The Accreditation Council for Continuing Medical Education includes sessions on AI at its annual meetings, focusing on how these technologies are shaping clinical practice and professional competencies [10]. Similarly, leading medical associations and scientific conferences now feature dedicated workshops, webinars, and online modules aimed at familiarizing clinicians with AI tools and their practical applications.

The American Medical Association offers CME-accredited courses that explore the clinical impact of AI, from diagnostic support to workflow efficiency and ethical considerations [11]. These programs play a vital role in helping healthcare professionals and faculty members adapt to new technologies, ensuring they can use AI effectively while maintaining high standards of care and professional judgment.

The authors of this chapter designed a faculty development AI training program at Tehran University of Medical Sciences. The topics developed through a census among AI experts are shown in Table 28.1.

In many medical schools, a common approach begins in the early years with foundational lectures on data science, algorithmic thinking, and the basics of machine learning, often introduced alongside subjects like biostatistics. As students move into the clinical phase, these concepts are reinforced through case-based discussions, where AI tools are presented in the context of diagnosis, treatment planning, or decision support. In the later years of training, students may have the opportunity to explore AI in greater depth through electives, research projects, or capstone experiences. These formats encourage hands-on application and independent inquiry, allowing learners to connect technical knowledge with real-world clinical challenges.

Table 28.1 Main topics of a comprehensive faculty development program

Title	Topics
Introduction and Overview of AI	General concepts, definitions, history, and applications of AI in medicine
A Global Perspective on University Responses to Chatbots	Evolution of natural and large language models
Machine Learning and Neural Networks	Fundamentals of machine learning and an introduction to neural networks
Natural Language Processing (NLP) – Part 1	Overview of large language models, their applications, and principles of effective prompt engineering
Natural Language Processing (NLP) – Part 2	Fine-tuning and model enhancement using Retrieval-Augmented Generation (RAG)
Image Processing and Its Applications	Image recognition techniques and their medical applications
Big Data and Data Analysis	Big data and analytical techniques in medicine and advanced tools for medical data mining
Clinical Applications of Artificial Intelligence	Use of AI in clinical practice
Applications of AI in Pharmaceutical Sciences and Biotechnology	Use of AI in drug development and biotech research
Applications of AI in Research	AI-driven approaches in scientific research
Applications of AI in Education	Integration of AI in teaching and learning environments
Ethics and Regulations in AI	Ethical issues and regulatory frameworks related to AI

To support this longitudinal integration, curriculum committees are increasingly turning to interdisciplinary faculty, including experts from computer science, engineering, and bioinformatics, to help ensure that AI content is thoughtfully sequenced and clinically relevant. A recent scoping review identified AI-related programs in a wide range of countries, such as the United States, Canada, Australia, Germany, and China. However, these initiatives often remain fragmented, with no single model or unified curriculum guiding implementation across regions [1].

28.4 Challenges to Implementing AI Education in Medical Schools

While there is growing interest in incorporating AI into medical education, turning that enthusiasm into practical curriculum changes is far from straightforward [12]. One of the most significant barriers is faculty readiness. Many educators today completed their training long before AI became relevant to clinical care. As a result, they may feel underprepared or lack confidence in teaching these topics. Meanwhile, students are often more familiar with digital tools and increasingly eager to explore AI, creating a noticeable gap between learner expectations and faculty expertise.

Curriculum overload is another key concern. Medical programs are already densely packed, leaving little room for new material. To manage this, some schools have chosen to embed AI concepts into existing courses, rather than adding standalone sessions. Others offer AI content as electives, micro-credentials, or optional certificate programs, allowing interested students to explore the topic in more depth without displacing essential content.

Resource availability can also limit implementation. Not all medical schools have access to high-performance computing infrastructure or AI labs. Institutions in low-resource settings may need to rely on affordable or cloud-based platforms to introduce AI education. Beyond infrastructure, local healthcare needs and systems vary, making a one-size-fits-all approach to curriculum design unlikely to succeed [2].

Finally, tools and platforms evolve quickly, and teaching materials can become outdated within months. For this reason, AI education should focus on core principles rather than specific software or tools. The goal is to equip students with adaptable skills that will remain relevant, even as the technology continues to evolve.

28.5 Instructional Methods

Considering the challenges and opportunities outlined above, effective teaching of AI in medical education often requires a combination of approaches. No single method is sufficient on its own. Key methods beyond lectures may include the following:

Blended learning modules: E-contents and interactive modules on AI basics let students learn at their own pace. These modules can free up in-class time for discussion.

Case-based learning and Problem-Based Learning: Embedding AI into clinical cases helps contextualize concepts. A problem-based learning scenario might present a patient and ask students how AI could assist in diagnosis or prognosis. Students learn by actively discussing the pros and cons of AI in that context.

Project work: Encouraging student projects or hackathons on real clinical data helps enhance skills. A project might involve evaluating a published AI tool or training a simple model on open datasets.

Interprofessional collaboration: Joint workshops with engineering or computer science departments build teamwork and bring technical expertise. A medical school might co-host a seminar series on AI with an engineering faculty.

Use of AI tools in teaching: Interestingly, AI itself can be used as a teaching aid. Some courses allow students to experiment with Chatbots or AI-based anatomy tutors under supervision. By treating AI as a digital study partner, educators can demonstrate its strengths and weaknesses in real time.

Institutions should invest in training faculty through seminars or sabbaticals in AI, too. Some schools have appointed new AI education leaders or committees to drive curriculum changes. Formalizing AI competencies in program objectives ensures accountability, and including AI knowledge in accreditation learning outcome documents elevates its priority.

28.6 Conclusion

AI has become an integral part of healthcare, influencing the delivery of care. As a result, medical education must evolve to prepare future clinicians for this new reality. Around the world, leading medical schools are shifting from concern about AI's impact to actively teaching its principles and applications [3]. A well-rounded AI curriculum is becoming essential at all stages of medical education.

Embedding AI into medical education requires a multidisciplinary approach, drawing on expertise from medicine, data science, and ethics. It also demands institutional commitment from updating content regularly to training faculty and building cross-departmental partnerships. When thoughtfully integrated, AI education empowers learners to engage with emerging tools in a way that enhances, rather than replaces, clinical judgment.

The goal is not to turn every student into a data scientist, but to ensure that all future clinicians are AI-literate: capable of understanding how AI works, evaluating its outputs critically, and using it responsibly to improve patient care [13]. Ultimately, AI literacy is becoming a core competency in the medical field. Through deliberate, forward-looking education, institutions can equip the next generation of physicians not only to keep pace with technological change, but also to lead it responsibly.

Acknowledgement We acknowledge the use of ChatGPT (OpenAI, July 2025 version, https://chat.openai.com) and Grammarly (https://www.grammarly.com/) for editing and refining the English language in this chapter. All suggestions were reviewed, and the final text reflects our scholarly voice.

References

1. Rincón EH, Jimenez D, Aguilar LA, Flórez JM, Tapia ÁE, Peñuela CL. Mapping the use of artificial intelligence in medical education: a scoping review. BMC Med Educ. 2025;25(1):526.
2. Schubert T, Oosterlinck T, Stevens RD, Maxwell PH, van der Schaar M. AI education for clinicians. EClinicalMedicine. 2025;79:102968.
3. Boyle P. Medical schools move from worrying about AI to teaching it. Association of American Medical Colleges (AAMC); 2025. [cited 2025 Aug 15]. Available from: https://www.aamc.org/news/medical-schools-move-worrying-about-ai-teaching-it.
4. Duan S, Liu C, Rong T, Zhao Y, Liu B. Integrating AI in medical education: a comprehensive study of medical students' attitudes, concerns, and behavioral intentions. BMC Med Educ. 2025;25(1):599.
5. Bouderhem R. Shaping the future of AI in healthcare through ethics and governance. Humanit Soc Sci Commun. 2024;11(1):1–2.
6. Ng FY, Thirunavukarasu AJ, Cheng H, Tan TF, Gutierrez L, Lan Y, Ong JC, Chong YS, Ngiam KY, Ho D, Wong TY. Artificial intelligence education: an evidence-based medicine approach for consumers, translators, and developers. Cell Rep Med. 2023;4(10):101230.
7. Tolentino R, Baradaran A, Gore G, Pluye P, Abbasgholizadeh-Rahimi S. Curriculum frameworks and educational programs in AI for medical students, residents, and practicing physicians: scoping review. JMIR Med Educ. 2024;10(1):e54793.
8. Lee YM, Kim S, Lee YH, Kim HS, Seo SW, Kim H, Kim KJ. Defining medical AI competencies for medical school graduates: outcomes of a Delphi survey and medical student/educator questionnaire of South Korean medical schools. Acad Med. 2024;99(5):524–33.
9. Car J, Ong QC, Fox TE, Leightley D, Kemp SJ, Švab I, Tsoi KK, Sam AH, Kent FM, Hertelendy AJ, Longhurst CA. The digital health competencies in medical education framework: an international consensus statement based on a Delphi study. JAMA Netw Open. 2025;8(1):e2453131.
10. CMEHappenings. The AI revolution: a hot topic @ ACCME's 2024 annual meeting. UConn Health; 2024. [cited 2025 Aug 15]. Available from: https://health.uconn.edu/continuing-medical-education/wp-content/uploads/sites/21/2024/07/CME-Newsletter_July-2024.pdf.
11. AMA. Advancing AI in medical education through ethics, evidence and equity. American Medical Association; 2023. [cited 2025 Aug 15]. Available from: https://www.ama-assn.org/practice-management/digital-health/advancing-ai-medical-education-through-ethics-evidence-and-equity.
12. Triola MM, Rodman A. Integrating generative artificial intelligence into medical education: curriculum, policy, and governance strategies. Acad Med. 2024;100:10–97.
13. Pucchio A, Eisenhauer EA, Moraes FY. Medical students need artificial intelligence and machine learning training. Nat Biotechnol. 2021;39(3):388–9.

29 Ethical Principles of the Use of AI in Teaching and Learning in Clinical Fields

Shabih Zaidi and Hasnain Zafar Baloch

Key Points

- Artificial intelligence in healthcare is aiding diagnoses and clinical practice.
- Moral integrity is an attribute of ethical practice reflecting steadfast adherence to moral standards.
- Safety and health refer to the actions taken for protection of health and wellness.
- Data safety refers to protecting data from loss, misuse, or threats.
- Social responsibility, accountability, and transparency are three pillars of fairness in distributive justice.

29.1 Introduction

The exponential growth of knowledge and skills in the last couple of decades has had a profound effect on medical sciences. One such transformative innovation is artificial intelligence. It is already embedded in medical education at all levels. Physicians can revolutionize patient care by integrating artificial intelligence (AI) into healthcare, enhancing diagnostic accuracy, and streamlining administrative processes, for example, AI assists administrators in scheduling appointments and recommending precise customized treatments and medications. In certain hospitals, management has been, with informed consent, using AI to transcribe conversations

S. Zaidi
al-Sadiq International Virtual University, London, UK

H. Z. Baloch (✉)
Digital Learning, Teaching and Learning, MILA University, Nilai, Malaysia

Medical Education and Emerging Technologies, Smart University of Medical Sciences, Tehran, Iran
e-mail: hasnainzafar@imu.edu.my

J. Sandars et al. (eds.), *Modern Medical Education*,
https://doi.org/10.1007/978-3-032-27958-3_29

between clinical staff and patients and then automating clinical documentation [1]. These systems can then translate records into local languages to improve understanding for patients and their families. These systems also allow clinicians to spend more time with patients.

However, this transformative technology raises significant ethical considerations that must be carefully addressed to ensure responsible and equitable use in both medical education and healthcare. The future promises extraordinary, even mind-boggling applications of AI in these fields. Combined with human intelligence, AI has the potential to alleviate numerous medical challenges. However, this makes incorporating ethics into the curricula more urgent than ever before.

Moral philosophy is the mother of ethics, which introduces and defines the doctrines and theories of doing good and avoiding evil. When applied to medicine, medical education, nursing care, and healthcare in general, it is called bioethics. The founding principles of medical ethics are universal such as truth, honesty, fair play, equity, equality, and justice. However, in certain situations, culture, faith, and local practices can impact ethical judgement. The four recognized normative principles of Western bioethics are autonomy, beneficence, nonmaleficence, and justice, as described by Beauchamp and Childress [2].

29.1.1 Autonomy

Autonomy is the first guiding principle in healthcare, which has increasingly gained importance since the appreciation and application of human rights in the last few decades. Informed consent is the backbone of autonomy. It becomes a complex issue in the context of AI in healthcare. AI platforms need to clearly state who is the owner of the information and the purpose for the collection of information and ensure that data is securely stored. The patients need to be adequately informed about how AI tools are used in their care, including the risks and benefits associated with these technologies. The challenge lies in explaining AI processes in a manner that is comprehensible to patients, who may not have a technical background. Ensuring that patients understand the implications of AI in their informed decision-making is vital for maintaining autonomy in their healthcare choices.

29.1.2 Human Dignity

The Human Rights Act 1998 asserts that every human being is fully entitled to possess a range of fundamental rights, including the rights to life, freedom from torture, slavery, and forced labor, the right to liberty and security, the right to a fair trial, and the right to work and education [3]—in one word, human dignity.

It is feared that the adoption of AI in education as well as healthcare can lead to concerns about the dehumanization of patient care. While AI can enhance efficiency and accuracy, there is a risk that the human touch in healthcare may be compromised. Patients often value empathy and understanding that come from human providers, and reliance on AI could lead to a more transactional approach to healthcare. Maintaining a balance between technological advancement and the humanistic aspects of patient care is crucial in preserving the quality of care. So, in matters related to end-of-life care, even the most seasoned physicians may find themselves cornered by family pressure, such as whether to assist the prolongation of life in a brain-dead patient. AI will fail to make decisions with empathy, sympathy, sensitivity, practicality, cost-versus-benefit analysis, emotional and economic matters, etc. If the medical students are not taught medical ethics at the undergraduate level, they may fail to appreciate the ethical use of AI in their practical life.

29.1.3 Beneficence and Nonmaleficence

In Eastern cultures, where a patient is an integral part of a family and not just a solitary individual, beneficence may precede autonomy. Therefore, many decisions are made collectively without the full informed consent of the patient. Nonmaleficence is a corollary of beneficence. The primary goal of a physician is to treat the patient without causing harm, i.e., maleficence. AI may be used for both these principles in clinical education. It may however find it difficult to prioritize beneficence over autonomy in certain situations, thus necessitating human intervention for nuanced decision-making.

29.2 Data Governance and Protection and Ethically Handling Clinical Data with AI

Data governance in the era of AI, especially when handling clinical data, is an important area that requires careful consideration of ethical principles to ensure patient privacy, data security, and compliance with regulations [1]. The following are some key principles and practices:

29.2.1 Patient Privacy and Confidentiality

Healthcare providers need to make sure that patient data is anonymized and that privacy is maintained in compliance with regulations mentioned in Health Insurance Portability and Accountability Act (HIPAA) for the USA, General Data Protection Regulation (GDPR) for Europe, or the Personal Information Protection and Electronic Documents Act (PIPEDA) for Canada.

29.2.2 Data Security

Healthcare providers need to use strong encryption methods to protect data at storage and in transfer and to regularly update security protocols to defend against cyber threats and hacking. In this respect, transparency is necessary; providing clear explanations to patients and stakeholders about how AI algorithms make decisions, including the data used, and elaborate the complete decision-making process is highly recommended. To avoid bias and fairness, it is recommended to audit the AI models regularly and ensure they do not discriminate against any group and use diverse datasets and repeatedly monitor model performance. It is recommended to establish accountability mechanisms for decisions made by AI systems; for this, human oversight may be necessary.

29.2.3 Data Governance Practices

Medical students must learn and healthcare providers need to be aware of updates with relevant regulations and standards, such as HIPAA, GDPR, and local data protection laws, and to ensure to comply with these rules. Compliance with regulations is therefore an essential component of the ethical use of AI. This may be carried out by appointing data stewards. One needs to minimize data collection and collect only the data necessary for the intended purpose.

29.2.4 Regular Audits and Assessments

Regular audits and risk assessments are needed to identify and mitigate potential issues in data handling and AI model performance. It can be best carried out by appointing Ethics Committees or Institutional Review Boards (IBR), a common practice in all institutions.

To ensure awareness, one needs to provide training programs at medical schools and healthcare facilities emphasizing the importance of data governance and maintaining ethical principles in handling clinical data.

29.2.5 Patient Engagement

Engaging with patients and the public helps understand their concerns and expectations regarding the use of their data and AI in healthcare. Adhering to these guiding ethical principles and governance practices helps organizations build trust with patients and stakeholders, ensure compliance with regulations, and utilize AI in healthcare responsibly [4].

29.2.6 Intellectual Property Rights and Content Generation

It is a good practice to remember the "3 Cs," which are copyright, citation, and circumspection regarding privacy and confidentiality policies and quality checking generated content. Users of these systems will need to consider ethical principles irrespective of the content they are creating or analyzing with generative AI tools. There have been multiple developments related to AI since November 2024, particularly related to copyright matters. The Copyright Offices in different parts of the world have released reports on copyright issues relating to AI, and several new models and services have come out that offer better privacy than regular models [5].

29.3 Monitoring and Evaluating Large Language Models

An important aspect of AI is machine learning (ML), especially large language models (LLMs) that can rapidly analyze large amounts of data. These LLMs have become increasingly used in teaching and learning, from generative AI (such as ChatGPT and Claude) to learning analytics that identify and track performance. There are concerns about the outputs from these models, including misinformation and bias, but also their privacy, copyright, and misuse. Safeguards can be implemented in response to these concerns, such as the OSI (Open Systems Interconnection) model. This model is a network communication hierarchy with seven distinct layers. Each of these layers is responsible for different aspects of data communication. These layers are physical, data link, network, transport, session, presentation, and application. The addition of an eighth layer can manage AI traffic and provide an essential safeguard.

The AI oversight layer encompasses a multifaceted framework designed to enhance the reliability, ethical integrity, and transparency of LLMs. Foremost, real-time monitoring facilitates the continuous evaluation of AI-generated responses, enabling the identification and flagging of outputs that may be inaccurate, misleading, or ethically questionable. Advanced content filtering mechanisms serve to restrict the production of harmful or inappropriate material, including outputs associated with illegal activities, discriminatory language, or other deleterious content, thereby reinforcing adherence to both ethical and legal standards. AI is known to hallucinate, so the authors have to be quite clear in ensuring the statements for accuracy. AI cannot be held responsible for a misstatement. It can however be used for language and grammar check as English may not be the first or even the second language of a writer.

Integration of bias detection tools allows for the identification and mitigation of discriminatory or prejudicial patterns within the model's responses, promoting fairness, equity, and inclusivity. Transparency and accountability are further strengthened by the explicit disclosure to users when they are interacting with an AI system rather than a human, alongside the maintenance of comprehensive interaction logs, which provide an auditable record of the LLM's decisions and actions. Finally, the system is designed to leverage user feedback and monitoring insights to support continuous learning and iterative improvement, encompassing algorithmic refinement, knowledge base updates, and the enhancement of contextual and ethical responsiveness.

Collectively, these mechanisms can establish a robust framework that ensures responsible, reliable, and ethically grounded AI-assisted interactions, thereby fostering trust and efficacy in AI and LLM deployment.

The gateway can ensure that the AI applications adhere to ethical guidelines and comply with relevant laws and regulations. This can include guidelines on privacy, data protection, and the ethical use of AI and LLM.

By implementing a proposed AI layer or gateway to monitor and evaluate prompts and responses, organizations can help ensure that their AI systems and applications provide accurate, reliable, and ethical assistance to users. This can help build trust in AI technologies and promote their responsible use.

29.4 Ethical Guidelines for Using AI

The future of AI in health and education is bewildering, as each day opens new pathways to excel. AI helps analyze health data and medical images, enhances diagnoses, and speeds up research [4]. Since COVID-19, telehealth and telemedicine have become essential parts of healthcare. There were many instances of data breach until the General Data Protection Regulation (GDPR) was introduced in the UK [7]. According to these regulations, all personal data and the activities of foreign communities and companies are processed by the union-based data processor or controller in order to protect the information of natural persons with sufficient protection [8, 9]. In the USA, the Genetic Information Nondiscrimination Act (GINA) is an organization that prohibits employers from discriminative decisions according to the genetic health information of individuals [10]. Any form of bias or discrimination is against the fundamental principles of human rights and a violation of human dignity.

29.4.1 Privacy and Confidentiality

Privacy in healthcare means a personal space allowing everyone to live free of encroachment on their personal space. Even a husband and wife are entitled to personal space. Confidentiality, on the other hand, means personal data, which may stretch from personal details to health information, investigations and diagnostic workup, past and current management to future plan, prognosis, and expected outcome.

One of the primary ethical concerns surrounding AI in healthcare is the issue of patient privacy and data security. AI systems often rely on vast amounts of patient data for training and functioning. This data may include sensitive health information, which, if mishandled or inadequately protected, could lead to breaches of confidentiality and privacy. Healthcare organizations must ensure that robust data protection measures are in place and that patient consent is obtained for the use of their data. Additionally, transparency in how AI systems use and store data is crucial to maintain trust between patients and healthcare providers.

29.4.2 Accountability and Liability

There is also the ethical dilemma surrounding accountability and liability when AI systems are used in clinical decision-making, for instance, when an AI tool provides a recommendation that results in a negative health outcome, it raises a critical question of responsibility: Should the blame lie with the healthcare provider, the AI developer, or the institution that deployed the technology?

So, for instance, if a surgeon is performing intricate surgery in a narrow space such as the skull base, a robotic hand may be more precise than a human hand but may encounter an aberrant artery not fed into the algorithm database of the controlling AI, resulting in uncontrollable hemorrhage. So, the question is who should be responsible for the damage, even a fatality. It is a moral question which needs addressing, as the machine will only do what it is taught to do.

Establishing clear guidelines and frameworks for accountability is therefore necessary to navigate these complex situations and ensure that patients receive appropriate recourse in cases of harm.

29.4.3 Data Bias

Another significant ethical consideration is the potential for bias in AI algorithms. AI systems are only as good as the data they are trained on. If the training data is biased or unrepresentative of the diverse patient population, the AI may produce skewed results that disproportionately affect certain demographic groups, for instance, algorithms developed primarily on data from one ethnic group may not perform as effectively for individuals from other backgrounds. This can exacerbate existing health disparities, leading to unequal treatment outcomes. It is essential for developers and researchers to actively work toward creating inclusive datasets and to continuously evaluate AI systems for fairness and equity.

29.4.4 Justice

It is a pillar of global ethics. It is displayed in many forms such as equality, i.e., distribution of services and resources across the board in a society as is the fundamental principle of social justice [11]. It may be sometimes modified to equity, i.e., to give according to the needs, thus maximizing the resources as was seen during the pandemic in the distribution of ventilators and oxygen following the principles of utilitarianism [12]. These are good examples of distributive justice seen in clinical education and health services. Sometimes, retributive justice is employed such as someone making a mistake or falling short of an accepted standard, requiring retraining or reeducation. Punitive justice, another form of justice, is seen in case of a mistake, a blunder, a technical glitch leading to liability and legal issues. The human mind can differentiate and execute these subtle applications of justice in healthcare. AI will need to be meticulously designed to do the same, raising many ethical questions as machines are emotionless.

29.4.5 Clinical Education

The integration of AI and online learning platforms in medical education presents various opportunities and challenges. As educators and institutions incorporate new technologies, understanding the ethical implications is essential for creating a responsible and effective learning environment.

Let us examine the ethical considerations associated with these advancements, highlighting the necessity of upholding integrity, equity, and patient-centered care in medical training.

Since the COVID-19 pandemic, traditional clinical education has shifted from face-to-face instruction and bedside teaching to simulations, flipped classrooms, and virtual methods. Artificial intelligence now supports these new approaches and is shaping the future of medical training, moving pedagogy toward "technology." Although AI is still developing, it has already changed clinical education and may eventually replace older practices. Health professionals must adapt to these technologies to stay relevant, and ethical guidelines to incorporate AI in healthcare are part of medical education.

With AI and online learning becoming integral to medical education, prioritizing data privacy, addressing algorithmic bias, and promoting equity are essential. While AI offers benefits such as personalized learning and advanced simulations, it also introduces challenges like protecting confidentiality and ensuring fair outcomes to avoid perpetuating disparities.

The principle of equity may be employed so that AI-assisted educational tools may reach out to the less advantaged pupils who may not have access or may not be so tech-savvy [6]. Medical educators should create a system that not only leverages cutting-edge technology but also remains committed to the foundational principles of healthcare, such as compassion, fairness, and integrity [5].

29.5 Conclusion

While the use of AI in medical education and its applied form in healthcare holds immense promises for improving patient outcomes and optimizing healthcare delivery, it is accompanied by a myriad of ethical challenges that must be addressed. Ensuring patient privacy, mitigating bias, obtaining informed consent, clarifying accountability, and preserving the human element in care are all critical considerations. As the healthcare landscape continues to evolve with the incorporation of AI technologies, stakeholders must engage in ongoing dialogue and collaboration to establish ethical frameworks that prioritize patient welfare and equity in healthcare. By doing so, clinicians can harness the power of AI responsibly and effectively, ultimately enhancing the quality of care for all patients. And in order to succeed in ethically harnessing the AI technology, it is essential that medical ethics is fully incorporated in undergraduate interprofessional curricula.

References

1. World Health Organization. Ethics and governance of artificial intelligence for health: guidance on large multi-modal models. World Health Organization; 2024. https://www.who.int/publications/i/item/9789240084759
2. Beauchamp TL, Childress JF. Principles of biomedical ethics. New York: Oxford University Press; 1979.
3. Human Rights Act 1998. London: The Stationery Office; 1998.
4. Smith H, Downer J, Ives J. Clinicians and AI use: where is the professional guidance? Journal of Medical Ethics. 2024;50(6):437–41.
5. Farhud DD, Zokaei S. Ethical issues of Artificial Intelligence in medicine and healthcare. Iran J Public Health. 2021;50(11):i–v. https://doi.org/10.18502/ijph.v50i11.7600. PMID: 35223619; PMCID: PMC8826344
6. Ministry of Science, Technology, and Innovation. Artificial Intelligence governance and ethics guidelines (AIGE): the national guidelines on AI governance and ethics; 2024. https://mastic.mosti.gov.my/publication/the-national-guidelines-on-ai-governance-ethics/
7. Health Education England, & NHS AI Lab. Understanding healthcare workers' confidence in AI. NHS Transformation Directorate; 2022.
8. World Health Organization. Regulatory considerations on artificial intelligence for health. World Health Organization; 2023. https://iris.who.int/handle/10665/373421
9. UNESCO. AI competency framework for teachers. 2024 [cited 2025 June 16]. Available from: https://doi.org/10.54675/ZJTE2084
10. European Parliament, Council of the European Union. Regulation (EU) 2016/679 of the European Parliament and of the Council of 27 April 2016 on the protection of natural persons with regard to the processing of personal data and on the free movement of such data, and repealing Directive 95/46/EC. 2016. Available from: https://eur-lex.europa.eu/eli/reg/2016/679/oj
11. American Society of Human Genetics. The Genetic Information Nondiscrimination Act (GINA) [Internet]. [cited 2025 June 17]. Available from: https://www.ashg.org/advocacy/gina/
12. Ekmekci PE, Arda B. Enhancing John Rawls's theory of justice to cover health and social determinants of health. Acta Bioeth. 2015;21(2):227–36. https://doi.org/10.4067/S1726-569X2015000200009. PMID: 27340331; PMCID: PMC4915381

Developing Contextual, Evidence-Based, and Consensus-Based Guidelines for the Judicious Use of AI in Medical Education

30

Lubna Ansari Baig, Mahwish Arooj, and Saima Chaudhry

Key Points

- Recommendation for the development of contextual and ethical AI policies for its judicious use.
- Involvement of all stakeholders is critical for policy development and its ownership.
- An eight-step model is proposed for developing policies using Nominal Group Technique.
- Policies should be evidence-based, inclusive, and reviewed periodically.

30.1 Introduction

With the massive development of artificial intelligence (AI) and its widespread use by healthcare practitioners and students, there is an urgent need to have policies ensuring safety of all [1]. We are living in the age of AI, moving from fourth to fifth industrial revolution where man and machine are working together for all practical purposes [2]. However, those who have actually worked with technology are now

L. A. Baig (✉)
University College of Medicine and Dentistry, The University of Lahore, Lahore, Pakistan

Department of Educational Development, The Aga Khan University, Karachi, Pakistan

M. Arooj
University College of Medicine and Dentistry, The University of Lahore, Lahore, Pakistan
e-mail: mahwish@uol.edu.pk

S. Chaudhry
Centre for Health Professionals Development and Lifelong learning, The University of Lahore, Lahore, Pakistan
e-mail: saima.chaudhry@chpl.uol.edu.pk

J. Sandars et al. (eds.), *Modern Medical Education*,
https://doi.org/10.1007/978-3-032-27958-3_30

wondering if we are placing AI too high on the intelligence ladder if we think it will replace natural intelligence [3]. This school of thought believes that all AI is capable of is augmenting the current intelligence of the collective and in turn leaving more time and space for creativity and innovation.

No matter which school of thought we approach the era of the AI, has proven to be influential in all fields including education [4]. History guides us that the impact can both be positive and negative and and harm can be mitigated by appropriate design strategies [5]. This has led to all involved in healthcare and health professions education to start a dialogue regarding the rules, regulations, policies, and procedures for the use of AI that is more beneficial than harmful. Healthcare professionals' training is grounded in mantras of patient safety and confidentiality which are the two most important areas that are expected to be threatened by the non-judicious use of AI [1, 2]. Training of health professionals directly impacts health care practices. A well trained, skilled, safe health care practitioners can raise the standard of care and minimize harm if technology is used judiciously; particularly in this era of massive explosion of AI. The term judicious use of AI, means careful, responsible, ethical and intelligible application of AI technologies for health professions education and health care. This involves aligning AI with societal values and ethical principles, ensuring that systems are valid and reliable [6].

Digital citizenship is a concept well understood in the global north while in the global south, most of the population have a limited comprehension of the importance of digital safety and accountability [7]. These concerns about digital safety have also become more to the foreground with the technology experts themselves calling for a 6 month ban to slow down the evolution of AI to be able to develop systems for enhancing its benefits and mitigating risks [8].

All professionals in healthcare and education must rise to this challenge and develop policies and guidelines based on their context to make the most efficient and effective use of AI. No matter which policy development framework is adopted, the commonality in all frameworks is the identification of the stakeholders, including technical experts both from computer sciences and health sciences, institutions, and the government [9]. This choice of stakeholders will determine the success of policy implementation since having the right team is essential to understand the contextual realities of AI [10], especially when AI and its potential impact on healthcare and education is unclear [11].

Healthcare professionals and health professions educators have realized that AI and more specifically Generative Artificial Intelligence (GenAI) is being extensively used by students, faculty and practitioners [12] therefore a proactive policy for judicious use of AI is urgently needed to be developed and updated frequently given the massive growth in AI. The term judicious use of AI as it pertains to medical education refers to careful responsible, ethical and intelligent application of AI technologies to education and health care. It involves deliberate process of aligning AI systems with the fundamental values of professional integrity and ethics.

Globally the academicians, policy makers, health care providers, and all other relevant stakeholders should be vigilant, for operationalization, of AI tolls, ensuring Judicious use of AI in their context. The development of policies and guidelines can use the UNESCO, WHO, and other policy frameworks for ensuring evidence based and contextual guidelines.

While often used interchangeably it is important to differentiate between policy and guidelines as they serve distinct purposes within an organization. A policy is a formal high level statement that defines an organization's principles and rules for a specific area of operation. It provides mandatory direction and is a mining framework that ensures compliance with laws and regulations that are typically developed and approved by senior leadership or governing bodies and often carry consequences. Whereas guidelines are a set of recommendations of best practices designed to help individuals or teams to achieve objectives of the policies. They provide flexibility and practical advice allowing for a degree of professional judgment in their applications. Guidelines are generally not mandatory as the policies are.

Most policy documents have discussed the ethical principles for the use of AI and more specifically Gen AI [13]. Floridi [14] elaborated on the ethical use of AI with five core principles; non-maleficence, beneficence, autonomy, justice, and explicability. As AI is an extension of the digital world, these principles could provide a solid conceptual basis upon which AI policy and governance could be based in order to confront the growing risks triggered by GenAI.

30.2 Types of Policies

Before moving towards development of policies, one needs to understand how many and what types of policies are suggested in the literature. The policies most relevant to healthcare and education can be classified by response and purpose, scope and function, impact, and timeframe.

30.2.1 Response and Purpose

- Reactive Policies: These are developed due to some urgency or situation like policies developed during the COVID-19 times. These policies mostly address immediate issues however if drafted carefully long-term sustainability may be built in these policies, which is often overlooked [1, 15].
- Proactive Policies: These are generally developed ahead of any expected situation like policies related to disaster management, heat stroke, environmental exigencies. Typically they are more thoughtfully prepared taking into account all possible situations and are considered more effective and sustainable [2, 16].

30.2.2 Scope and Function

- Organizational Policies: These are mostly developed by the management of an organization and are related to internal operations, code of conduct, processes, and procedures [6].
- Regulatory Policies: They are mostly developed by higher authorities, regulatory, accrediting and controlling authorities like Pakistan Medical & Dental Council (https://pmdc.pk), Higher Education Commission (https://www.hec.gov.pk/english/Pages/default.aspx), to ensure compliance with laws and standards.

30.2.3 Impact and Timeframe

- Major Policies: These are the policies that are developed by Government or any other organization which may have a major impact on community, society, or organization. These policies are mostly long term except when it is an emergency effecting large population [15, 16].
- Minor Policies: These are developed for issues with limited impact and are mostly short termed; however they can also be long-term depending on the scope of the policy [15, 16].

30.3 Policy Development

Various models of policy development have been known for a while like, the James Anderson's Model and the Bridgman and Davis model [15, 16]. The Anderson model includes agenda setting, formulation, decision-making, implementation, and evaluation. The Bridgeman and Davis model includes: analysis, consultation, development, coordination, and evaluation. For consensus meetings Nominal group technique could be employed to ensure the scientific rigor during policy development particularly with reference to AI [17]. The model for policy development based on evidence that we are suggesting includes the following eight steps:

1. Developing a core team/steering committee for policy formulation
2. Stakeholder involvement
3. Situation analysis and evidence-based approach
4. Analysis of existing relevant policies
5. Consensus building
6. Documentation and policy formulation
7. Dissemination and operationalization
8. Review and evaluation plan

The eight steps for policy formulation are given in Fig. 30.1. For clarity of understanding the application of eight steps, we are using a case study from Pakistan as an example for development of proactive policy for the Judicious use of AI.

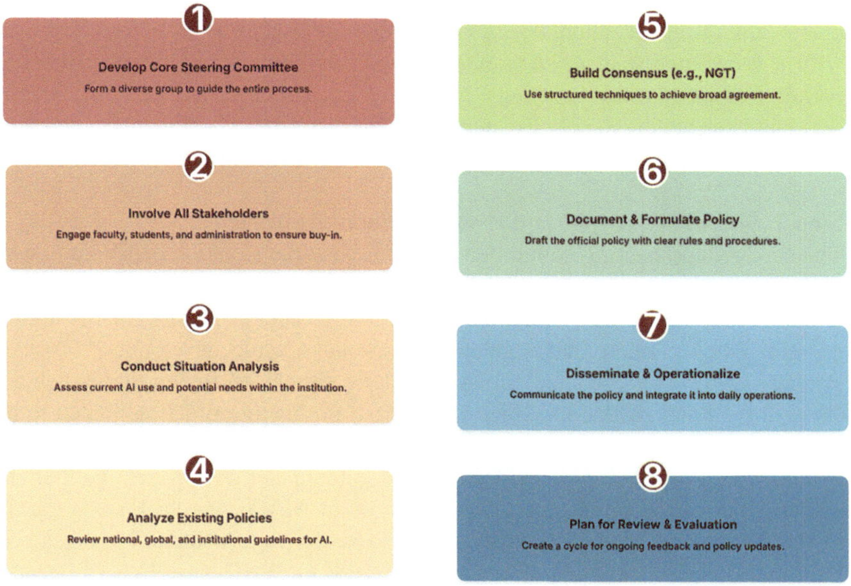
1
Develop Core Steering Committee
Form a diverse group to guide the entire process.
2
Involve All Stakeholders
Engage faculty, students, and administration to ensure buy-in.
3
Conduct Situation Analysis
Assess current AI use and potential needs within the institution.
4
Analyze Existing Policies
Review national, global, and institutional guidelines for AI.
5
Build Consensus (e.g., NGT)
Use structured techniques to achieve broad agreement.
6
Document & Formulate Policy
Draft the official policy with clear rules and procedures.
7
Disseminate & Operationalize
Communicate the policy and integrate it into daily operations.
8
Plan for Review & Evaluation
Create a cycle for ongoing feedback and policy updates.

Fig. 30.1 An eight-step framework for Generative AI Policy development in HPE

Step 1: Developing a Core Team/Steering Committee for Policy Formulation
A steering committee inclusive of relevant experts should be identified, who will take the responsibility of organizing meetings, policy review, consensus building and finalizing the policy. Before moving on to consensus building this team should develop a plan for consensus meetings and identify all major stakeholders relevant to the policy.

Example: For developing guidelines for use of AI by the Pakistan Association of Private Medical & Dental Institutions (PAMI) the core team was identified which, included professionals with major degrees in Health Professions Education and experience of over 20 years in policy development.

Step 2: Involvement of Stakeholder
Involvement of stakeholders is crucial particularly in policy development related to health care and education. (https://unesdoc.unesco.org/ark:/48223/pf0000381137). It has been mentioned in most policy development guidelines to involve stakeholders from the beginning for developing consensus-based guidelines [6, 16]. Involvement of stakeholders is essential for getting their valued opinions and later for buy-in into the policy. (https://www.who.int/publications/i/item/9789240029200) The stakeholders should include all relevant academics, experts in the relevant field henceforth, for AI it should include software engineers, programmers, developers of AI models, health care providers, and academics.

Example: For developing judicious use of AI policy, the steering committee held an initial meeting via zoom with major stakeholders from medical schools across all four provinces of Pakistan and the federal capital. These stakeholders included chairs of medical education departments with more than 10 years of experience and with a keen interest in AI. The relevant stake holders as described above were invited to the consensus meetings. Nominal Group Technique (NGT) was chosen for consensus building [17]. Broad areas for discussion and documents to be shared with the participants 1 week before the face-to-face interaction were identified.

Step 3: Situation Analysis and Evidence-Based Approach
The core groups/steering committee should review the situation depending on the policy to be developed. This aspect is often ignored in policy development as it relates to existing pending situations like cultural acceptance, political environment, present policies, rules, and regulations especially while developing "Proactive Policies" [15]. The evidence across the globe should be reviewed for policies, issues, researches related to subject of interest, in this this situation related to use and misuse of AI.

Example: For developing evidence based guidelines by PAMI, as the first step evidence across the globe regarding ethical use of AI was searched, using the following major key terms: Guidelines, Policy Development, Artificial Intelligence on PubMed, Google Scholar. The websites of UNESCO, WHO, and Higher Education Commission Pakistan were explored for general guidelines and policies. Two relevant documents were identified for providing context to participants' before the face to face meetings.

Step 4: Analysis of Existing Relevant Policies
The steering committee/core group should review all the existing policies related to: the urgency, (reactive or proactive), type of policy (major, minor), or organizational or regulatory policy. This review assists the authors to get insight in the existing policies inclusive of scope and vision of the policies and the methodologies used for development. (https://www.who.int/publications/i/item/9789241548960). The responsibility of critically reviewing the policies should be of the core group/steering committee as they are the ones ensuring scientific rigor of policy development. Once that is done it is crucial to send the reference material to the experts before the consensus meeting.

Example: For policy review the core group responsible for developing AI guidelines reviewed multiple policies and selected two documents for sharing with participants' of the consensus meeting which were most relevant. These documents included the UNESCOs document on policy guidelines (https://unesdoc.unesco.org/notice?id=p::usmarcdef_0000381137) and the Pakistan policy (https://moitt.gov.pk)) on use of AI.

Step 5: Consensus Building
There are various methods that have been used for consensus building. The core group/steering committee can decide based on their context and ease of application the moist suitable one [17]. Our suggestion is that using NGT for consensus

building is appropriate for policy development. In the NGT the following steps are to be followed:

1. Develop a core group
2. Identify the panel for consensus meetings
3. Send documents for review before the consensus meeting
4. In the meeting:
   (a) Introduction of all participants' is done with explanation of the process. The facilitator should explain the purpose of the session and explain the steps of NGT.
   (b) Silent idea generation: the participants are asked to independently write down their ideas or topics related to policies with no discussion.
   (c) Round Robin sharing of ideas: facilitator goes from one participant to another in a round robin manner and each participant gives one idea only. The process is followed for 2–3 rounds if required or any new ideas are still coming up.
   (d) Discussion and clarification of ideas: ideas are discussed for clarity and then grouped together wherever appropriate. The facilitator ensures that all participants' can clarify and also voice their views.
   (e) Ranking/voting: A criterion for ranking is agreed upon (importance, feasibility, urgency), and then voting is done either electronically or on cards.
   (f) Discussion on rankings: discussion is done openly on the rankings and adjustments can be made accordingly if required.
   (g) Final consensus: this can be done by ranking again which can be done openly as well, depending on group dynamics. The facilitator then finalizes the group consensus and shares with the group.
   (h) Report writing and documentation: The core group then finalizes the policy document and shares with the group for further clarification and confirmation. In some situation it is only shared before operationalizations.

Example: In development of the policy guidelines for AI by PAMI four consensus meetings were held in the same manner using all the above steps. An agreement of 90% of the panel was considered as a final consensus on the relevant items. The guidelines document was finalized and shared with the participants of the four panels.

Step 6: Documentation and Policy Formulation

The final document should be shared with the participants of the panel that participate in the consensus meetings, inclusive of all. Stakeholders. If no disagreements are highlighted or clarifications requested the document is finalized. In case of disagreements or clarifications, online meetings can be held for finalizing the policy document. This ensures rigor in the process and ensures that accurate information has been added as suggested in the meetings.

Example: The final policy document developed by core group of PAMI was shared with the major stakeholders, accrediting and regulating bodies inclusive of HEC and PM&DC. Following is an abridged version of those guidelines for developing policies for Judicious use of AI inclusive of suggestions for vision and scope:

Vision: To harness the transformative power of Artificial Intelligence to revolutionize healthcare and academic excellence while ensuring its responsible and ethical use.

Scope: The policy framework should provide key areas related to judicious use of AI by health care students, faculty and health care institutions (inclusive of nursing, allied health, medical and dental teaching colleges and related universities).

The guidelines for policy development had two aspects' one for the accrediting and regulating bodies and the other for institutions to develop their own contextual policies and guidelines for judicious use of AI. For regulating and accrediting bodies the suggestion was to ensure that AI based standards are added to the national accreditation framework. For the institutions the suggestion was to first develop infrastructure and acquire sufficient trained faculty competent in the use of AI, then incorporate AI detection and plagiarism tools and disclose use of AI tools. The suggestions for developing policies and guidelines for the academic and health care institutions identified the following areas that need to be targeted for judicious use of AI:

A. Curriculum framework
B. Faculty/Staff capacity Building
C. Data Governance and E-support
D. Research and Scholarship

Step 7: Dissemination and Operationalization

After finalization of the policy document, it should be shared with the stakeholders, major policy makers and implementers. World Health Organization (WHO) has recommended guiding principles for health care institutions in the member countries that focus on protecting human autonomy, promoting human safety, ensuring transparency, fostering accountability, ensuring inclusiveness and promoting AI that is sustainable (https://www.who.int/news/item/28-06-2021-who-issues-first-global-report-on-ai-in-health-and-six-guiding-principles-for-its-design-and-use). By disseminating the policy document, its transparency is ensured and more stakeholders can utilize it for the protection of health care and academics.

Example: The guidelines for developing policies for judicious use of AI were disseminated through a conference on AI jointly organized by all medical and dental colleges members of PAMI. The heads of the accrediting, regulating, and controlling authorities were invited to the conference and presented the document for operationalization. The public and private health care institution's vice chancellors, rectors, and presidents were invited for ensuring that they develop their own contextual policies and guidelines.

Step 8: Review and Evaluation Plan

Once a policy is developed it is important to ensure that an evaluation plan is built into it for quality assurance [15]. Most policies include preferable review time which is mostly 3–5 years; however for policies on AI as it is still a reactive and major policy it has to be reviewed more frequently than 3 years as the growth of AI is in leaps and bounds.

30.4 Global Applications of the Guidelines

While the eight-step model presented in this chapter uses the case of Pakistan for contextualization, its core principles and methodology are globally applicable for any institution seeking to formulate AI policies. Strength lies in its adaptability and its emphasis on a scientific consensus-based approach that transcends geographic and cultural boundaries. For instance, in regions with developing digital infrastructure, proactive policy would first need to focus on foundational digital literacy and capacity building before moving to more advanced governance principles. The process of stakeholder involvement must be sensitive to local power dynamics, cultural norms and diverse community structures. Furthermore, the emphasis on an evidence-based approach means that each region would need to conduct its own thorough analysis of its unique situation. The analysis of existing policies would, similarly, be a contextual exercise where country's national AI strategy and its broader healthcare and education regulations must be carefully considered. The consensus building method of nominal group technique is particularly valuable for its universal applicability and shows that every stakeholder regardless of their position or cultural background has an equal voice in the process. Developed under these steps, the final policy document while informed by global frameworks from organizations like UNESCO and WHO, will be a direct reflection of local needs values and priorities ensuring that it is not merely a borrowed solution but a genuine locally owned agenda. The inherent design of the framework from its focus on situation analysis to its built-in review mechanism makes it excellent and effective tool for any country or organization looking to navigate the complex and rapidly evolving landscape of AI and medical education.

30.5 Summary

World is seeing a major shift with the advancement in machine learning and generative AI models that is seeping through all systems of health professions education [18], and healthcare delivery [19] starting from basic education to advanced, basic research to clinical studies and hospital-based healthcare delivery to remote devices and home health services and monitoring. This chapter gave eight steps for developing evidence and consensus based guidelines for policy development particularly with reference to judicious use of AI in HPE.

References

1. Alowais SA, Alghamdi SS, Alsuhebany N, Alqahtani T, Alshaya AI, Almohareb SN, et al. Revolutionizing healthcare: the role of artificial intelligence in clinical practice. BMC Med Educ. 2023;23(1):689. https://link.springer.com/article/10.1186/s12909-023-04698-z.
2. Ziatdinov R, Atteraya MS, Nabiyev R. The fifth industrial revolution as a transformative step towards society 5.0. Societies. 2024;14(2):19. https://doi.org/10.3390/soc14020019.
3. Hassani H, Silva ES, Unger S, TajMazinani M, Mac FS. Artificial intelligence (AI) or intelligence augmentation (IA): what is the future? AI. 2020;1(2):8. https://doi.org/10.3390/ai1020008.
4. Sætra HS. Generative AI: here to stay, but for good? Technol Soc. 2023;75(1):102372. https://doi.org/10.1016/j.techsoc.2023.102372.
5. Kamalov F, Santandreu Calonge D, Gurrib I. New era of artificial intelligence in education: towards a sustainable multifaceted revolution. Sustainability. 2023;15(16):12451. https://doi.org/10.3390/su151612451.
6. Dignum V. Responsible artificial intelligence, from principles to practice: a keynote at the Web Conf 2022. ACM SIGIR Forum. 2023;56(1):1–6. https://doi.org/10.1145/3582524.358252.
7. Yu D, Rosenfeld H, Gupta A. The 'AI divide'between the Global North and Global South. In: World economic forum; 2023.
8. Leslie D, Perini AM. Future shock: generative AI and the international AI policy and governance crisis. Harvard Data Sci Rev. 2024;(Special Issue 5)
9. Vo V, Chen G, Aquino YS, Carter SM, Do QN, Woode ME. Multi-stakeholder preferences for the use of artificial intelligence in healthcare: a systematic review and thematic analysis. Soc Sci Med. 2023;338(1):116357. https://doi.org/10.1016/j.socscimed.2023.116357.
10. Hogg HD, Al-Zubaidy M, Technology Enhanced Macular Services Study Reference Group, Talks J, Denniston AK, Kelly CJ, Malawana J, Papoutsi C, Teare MD, Keane PA, Beyer FR. Stakeholder perspectives of clinical artificial intelligence implementation: systematic review of qualitative evidence. J Med Internet Res. 2023;25(1):e39742. https://preprints.jmir.org/preprint/39742.
11. Bekbolatova M, Mayer J, Ong CW, Toma M. Transformative potential of AI in healthcare: definitions, applications, and navigating the ethical landscape and public perspectives. Healthcare. 2024;12(2):125. https://doi.org/10.3390/healthcare12020125.
12. Sauder M, Tritsch T, Rajput V, Schwartz G, Shoja MM. Exploring generative artificial intelligence-assisted medical education: assessing case-based learning for medical students. Cureus. 2024;16(1):124. https://doi.org/10.7759/cureus.51961.
13. Sam AK, Olbrich P. The need for AI ethics in higher education. In: AI ethics in higher education: insights from Africa and beyond, vol. 21; 2023. p. 3–10.
14. Floridi L, Cowls J. A unified framework of five principles for AI in society. Mach Learn City: Appl Archit Urban Des. 2022;1(1):535–45. https://doi.org/10.1002/9781119815075.ch45.
15. Anderson JE. Chapter 1, The Study of Public Policy. In: Public policymaking: an introduction. Boston: Houghton Mifflin Company; 2003. p. 1–34.
16. Bridgman P, Davis G. The Australian policy handbook. 3rd ed. Crows Nest (AU): Allen & Unwin; 2004.
17. McMillan SS, King M, Tully MP. How to use the nominal group and Delphi techniques. Int J Clin Pharm. 2016;38(3):655–62. https://link.springer.com/article/10.1007/s11096-016-0257-x.
18. Patino GA, Amiel JM, Brown M, Lypson ML, Chan TM. The promise and perils of artificial intelligence in health professions education practice and scholarship. Acad Med. 2024;99(5):477–81. https://doi.org/10.1097/ACM.0000000000005636.
19. Zhang P, Kamel Boulos MN. Generative AI in medicine and healthcare: promises, opportunities and challenges. Futur Internet. 2023;15(9):286. https://doi.org/10.3390/fi15090286.

The Role of Artificial Intelligence in Medical Education in the Future: A Teacher or a Tool?

31

Yadolah Zarezadeh, Hasnain Zafar Baloch, and Farzad Parvizpour

Key Points

- AI is revolutionizing medical education by enhancing learning efficiency and diagnostic accuracy.
- AI technologies like machine learning, NLP, and computer vision are reshaping training for healthcare professionals.
- AI-driven adaptive learning environments personalize education based on individual learner needs.
- Ethical considerations and interdisciplinary collaboration are crucial for responsible AI integration in medical education.
- The future of AI in medical education includes AI-enabled audio learning and the rise of large language models.

31.1 Introduction

Education and technology have always been in a reciprocal relationship of shaping and reshaping one another so that it seems they are inherent parts of each other. Artificial Intelligence (AI) emerged as a technology like other promising technologies but on the contrary to its ancestors it has rapidly evolved from a theoretical concept to a practical tool revolutionizing life and all types of industries worldwide.

Y. Zarezadeh (✉) · F. Parvizpour
Department of Medical Education, Kurdistan University of Medical Sciences, Sanandaj, Iran
e-mail: farzad.parvizpour@muk.ac.ir

H. Z. Baloch
Digital Learning, Teaching and Learning, MILA University, Nilai, Malaysia

Medical Education and Emerging Technologies, Smart University of Medical Sciences, Tehran, Iran
e-mail: hasnainzafar@imu.edu.my

J. Sandars et al. (eds.), *Modern Medical Education*,
https://doi.org/10.1007/978-3-032-27958-3_31

People are increasingly using, discussing and investing on AI almost everywhere. AI is becoming the episteme of our time. Epistemes, according to Foucault (1978) [1] are implicit "rules of formation" which determine what constitutes accepted forms of knowledge for a specific cultural period. It seems Knowledge generated by AI is becoming the most valid and accepted form of knowledge in our time. Medical education is the art and science of training healthcare providers that are aimed to be able to work in the most complex situations on the most complex entities, human body, and mind. In order to overcome these complexities, medical education has always embraced new methods and technologies. This chapter explores the current and future impact of AI in medical education, highlighting key trends, innovations, and ethical considerations that will shape the next generation of healthcare training.

31.2 The Role of AI in Medical Education

AI encompasses a broad spectrum of technologies, including machine learning (ML), natural language processing (NLP), computer vision, predictive analytics, intelligent data retrieval, and more, all of which contribute to more efficient, personalized, and scalable medical education therefore it is reshaping how future physicians, nurses, and allied health professionals are trained.

The integration of AI in medical education is not a distant possibility; it is already transforming curricula, assessments, and preclinical and clinical training. The gap between theory and practice has always been one of the main concerns of medical educators [2]. By leveraging AI, educators can enhance learning efficiency, improve diagnostic accuracy, and provide immersive, real-world simulations that bridge the gap between theoretical knowledge and practical application.

31.3 The Foundation of Intelligent Systems

At its core, AI relies on algorithms and computational models that mimic human cognitive functions such as learning, reasoning, and decision-making. The most prominent AI techniques in medical education include:

1. Machine Learning (ML): ML algorithms analyze vast datasets to identify patterns, predict outcomes, and adapt over time without explicit programming. In medical education, ML can assess student performance, recommend tailored study materials, and predict areas where learners may struggle.
2. Natural Language Processing (NLP): NLP enables AI to understand, interpret, and generate human language. This is particularly useful in medical education for automated grading of essays, extracting insights from medical literature, and powering AI-driven tutoring systems that answer student queries in real time.
3. Computer Vision: AI-powered image recognition assists in diagnostic training, allowing students to analyze radiology scans, pathology slides, and other medical images with AI-guided feedback.

4. Predictive Analytics: By evaluating historical and real-time data, AI can forecast student performance, optimize curricula, and identify at-risk learners who may need additional support.

A major aim of medical education is to create Adaptive Learning Environments (ALE), which ensure optimal learning success opportunities for most students through intended and planned adaptive instructions [3]. These AI technologies work synergistically to create adaptive learning environments, where AI continuously refines educational approaches based on individual learner needs.

31.4 AI's Current Role in Medical Education

AI is already making significant contributions across multiple facets of medical education:

1. Personalized Learning Paths

Traditional medical education follows a one-size-fits-all approach, but AI enables adaptive learning systems that customize content based on a student's strengths and weaknesses. By analyzing performance data, AI can:

- Recommend specific study materials (e.g., focusing on cardiology for a student struggling with EKG interpretation).
- Adjust difficulty levels in real time to match the learner's progress.
- Predict knowledge gaps and provide targeted remediation.

2. Enhancing Diagnostic and Clinical Reasoning Skills

Acquiring knowledge, skills, and attitudes for all healthcare professionals in a safe and efficient environment has always been perused by medical educationalists [4]. AI-driven platforms like virtual patient simulations and diagnostic decision-support tools allow students to practice clinical reasoning in a risk-free environment. Examples include:

- AI-generated case studies that evolve based on student input
- Virtual standardized patients that respond dynamically to student interactions
- Automated feedback systems that highlight diagnostic errors and suggest improvements [5]

3. Self-Directed Learning and AI Tutors

AI-powered virtual tutors, such as chatbots and intelligent tutoring systems, provide instant explanations, quiz students, and guide them through complex topics. These systems use NLP to answer questions in natural language, making them accessible and intuitive [6, 7].

4. Automating Administrative Tasks

AI reduces the administrative burden on educators by:

- Grading exams and assignments automatically
- Managing student attendance and performance tracking
- Generating personalized feedback reports

This allows faculty to focus more on interactive teaching and mentorship rather than repetitive tasks [8].

31.5 The Future of AI in Medical Education

As AI technology advances, several key trends will shape its future in medical education:

1. AI-Enabled Audio Learning

Voice-assisted AI (e.g., AI-powered audiobooks, podcasts, and interactive voice response systems) will make medical education more accessible. Students can engage in hands-free learning during commutes or clinical rotations, reinforcing knowledge through auditory reinforcement [9–11].

2. Ethical and Responsible AI Integration

The increasing reliance on AI raises ethical concerns, including:

- Data privacy and security (ensuring student and patient data is protected)
- Algorithmic bias (preventing AI from perpetuating disparities in medical training)
- Professionalism in AI-augmented learning (maintaining human oversight in clinical decision-making)

Developing ethical guidelines and governance frameworks will be crucial to ensure AI is used responsibly in medical education [10, 12].

3. Interdisciplinary Collaboration for AI Implementation

Successful AI integration requires collaboration between:

- Medical educators (to define learning objectives)
- Computer scientists (to develop robust AI models)
- Ethicists and policymakers (to establish regulatory standards)

A unified approach will ensure AI tools align with educational goals while maintaining ethical integrity.

4. Investment in AI Literacy for Medical Professionals

Future healthcare providers must be proficient in AI-assisted diagnostics and treatment planning [10]. Medical schools must incorporate AI literacy into curricula, teaching students:

- How to interpret AI-generated insights
- When to rely on AI versus human judgment
- The limitations and potential biases of AI systems

5. The Rise of Large Language Models (LLMs) and Agentic AI

- Large Language Models (LLMs): Models like GPT-4 and Med-PaLM can summarize medical literature, generate case-based questions, and simulate patient interactions, providing students with an interactive learning experience [13–15].
- Agentic AI: Autonomous AI agents could soon act as virtual mentors, guiding students through clinical scenarios, offering real-time feedback, and even assisting in research by synthesizing medical data.
- Decentralization of medical education is an area where medical educators and course designers can use AI. Decentralized training courses such rural, community based, and longitudinal rural can be facilitated by AI.
- Medical education schools of thoughts, theories, models and pedagogical approaches have so far been based on human intelligence, cognition and psychology. AI can transform and expand this landscape. We may need new theories to understand and predict human–AI interaction in medical and clinical education.
- AI has started and will continue to help us to pass the language barriers. Although the publications will continue in dominant national and international languages but reading through AI translations will help all to benefit from a worldwide shared platform of knowledge [15].

31.6 Conclusion

The future of AI in medical education is not about replacing educators but augmenting their capabilities to create a more efficient, personalized, and immersive learning experience. This is what we, medical educators, like to happen. By embracing AI-powered adaptive learning, virtual simulations, and intelligent tutoring systems, medical schools can produce better-prepared, tech-savvy healthcare professionals.

However, this transformation must be approached thoughtfully, with strong ethical frameworks, interdisciplinary collaboration, and continuous investment in AI training. As AI evolves, so too must medical education—ensuring that the next generation of healthcare providers is equipped not only with medical expertise but also with the skills to harness AI's full potential responsibly. This conclusion is what we, as human medical educators and educationalists, like to happen. However the journey has just begun and the possibilities are limitless.

AI is not just the future of medical education—it is the key to unlocking a new standard of excellence in healthcare training, and like it or not, it's the future shaper of all industries including medical education. Considering the trend of evolving AI from a tool to a very sophisticated technology, in a relatively short period of time, it is predicted that AI becomes even more and more independent of human brain and command. It is likely that a form of recursive self- improvement happens in AI. There is a possibility that AI becomes a shareholder who owns part of medical education through shares of educational stocks, this may go in different directions. Based on our current understanding of the medical education and AI, there will be real challenging ethical issues to think and address in addition to moral and legal issues that need proper attention as soon as possible.

References

1. Nola R. Knowledge, discourse, power and genealogy in Foucault. Crit Rev Int Soc Pol Phil. 1998;1(2):109–54.
2. Roth WM, Mavin T, Dekker S. The theory-practice gap: epistemology, identity, and education. Education. 2014;56:521.
3. Evans-Wilson S. Examining teacher self-efficacy, collective efficacy, and job satisfaction of elementary school teachers. Wilmington University; 2021.
4. Topol EJ. Deep medicine: how artificial intelligence can make healthcare human again. Basic Books; 2019.
5. Wartman SA, Combs CD. Medical education must move from the information age to the age of artificial intelligence. Acad Med. 2018;93(8):1107–9.
6. Paranjape K, Schinkel M, Nannan Panday R, Car J, Nanayakkara P. Introducing artificial intelligence training in medical education. JMIR Med Educ. 2019;5(2):e16048.
7. Masters K. Artificial intelligence in medical education. Med Teach. 2019;41(9):976–80.
8. Kolachalama VB, Garg PS. Machine learning and medical education. NPJ Digital Med. 2018;1(1):54.
9. Lupton D. AI in the clinic: how artificial intelligence is transforming healthcare. MIT Press; 2021.
10. Chan KS, Zary N. Applications and challenges of artificial intelligence in medical education: a systematic review. JMIR Med Educ. 2019;5(2):e13930.

11. Blease C, Kharko A, Bernstein M, Bradley C, Houston M. Machine learning in medical education: a survey of the experiences and opinions of medical students in Ireland. BMJ Health & Care Inform. 2021;28(1):e100357.
12. Holmes JH, Sacchi L. Artificial intelligence in medical education: ethical considerations. Camb Q Healthc Ethics. 2022;31(2):278–86.
13. Esteva A, Chou K, Yeung S, Naik N, Madani A, Mottaghi A, et al. Deep learning-enabled medical computer vision. NPJ Digital Med. 2021;4(1):1–9.
14. Sutton RT, Pincock D, Baumgart DC, Sadowski DC, Fedorak RN, Kroeker KI. An overview of clinical decision support systems: benefits, risks, and future directions. Front Digital Health. 2020;2:61.
15. Graber ML, Byrne C. The future of AI in medical diagnosis and education. JAMA. 2023;329(10):827–8.

32 Clinical Supervision in the Era of Technology and Innovation: The InnoVISION-Framework Applied to Competency/Outcome-Based Model of Clinical Supervision (COBECS)

Tabassum Zehra

Key Points

- The advancement of technology requires clinical supervisors to engage with it as an integrated ecosystem; shaping communication, interaction, and creating new opportunities for learner growth, rather than viewing it as a set of isolated tools.
- AI Integration in clinical supervision is essential to promote digital learning environment and equip supervisors with essential digital competencies for better patient outcomes.
- The InnoVISION-COBECS framework for AI-augmented clinical supervision supports multiple dimensions of learner development and competency achievement.
- Clinical AI support tools to enhance learner performance face significant challenges including the humanistic approach to patient care and student wellbeing.
- AI augmented clinical supervision demands intentional effort and the integration of humanistic principles, which can be nurtured through diverse and well-designed combination of learning experiences.

32.1 Introduction

Clinical supervision represents a cornerstone of medical education, serving as a vital process through which medical trainees learn their profession through clinical practice alongside experienced physicians who ensure safe and timely care delivery. It involves providing structured guidance and feedback that support the trainee's personal,

T. Zehra (✉)
Medical Education and Informatics Department, College of Medicine and Health Sciences, Sultan Qaboos University, Muscat, Oman
e-mail: z.tabassum@squ.edu.om

J. Sandars et al. (eds.), *Modern Medical Education*,
https://doi.org/10.1007/978-3-032-27958-3_32

professional, and educational development, all within the context of delivering safe and appropriate patient care [1]. In medical settings, clinical supervision takes various forms, from brief discussions during ward rounds to extended reflective discussions of complex cases, encompassing day-to-day clinical case management and arising issues [2].

The conceptual framework of clinical supervision encompasses three interrelated functions that operate in tandem: the educational or formative function, which promotes learning and skill development; the supportive or restorative function, which addresses the emotional well-being and resilience of supervisees; and the managerial or normative function, which upholds the quality, accountability, and ethical standards of clinical practice. Together, these functions interact dynamically to ensure that supervision not only facilitates professional growth but also maintains safe and effective patient care [1]. Current perspectives advocate that effective supervision should be integrated into clinical care activities, adapted to the specific context of practice, rather than treated as a process separate from patient care [2, 3].

The gap in supervisor training is compounded by limited and inconsistent research, with varying definitions of clinical supervision hindering consensus and scholarly advancement. Concurrently, the field is evolving conceptually, with emerging frameworks integrating traditional supervision principles and systems psychodynamics to better support role transitions and advanced practice in complex healthcare systems. These developments underscore that clinical supervision is faced with individual and systemic challenges that continue to evolve as healthcare practice becomes increasingly complex and specialized [4].

Beyond the immediate effects of the COVID-19 pandemic, clinical supervision continues to face a range of emerging challenges that mirror the evolving landscape of healthcare practice and professional development. A key issue is the adaptation of clinical supervision model that align with the unique supervisory roles and learning preferences of the learner in the modern era. Across the literature, recurring concerns include variations in how supervision models are interpreted and the practical barriers encountered in their application [5].

Literature reports the importance of employing diverse educational modalities to promote the development of shared values, knowledge, and skills necessary for effectively working with medical students. Fostering a person-centered learning environment that addresses learners' needs, experiences, and goals is essential for cultivating patient-centered care. By actively engaging learners, respecting their perspectives, and tailoring clinical supervision to support growth, educators model empathy, collaboration, and respect; core principles of patient-centered practice. Nevertheless, evidence on patient-centered, contextually situated education for clinical supervisors remains limited [6].

32.2 Building Blocks of a Competency-Based Clinical Supervision Model

The construction of competency-based supervision models relies on established research approaches that integrate theory with practice. Studies conducted in clinical settings with learners and practicing professionals (supervisors) provide real-world insights into supervisory practices. Needs assessments within clinical contexts further identify supervision requirements by engaging professionals to reflect on current practices and articulate areas for improvement, often in a confidential manner to ensure openness. Quantitative methods, such as surveys, complement qualitative findings and enable triangulation. The most robust models synthesize evidence from these diverse sources, combining theoretical foundations with practical perspectives from both supervisors and supervisees. This multi-method approach captures the complexity of clinical supervision, linking supervisory practices to supervisee's development and patient outcomes while aligning with the principles of competency-based education [6, 7].

Competency-based clinical supervision models should be grounded in clearly defined competency frameworks that articulate learner outcomes while also setting benchmarks for supervisor development. Within this context, supervisor training is pivotal for translating competencies into effective supervisory practice, particularly through the provision of competency-focused feedback. Although frameworks such as CanMEDS and the ACGME specify the competencies residents are expected to achieve, these alone do not ensure that supervisors can provide meaningful, actionable feedback. Hence, robust supervisor training is essential. Resources like the National Clinical Supervision Competency Resource offer structured benchmarks that support both individual supervisor development and broader institutional training needs. This enables institutions to benchmark supervisor performance, diagnose individual and organizational learning needs, and design targeted training programs. In this way, the integration of structured competency frameworks into clinical supervision supported by systematic supervisor training and guided feedback processes creates a model that is both outcome-driven for learners and capacity-building for supervisors, thereby ensuring the effective implementation of competency-based residency training [5–7].

Although structured, evidence-informed, and multi-phase methodologies incorporating evidence synthesis, learner input, goal setting, design, implementation, evaluation, and feedback have been proposed, their consistent application in supervision remains limited.

32.3 The COBECS Model: Foundations and Principles

The landscape of clinical supervision is increasingly complex, with approximately 52 models currently in use [7]. However, many of these models offer limited guidance regarding their practical implementation and functioning within clinical contexts. The rapidly evolving landscape of healthcare education necessitates reimagining clinical supervision to align with technological advancements and competency-based frameworks.

The Competency/Outcomes-Based Effective Clinical Supervision (COBECS) model, along with its operational framework, was developed through the integration of findings from six key perspectives: (i) cross-sectional surveys to gather information on needs assessment, enablers and barriers in clinical supervision *(residents enrolled in postgraduate clinical specialties, clinical supervisors at Aga Khan University, Pakistan)*; (ii) focus group discussions *(residents)* (iii) clinical supervisor self-assessment of competencies (iv) extensive review of the relevant literature;

(v) resident and supervisor evaluations (vi) theoretical alignment with Socio-Cognitive Theory and Proctor's Model of Clinical Supervision (Fig. 32.1) [8].

The COBECS clinical supervision can be used to align programatic expected outcomes for the resident's level of training, fostering appropriate performance that ultimately enhances patient care. Socio-structural factors can either facilitate or impede the supervision process, influencing both resident personal and professional development and performance. The operational model of COBECS provides a structured approach that can be applied and tailored to contextual relevance and

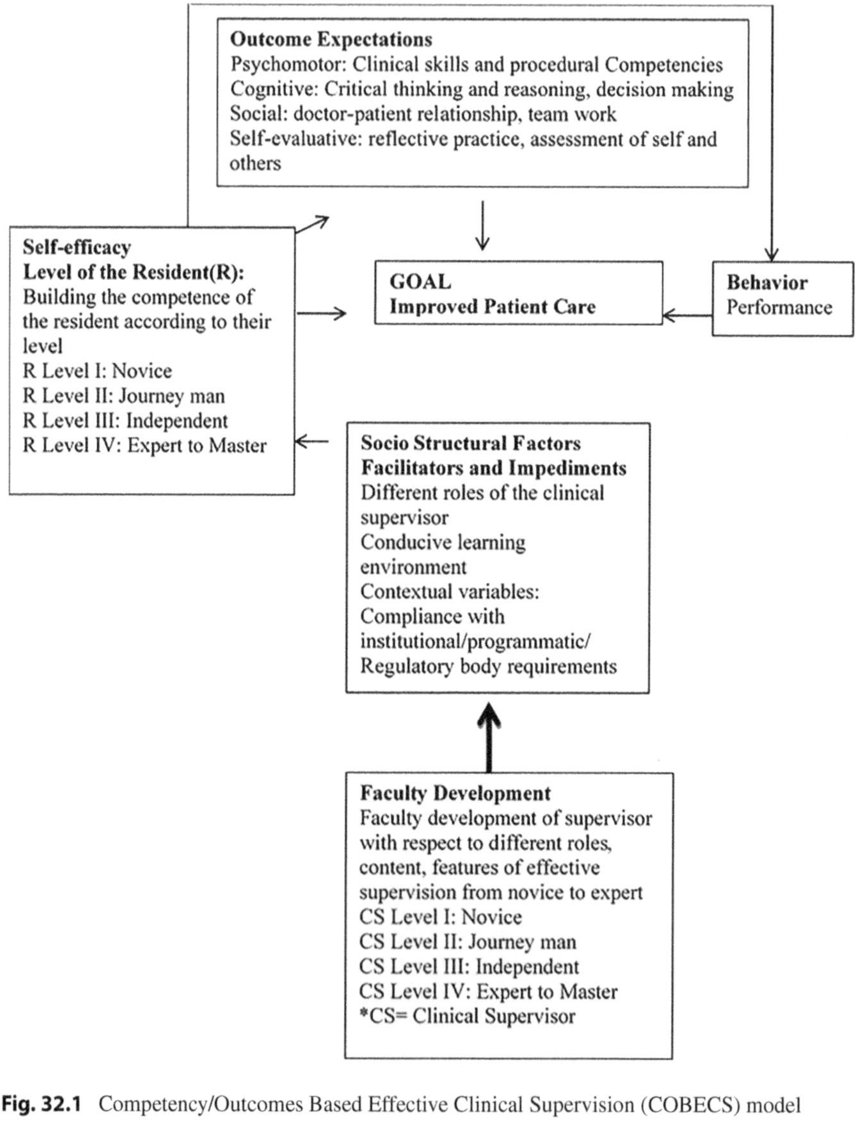

Fig. 32.1 Competency/Outcomes Based Effective Clinical Supervision (COBECS) model

programatic requirements. The implementation of clinical supervision proceeds through structured, sequential phases.

The operational model of COBECS (Fig. 32.2) is based on five main pillars of the five-dimension modeling: (I) Faculty Development of Supervisors (II) Resident-Supervisor Relationship (III) Effective Clinical Supervision Practices through assessment of resident competence with feedback, within the (IV) Socio-Structural Factors and the overall Learning Environment and (V) Self-Efficacy.

Established frameworks outline eight steps: building the supervisor–supervisee relationship, collaborative planning with the teacher, designing the observation strategy, observing instruction, analyzing the teaching–learning process and engaging in renewed planning.

Assessment tools can be utilized in the development of resident portfolios to systematically evaluate performance, monitor the attainment of expected competencies, and track progress over time aligned with competency framework. Such portfolios not only enable residents to engage in self-reflection on their performance but also provide supervisors with structured opportunities for periodic review of competence and the delivery of constructive feedback to support personal and professional growth. This process fosters a stronger resident–supervisor relationship, and collectively contributes to enhancing residents' self-efficacy.

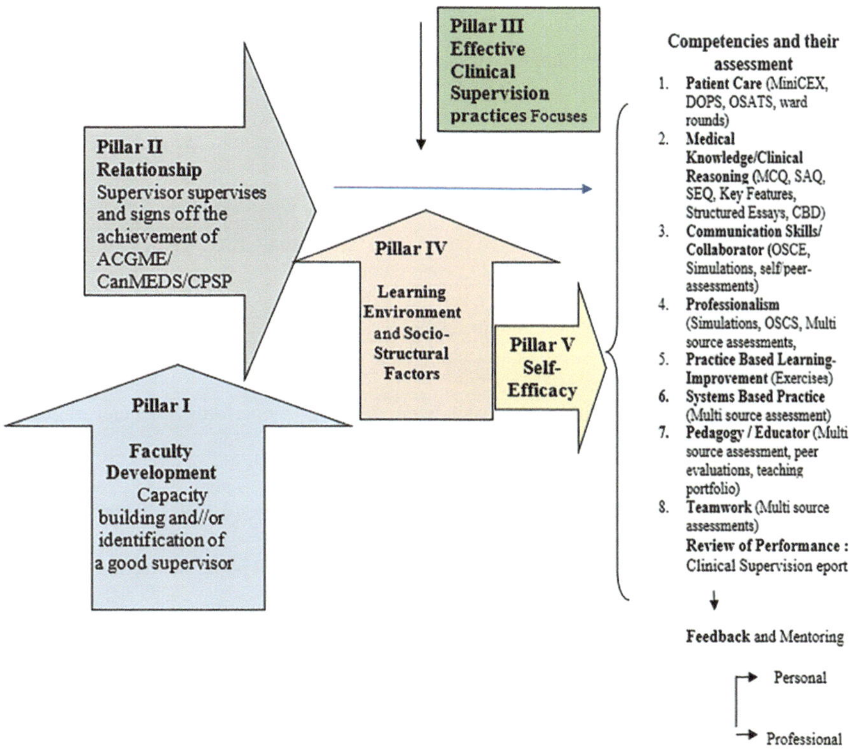

Fig. 32.2 Operational model of COBECS

32.4 COBECS Model Operational Roadmap: Practical Implementation for Clinical Supervision

The stepwise roadmap offers a structured framework for competency-based clinical supervision, integrating supervisory goals, faculty development, and assessment practices, while considering the impact of the learning environment and supervisory relationships on resident competency development and performance. This framework can be adapted to suit contextual needs and relevance.

Step 1: Faculty Development of Supervisors

Training programs	Workshops on competency-based supervision, assessment, and feedback.
Mentorship	Pair novice supervisors with experienced faculty for guidance and observation.
Continuous professional development	Online modules, reflective practice sessions, peer review.

Step 2: Strengthen Resident–Supervisor Relationships

Set clear expectations	Define roles, responsibilities, and learning goals.
Structured check-ins	Regular meetings for progress review, challenges, and guidance.
Trust-building	Promote open dialogue and psychological safety for honest feedback.

Step 3: Implement Effective Clinical Supervision Practices

Direct observation	Use structured observation tools (mini-CEX, DOPS, Case based Discussions) to assess competence.
Competency-based feedback	Deliver timely, specific, actionable feedback aligned with CanMEDS/ ACGME competencies.
Assessment integration	Use EPAs, milestones, and workplace-based assessments to monitor progress
Adaptive supervision	Tailor supervision intensity to resident performance and learning needs.

Step 4: Optimize Socio-Structural Factors and the Learning Environment

System evaluation	Review workload, staffing, and institutional policies affecting supervision.
Supportive culture	Promote teaching, collaboration, and continuous improvement.
Resource allocation	Ensure availability of clinical and educational resources.

Step 5: Promote Self-Efficacy

Supervisor development	Reflective practice, peer feedback, and skill-building exercises.
Resident empowerment	Goal-setting, self-assessment, and reflective learning
Joint reflection	Structured sessions to enhance self-awareness and professional growth.

Step 6: Integrate Assessment Tools into Learning Portfolios

Portfolio building	Residents collect workplace-based assessments (Mini-CEX, DOPS, Case based Discussions), reflective logs, and feedback notes.
Personal and professional development	Portfolios provide evidence of progress, identify gaps, and guide individualized learning plans.
Feedback loops	Supervisors review portfolios to provide targeted feedback and track competency achievement over time

Step 7: Continuous Monitoring and Evaluation

Evaluate supervision effectiveness via resident and supervisor feedback.
Track resident performance and portfolio growth to refine supervision practices.
Adjust faculty development and supervision strategies based on evaluation outcomes.

32.5 Adapting COBECS to the Digital Age: The InnoVISION Approach

The landscape of clinical supervision underwent a dramatic transformation with the onset of the COVID-19 pandemic, which necessitated a swift overnight shift from traditional in-person healthcare and training systems to telebehavioral health (TBH) platforms. The pandemic experience prompted an unprecedented and rapid shift to virtual service delivery and supervision across healthcare settings. This transition to technology-based platforms compelled healthcare organizations and educational institutions to re-evaluate traditional approaches, necessitating adaptations such as videoconferencing for establishing therapeutic alliances, supervising learners in clinical settings, conducting assessments, delivering treatment, and teaching clinical skills [9]. Given its demonstrated benefits and sustained use during the pandemic, technology-based supervision is likely to persist and expand rapidly. The advancement of technology necessitates that supervisor engage with it not merely as a collection of tools, but as an integrated technology ecosystem that shapes communication, interaction, and opportunities for learner growth [10].

Moving forward, it is essential to consolidate best practices for AI driven distance supervision, addressing ethical considerations such as competency, informed consent, and evidence-based practice, while recognizing that effective clinical supervision can occur in face-to-face, online, and hybrid formats [11].

The InnoVISION extension of the Competency/Outcomes-Based Effective Clinical Supervision (COBECS) model delineates a structured framework that foregrounds Collaboration, Observation, Feedback, Evaluation, Communication, and Support as essential components of effective, competency-oriented supervision, while integrating digitally mediated approaches to enhance accessibility, interactivity, and real-time feedback in contemporary clinical learning environments.

32.6 Operationalization of the Six Pillars in InnoVISION-COBECS

The integration of technology into healthcare ecosystems requires comprehensive change management that goes beyond the adoption of digital tools to address the broader context of healthcare delivery, including clinical pathways, healthcare professionals, patients and families, regulatory standards, and health data sharing. Aligned with the principles of the Competency/Outcomes-Based Effective Clinical Supervision (COBECS) model, this process can be conceptualized through its six core elements (Table 32.1):

1. *Collaboration*: fostering shared ownership of digital health adoption among patients, learners, healthcare providers, and other stakeholders (*virtual and AI-supported teamwork*)
2. *Observation*: monitoring how digital solutions are applied within real-world clinical pathways and care processes (*digital tracking, real-time analytics, and AI assistance*)
3. *Feedback*: engaging patients, families, learners and professionals in iterative dialogue to refine usability and effectiveness (*structured, timely, and personalized using digital tools*)
4. *Evaluation*: systematically assessing outcomes to ensure alignment with clinical standards, patient safety, and competency expectations (*competency-based assessments augmented with AI insights*)
5. *Communication*: ensuring transparent information exchange across all stakeholders, including regulatory bodies and health services (*maintaining effective human-centered interactions*)

Table 32.1 Digital enablers aligned with the InnoVISION-COBECS pillars for use in medical education

InnoVISION-COBECS pillars aligned with digital enablers	
Collaboration	Virtual patients and AI supported teamwork
Observation	Digital; tracking, real-time analytics and AI assistance
Feedback	Structure, timely, personalized feedback via digital tools
Evaluation	Competency-based assessments with AI insights
Communication	Maintaining effective human-centered interactions
Support	Digital mentorship, guidance, and scaffolding

6. *Support*: sustaining adoption through continuous healthcare system engagement, integration within procurement systems, and provision for reimbursement and long-term maintenance (*digital mentorship, guidance, and scaffolding*)

Within this technology-integrated ecosystem, advanced tools for diagnosis, treatment, and disease management are envisioned to operate in a coordinated and seamless manner, supporting the full spectrum of care from hospital to community to home. AI-assisted diagnosis, care robots, wearable devices, virtual consultations, and remote monitoring are becoming increasingly integrated, with significant potential to enhance not only patient care but also clinical learning environments by providing learners with real-time, data-driven insights and immersive, technology-enabled learning experiences [12, 13].

Effectively adapting the InnoVISION-COBECS pillars to medical education and the learner's level requires careful deliberation. Aligned with the operational principles of the COBECS model and the ACGME competency framework, the InnoVISION approach offers a conceptual structure that leverages technology to enhance competency development and optimize learning outcomes. This framework supports progression across both undergraduate and postgraduate medical education, accelerating the learner's overall development trajectory (Table 32.2).

Table 32.2 InnoVISION-COBECS aligned with technology, learner level, competency framework

InnoVISION-COBECS Pillars	Technology tool (examples)	Level of learner	ACGME Competency Framework
Collaboration *Team-based* *Interprofessional* *Shared decision making*	Learning Management System (MOODLE, Canva), Microsoft Teams, Slack clinical case discussions	Undergraduate Medical Education (Years 1–6) *(Novice to advance beginner)* Postgraduate/ Fellowship *(Advance Beginner to Master)*	System-based Practice, Interpersonal and Communication Skills, Professionalism
Observation (structured) *Real-time clinical assessment, observation, insights for learner and faculty development*	Video-based assessments (e.g., VEO or Qpercom), AR/VR simulations for remote observations	-do-	Patient Care, Medical Knowledge, Practice Based Learning and Improvement
Feedback *Timely Technology facilitated Reflection*	Digital feedback platforms (Mentimeter, Formative, MedEd portal for peer feedback)	-do-	Interpersonal and Communication Skills, Practice Based Learning and Improvement

(continued)

Table 32.2 (continued)

InnoVISION-COBECS Pillars	Technology tool (examples)	Level of learner	ACGME Competency Framework
Evaluation *Faculty effectiveness, Competency milestones, Performance tracking*	Online assessment Tools (ExamSoft, MinCEX, OSCE Checklist on mobile apps)	-do-	Medical Knowledge, Patient Care, Practice Based Learning and Improvement
Communication *Faculty -trainee communication, culture of respect*	Asynchronous discussion boards, AI-driven chatbots for clinical Q&A, Mobile App	-do-	Interpersonal and Communication Skills, Professionalism
Support *Safe learning environments Institutional support system*	Virtual mentoring (ZOOM, MS Teams), Well-being Apps for mental health support in clinical training	-do-	Professionalism, System-based Practice, Patient Care

32.7 Challenges and Considerations

The evolution of clinical technology ecosystems is shifting toward care delivery models in which technology is central rather than peripheral. Within this technology-integrated ecosystem, advanced tools for diagnosis, treatment, and disease management are envisioned to operate in a coordinated and seamless manner, supporting the full spectrum of care from hospital to community to home [12]. The development and use of clinical AI support tools to enhance learner performance face significant challenges. In the modern era, effective clinical supervision is increasingly intertwined with digital health infrastructures. The lack of physical presence also removes opportunities for immediate, tactile support, which supervisors traditionally use to comfort learners. As reported in a study by Schmittel et al. (2022), a supervisor described losing *that ability to just put a hand on their arm or hand them a tissue* during difficult moments, instead virtual settings require conveying support solely through facial expressions and language [13].

Digital literacy gaps between clinical supervisors and learners span multiple dimensions, creating disparities in technological competency. A pronounced generational divide contributes significantly, with trainees often functioning as "digital natives" fluent in technology, while many educators are "digital immigrants" with varying degrees of technological proficiency. Technical limitations of virtual platforms can reduce engagement and trust during collaborative learning [12, 14].

Clinical supervisors face particular challenges in fulfilling their educational roles while managing their own digital literacy limitations. Gaps in supervisors' digital literacy or poorly designed tools can hinder their ability to provide timely feedback, model digital professionalism, and scaffold competency development in line with COBECS framework and the ACGME competencies. Consequently, the effectiveness of technology-enhanced clinical supervision depends not only on the availability of digital tools but also on the capacity of supervisors to integrate them into structured, supportive, and safe learning environments [14].

These gaps are also evident in specialized clinical contexts. In a study reported by Noori et al. (2022), over 90% of psychiatry professionals reported that limited knowledge of digital app appraisal constrained their clinical use, despite more than half having recommended digital interventions to patients. More broadly, over one-third of clinicians express only moderate comfort with digital devices and the Internet, with older and rural practitioners facing the greatest challenges [15]. Collectively, these deficiencies highlight the lack of structured strategies for integrating technology with clinical teaching, leaving educators to pursue individual rather than collaborative digital professional development. Without addressing these gaps, healthcare graduates risk entering practice without essential digital competencies, potentially limiting their contributions to technological innovation and affecting patient outcomes [14].

32.8 Recommendations and Best Practices

The effectiveness of technology-mediated clinical supervision relies on careful alignment between clinical supervisors' digital competence, level of the learner, and appropriate use of digital to tool to match with expected competency.

The integration of AI in clinical supervision calls for a fundamental curricular transformation, emphasizing not only AI literacy (supervisor /supervisee) but also critical appraisal, human-AI collaboration, and communication skills. Future training should foster competencies that enable clinicians to use AI synergistically, recognize its limitations, and apply human judgment effectively in patient care.

Human-AI synergy is increasingly recognized as the preferred model for future implementation. While adaptation is possible, authentic connections in virtual supervision require deliberate effort, and a humanistic approach that can be fostered through a combination of learning experiences.

Future implementation should prioritize collaborative frameworks grounded in human-AI synergy. AI ought to complement, not replace, human expertise by enabling dynamic task allocation, shared decision-making, and adaptive interfaces that support both clinicians and learners, fostering competency development, critical judgment, and effective engagement across diverse clinical and educational contexts.

32.9 Conclusion

The COBECS roadmap and model can be adapted to the digital age by incorporating technology-enhanced teaching, assessment, and feedback strategies, with modifications tailored to contextual needs, learning environments, and evolving supervisory practices.

InnoVISION-COBECS provides a foundational framework that, with appropriate modifications, can be leveraged to advance AI-driven clinical supervision. By adopting the InnoVISION-COBECS model with technological innovation and advancements, clinical supervision can evolve to meet the demands of modern healthcare education, ensuring that learners are well-equipped to navigate the complexities of contemporary clinical environments.

References

1. Ahmady S, Minouei MS. Explanation of medical students' experiences of educational clinical supervision: a qualitative study. J Educ Health Promot. 2021;10:12.
2. Herlambang H, Fitri AD, Shafira NN, Puspasari A, Tarawifa S. The role of clinical supervision: teaching basic obstetric ultrasound for undergraduate medical students. Indonesian Res J Educ |IRJE|. 2020;4:556–68.
3. Noble C, Hilder J, Billett S, Teodorczuk A, Ajjawi R. Supervisory knowing in practice across medical specialities. Adv Health Sci Educ. 2023;29:107–28.
4. Masamha R, Alfred L, Harris R, Bassett S, Burden S, Gilmore A. Barriers to overcoming the barriers': a scoping review exploring 30 years of clinical supervision literature. J Adv Nurs. 2022;78:2678–92.
5. Rocha I, Pinto CM, Carvalho AL. Impact of clinical supervision on job satisfaction and emotional competence of nurses. Rev Bras Enferm. 2021;74(6):e20210125.
6. Gordon SP. Integrating the experiential learning cycle with educational supervision. J Educ Superv. 2022;5(3):1–34.
7. Wells R, et al. Testing the effectiveness and acceptability of online supportive supervision for mental health practitioners in humanitarian settings: a study protocol for the caring for carers project. BMC Psychiatry. 2023;23:884.
8. Doody O, Markey K, Turner J, Donnell CO, Murphy L. Clinical supervisor's experiences of peer group clinical supervision during COVID-19: a mixed methods study. BMC Nurs. 2024;23:612.
9. MacMahon ST, Richardson I. Pathways, technology and the patient—connected health through the lifecycle. Front Digit Health. 2023;5:1057518.
10. Hartley MT, Bourgeois PJ, Clarke B. Ethics of technology practice: beliefs and behaviors of certified rehabilitation counselors during the COVID-19 pandemic. Rehabil Couns Bull. 2023;66:244–56.
11. Ishii-Rousseau JE, Seino S, Ebner DK, Vareth M, Po MJ, Celi LA. The "Ecosystem as a Service (EaaS)" approach to advance clinical artificial intelligence (cAI). PLOS Digital Health. 2022;1:e0000011.
12. Schmittel E, Lettenberger-Klein C, Oliver T, Butterfras RF, Adamson D. Intentionality in academic telesupervision: a phenomenological study of faculty telesupervisors' experiences. Contemp Fam Ther. 2021;45:61–74.
13. Borycki E, Kushniruk AW. Health technology, quality and safety in a learning health system. Healthc Manage Forum. 2022;36:79–85.
14. Noori S, Khasnavis S, DeCroce-Movson E, Blay-Tofey M, Vitiello E. A curriculum on digital psychiatry for a US-based psychiatry residency training program: pilot implementation study. JMIR Format Res. 2022;8:e41573.
15. Le JT, Mahoney A, Court JL, Shiner CT. Barriers and facilitators of digital mental health use in regional, rural, and remote Australia: a comparison of clinician and consumer perspectives. Aust J Rural Health. 2025;33:e70011.

Education in Adult Congenital Heart Disease (ACHD): Building Competence, Confidence, and Capacity

33

Aysha N. Malik and Ali N. Zaidi

Key Points

- Adult congenital heart disease (ACHD), also referred to as grown-up congenital heart disease (GUCH), continues to grow exponentially due to the success of pediatric cardiology and congenital cardiac surgery.
- ACHD education requires dedicated training in imaging, intervention, high-risk pregnancy, pulmonary hypertension, and heart failure management, with a focus on competency-based learning.
- Postgraduate programs should adapt curricula to the trainee's background since trainees may come from either adult or pediatric cardiology, to address differing foundational skill sets.
- Awareness and exposure to ACHD should begin in medical school, residency, or general cardiology fellowship to attract and prepare future ACHD cardiologists.
- Educational progress should be assessed through defined milestones and competencies to ensure readiness for independent ACHD practice.

33.1 Introduction

The epidemiology of adult congenital heart disease (ACHD) has changed in the past 50 years with an increase in the prevalence and overall survival rate of children born with congenital heart disease (CHD) [1], as a result of more timely diagnosis and

A. N. Malik
Mount Sinai Adult Congenital Heart Disease Center, Mount Sinai Fuster Heart Hospital, Icahn School of Medicine at Mount Sinai, New York, NY, USA
e-mail: aysha.malik@mountsinai.org

A. N. Zaidi (✉)
Mount Sinai Adult Congenital Heart Disease Center, Mount Sinai Fuster Heart Hospital, New York, NY, USA
e-mail: ali.zaidi@mountsinai.org

J. Sandars et al. (eds.), *Modern Medical Education*,
https://doi.org/10.1007/978-3-032-27958-3_33

with the progress of interventions in CHD. As patients with CHD age, the disease burden shifts away from the heart and more toward acquired cardiovascular and systemic complications with rapidly increasing cohort of adults with CHD. However, the field of ACHD, both in the United States and even in European countries, is facing a significant shortage of healthcare professionals to meet the rising demands of a complex and aging patient population [1–3]. In 2008, Marelli et al. estimated that there were approximately 1.5 million adults with CHD in the United States, nearly half with moderate or complex lesions [4]. With a projected annual growth rate of 4.5%, the current ACHD population is estimated at 2.3 million individuals, including 1.15 million with moderate-to-complex disease, with adults clearly outnumbering children with CHD by approximately 2:1 [4]. To keep pace with this growing ACHD patient population, dedicated education and earlier workforce modeling in 2005 had projected that at least 250 full-time ACHD cardiologists would be required to adequately serve this population, corresponding to roughly 1032 patients per ACHD cardiologist [5]. This suggests that more cardiologists need to be trained and educated in ACHD as a specialized training track in order to meet these growing needs. It is recommended that one regional ACHD program per 2 million people is needed, each staffed by at least three ACHD-trained cardiologists, corresponding to approximately 666 patients per ACHD cardiologist [6, 7]. More recent estimates suggest that three to six ACHD cardiologists are required to serve a population of 1 million, among whom 3000–4000 are adults with CHD [2]. Clearly, the need for training and education ACHD cardiologists is of the essence and needs to be acted upon with due haste to meet these rising demands.

33.2 Historical Perspectives on ACHD Education

The education of physicians in ACHD has evolved in parallel with the remarkable advances in the field of pediatric cardiology (PC) over the past half century. In the early decades, CHD was viewed almost exclusively as a pediatric condition, with education and training concentrated within pediatric cardiology, with the thought that only a few of these children with moderate or severely complex CHD would make it into adulthood. Surgical techniques were evolving and interventional cardiac catheterization was developing as a subspecialty. Surgical and medical advances beginning in the 1940s dramatically improved survival into adulthood, yet formal training in the care of these survivors was virtually absent. As the decades progressed, slowly these children with repaired or palliated lesions started to reach adulthood. Over the last few decades, this cohort continues to age, and an increasing number of children with CHD transition into adulthood, with unique medical, surgical, and psychosocial needs which have exposed a significant educational gap for the clinical cardiologist taking care of this cohort. Early efforts to bridge this gap relied on informal collaborations between pediatric cardiologists, adult cardiologists, and cardiac surgeons, with knowledge transfer occurring largely through mentorship and anecdotal experiences and ad hoc clinical exposure rather than through structured curricula, which continues for several decades.

The roots of ACHD as a discipline lie in the pioneering work of Dr. Helen B. Taussig at Johns Hopkins in the 1930s and 1940s. Often considered the founder of pediatric cardiology, Dr. Taussig studied the physiology and natural history of cyanotic congenital heart lesions at a time when survival into adulthood was rare. Her landmark textbook, *Congenital Malformations of the Heart* published in 1947, provided the first complete clinical framework for understanding these conditions and set the stage for pediatric cardiology as a field. Working alongside surgeon Dr. Alfred Blalock and Dr. Vivien Thomas, they were responsible for the origins of the systemic-to-pulmonary artery shunt, first performed in 1944 and later known as the Blalock-Taussig-Thomas shunt. This historic procedure transformed the lives of children with cyanotic congenital heart disease including tetralogy of Fallot, marking the beginning of modern congenital heart surgery and creating, for the first time, a population of survivors who would live into adulthood.

By the 1970s, the number of adults living with repaired or palliated congenital heart disease had grown substantially, exposing a critical gap in specialized care [8]. Dr. Jane Somerville at the National Heart Hospital in London was the first to formally address this need by establishing a "Grown-Up Congenital Heart" (GUCH) unit—an innovative model of care dedicated to this unique population [9]. Dr. Somerville recognized that CHD did not end with just pediatric surgical repair, but rather carried lifelong consequences that required specialized, multidisciplinary follow-up, asides from the education and teaching of cardiologists who would eventually take care of these growing cohort. She not only developed systems of care but also coined the terminology and created a culture of recognition that ACHD or GUCH was its own distinct entity and not merely an extension of pediatrics or adult cardiology. Through her education, teaching and mentorship, Dr. Somerville inspired a generation of clinicians who specialized in the care of adults with CHD are now called "Unicorns", solidifying London as a global hub for ACHD expertise, which has remained true to its cause.

In parallel, in the United States, Dr. Joseph K. Perloff became the pivotal figure in the development of ACHD as a subspecialty in North America. At UCLA in 1980, he founded one of the first dedicated ACHD centers in the United States, integrating clinical care, education, and research in a way that was unprecedented at the time. His textbook, The Clinical Recognition of Congenital Heart Disease (first published in 1970 and later expanded through multiple editions), became an educational foundation for clinicians worldwide, linking pediatric and adult perspectives with unmatched clarity. Together, Dr. Somerville and Dr. Perloff transformed ACHD from an overlooked population in the 1970s into a recognized field of cardiology, laying the groundwork for later developments such as the Bethesda Conference statements, ACC/AHA guidelines, ABIM board certification, and ACGME fellowship accreditation.

33.3 Why Education and Training in ACHD Matters: Now More Than Ever

Adults now outnumber children living with CHD with long-term care shifting from episodic pediatric surgery to lifelong, complex adult management, across multiple domains including but not limited to high-risk pregnancy, complex arrhythmias, advanced heart failure/cardiac transplantation, advanced imaging, and re-intervention via transcatheter and surgical domains. Outcomes are better now than ever before, especially when patients receive care in specialized ACHD programs around the world, underscoring the need for purpose-built education and training for cardiologists. It is now unequivocally clear that the rapidly expanding and aging ACHD population driven by its complex healthcare needs has created a rising demand for skilled ACHD cardiologists who can provide care for the ACHD patient from teenage to geriatric ACHD. Yet the field faces significant challenges to meet this growing demand [10, 11] intensifying the focus on the education and training of the ACHD physician not just in the United States but all over the world.

Since the initial work by Dr. Somerville in the United Kingdom and Dr. Perloff in the United States, over the last three decades, through the efforts of multiple stakeholders and professional societies, significant milestones have been met regarding dedicated training in ACHD in the United States leading to the approval of an initial board certification exam via the American Board of Internal Medicine (ABIM) in 2015 [12]. With sustained efforts, another major milestone was achieved in 2016 with the approval of a 2-year Accreditation Council for Graduate Medical Education (ACGME)-accredited ACHD fellowship [13]. Since the inception of the 2-year ACGME fellowship in 2016, US training programs have graduated a variable number of fellows each year, ranging from 6 to 16 per year in the United States, though the small number of graduating fellows remains a cause of concern. However, despite the growing number of ACHD patients both in the United States and around the world, the number of ACHD-trained cardiologists has continued to be scarce, with only a handful ACHD cardiologists graduating annually. This is the crux of why education and training in ACHD needs to be of extreme importance to ensure that the supply-demand mismatch does not continue in the years to come.

33.4 Educational Competencies in ACHD: Defining, Aligning, and Measuring Standards for Training

In the early era of ACHD care, physician training was largely informal, rooted in mentorship and ad hoc exposure within pediatric or adult cardiology programs, without defined competencies. In 1999, the ACGME in the United States established six core competencies as defined by (1) medical knowledge, (2) patient care/procedural skill, (3) practice-based learning and improvement, (4) systems-based practice, (5) interpersonal/communication skills, and (6) professionalism as the foundation for standardized training and assessment. These core competencies are required to train ACHD cardiologists in the United States and around the world. Over the past three decades, ACHD has matured into a recognized cardiovascular subspecialty as professional societies have established ACGME-aligned competency standards and embedded them into fellowship training through key milestones. A formal measure of competence in ACHD fellowship training is eventual board certification, administered by the ABIM, which emphasizes lifelong learning through maintenance of certification (MOC). It was the 32nd Bethesda Conference,

Care of the Adult with Congenital Heart Disease (2000) the first to propose ACHD-specific competencies [10]. Yet, these recommendations remained largely aspirational until 2015, when they were incorporated into more formal training statements [11, 12], aligning ACHD training with the competency-based approach guiding the rest of cardiology [14]. While taking somewhat different approaches, these training documents addressed the six core competencies outlined by the ACGME and endorsed by the ABIM and ABP. Building on this development, ACHD training was further standardized in 2016 with the establishment of a dedicated 2-year ACGME-accredited fellowship pathway. Until 2019, a practice pathway was available for ABIM diplomates in cardiovascular disease (CVS) and American Board of Pediatrics (ABP) diplomates in pediatric cardiology (PC) who had not completed formal ACHD training but met practice thresholds as either full-time or part-time physicians [3]. Notwithstanding the progress over the last two decades, thoughtful discussions were whether ACHD competency standards can be achieved within a shortened training pathway without compromising preparedness and the competence of graduating ACHD fellow. It was agreed that any consideration of abbreviated fellowship models should be guided by robust outcomes data and shared input from trainees, program leaders, and certifying bodies, with safeguards to preserve clinical exposure, mentorship, and procedural proficiency and with patient safety and quality of care as the central priority, which has been at the core of ACHD ACGME-accredited fellowship programs since 2016.

33.5 The Divergent Approaches Between Adult and Pediatric Cardiology Training

Education in ACHD is distinct among cardiology subspecialties in that fellows may enter the fellowship after completing either an adult CVD or a PC fellowship, resulting in differing competency frameworks at entry. Both CVD and PC fellowships adopt the six ACGME core competencies but differ in structure. Adult CVD employs a tiered system (Levels 1–3), whereas PC uses a dichotomous model (Core vs. Advanced) in their educational framework for fellowships. This divergence in educational structure creates challenges in aligning competency assessment and expectations across eventual ACHD fellowship training since these fellows have to be deemed competent in taking care of adults with all forms of CHD. It should be understood that in ACHD fellowship *one size does not fit all* and these fellowships have to be tailored to the needs of the fellow, i.e., based on their prior background, either from adult CVD or PD. Currently, advanced (Level 3) training in ACHD in the United States requires an additional 2 years of fellowship training. However, with only a handful of ACHD fellows graduating annually, one potential avenue to improve access to high-quality ACHD care maybe to strengthen Level 2 ACHD training which allows a general cardiologist to have more dedicated ACHD education/experience but not having to complete two dedicated ACHD fellowship years. This approach would necessitate careful consideration and significant discourse with multiple stakeholders, boards, and multiple professional societies before any implementation could even be pursued.

33.6 Competency-Based Medical Education for ACHD: Addressing the "Time"-Based Training Concept

Much debate continues regarding the traditional postgraduate medical education which has relied on fixed training durations across all specialties and subspecialties including ACHD. However, over the past decade, the graduate medical education (GME) community at large has increasingly debated a shift toward competency-based medical education (CBME), in which progression depends on achievement of defined competency-based education rather than teaching over a fixed time. It should be highlighted that though this remains a cornerstone for discussion, it has not led to any changes in fellowship structure at the current time. Such flexibility though possible must be anchored in rigorous competency assessment, not "assumptions" based on prior rotations. This would allow shorter training tracks which may enable fellows to accumulate competencies earlier, potentially reducing training length and cost, though this comes with the understanding that reduced exposure to broader general cardiovascular medicine may be detrimental to a fellow in training. While this model offers adaptability and efficiency, it must be balanced against the value of broader cardiology exposure, education, and training, which remains critical for many ACHD cardiologists who also practice general cardiology aside from ACHD.

33.7 Measurement of Competencies: Fundamental for ACHD ACGME Fellowship Education

While existing tools such as in-training examinations, portfolios, and self-assessments align with ACHD ACGME milestones which has been described and incorporated by ACHD fellowship programs in the United States, additional methods may enhance consistency across the specialty. Since fellows may enter ACHD fellowship either from adult CVD or PC fellowships, standardized modules or assessments could provide objective measures of a fellows' development catered to their prior cardiology training. A structured evaluation of trainee progress through their fellowship is of essence to establish adequate and reliable competency assessment in order to maintain quality of ACHD fellowship training. As the ACHD population becomes more complex, the ACGME-accredited ACHD fellowship training programs must continue to evolve to address these challenges. Continuous refining of training pathways and educational curriculum will create a more effective educational structure. While ABIM ACHD board certification is valuable, in isolation, it does not fully capture a cardiologist's ability to thrive in the dynamic, long-term care environment of ACHD. Ongoing formative evaluations are essential to assess the readiness of an ACHD fellow for eventual clinical practice. At the time of writing, the American College of Cardiology (ACC) is working on an Advanced Training Statement (ATS) addressing the core competencies required of ACHD physicians and provides examples of appropriate measures for assessing competence in the context of ACHD fellowship training, which may become the benchmark for competency-based ACGME ACHD fellowship training.

33.8 Fellowship Training in Adult Congenital Heart Disease: The Core Essentials

In the United States, the ACHD fellowship curriculum is designed in accordance with the ACGME, the ACHD Milestones Project, and the ABIM ACHD Certification Exam Blueprint. The educational framework during ACHD fellowship has to ensure that fellows have achieved competency in all the nuances of CHD. This includes but not limited to morphology and physiology of repaired and unrepaired congenital heart lesions, the natural history of CHD, and recognition of late sequelae of surgical repair. Fellowship training emphasizes advanced imaging modalities including transthoracic and transesophageal echocardiography (including 3D), cardiac magnetic resonance imaging, and cardiac computed tomography (CT) with attention to indications, interpretation, and patient safety. Cardiac hemodynamics are at the very core of ACHD education and are addressed through exposure to cardiac catheterizations where significant emphasis is placed on understanding and analysis hemodynamics, shunts, pulmonary and systemic flow ratios, pulmonary and systemic vascular resistance calculations, and evaluation of pulmonary hypertension. Further domains include diagnosing and managing cardiac arrhythmias, with a basic understanding of pacemaker and ICD therapies. Educational curriculum has to focus on diagnosing and managing advanced heart failure, understanding heart failure therapies, mechanical circulatory support (MCS), and indications for cardiac transplantation. Fellowship education includes an in-depth understanding of reproductive health with high-risk pregnancy risk stratification and delivery planning, genetics and syndromic CHD, periprocedural and noncardiac surgery risk assessment, and structured transition of care from pediatric to adult programs. ACHD fellowship education includes completing 6–8 months in ACHD longitudinal ACHD clinic to ensure continuity and graduated responsibility to learn ambulatory management of all forms of CHD. Imaging expertise is developed over 3–4 months of ACHD-focused transthoracic echocardiography, transesophageal echocardiography, and on cardiac MRI and CT interpretation in ACHD. Two to three months are dedicated to diagnostic and interventional catheterization with integration into surgical case management conferences where the fellows learn on how to diagnose and manage complex clinical scenarios. Focused training in electrophysiology for management of atrial and ventricular arrhythmias and basic understanding of device management is key. Advanced heart failure/MCS, cardiac ICU, and cardiac transplant experiences span 1–2 months, and high-risk pregnancy provides 1 month of ACHD-OB comanagement and delivery planning. Fellows should be allowed 3–6 months devoted to electives, research, and quality improvement, tailored to institutional strengths and fellow career trajectories so they may focus on a discipline of their choosing within the field of ACHD.

33.9 Core Topics in ACHD Medical Education

As outlined above, training in ACHD requires a comprehensive and multidisciplinary curriculum that spans multiple domains in a systems-based practice. The educational framework must prepare clinicians not only to understand the complexities of congenital anatomy but also to manage the lifelong sequelae of disease and repair while integrating psychosocial and systems-level considerations. Five broad domains are highlighted below.

(a) *Morphology, Physiology, and Natural History*

Foundational to ACHD education is command of congenital cardiac morphology, including the native anatomy of unrepaired lesions as well as their repaired and palliated forms. Trainees must understand the physiology of shunt lesions, congenital obstructive lesions, cyanotic states, and single-ventricle palliation. Equally important is understanding the natural history of these conditions and the long-term sequelae encountered in adult survivors, such as arrhythmias, valvular dysfunction, heart failure, pulmonary vascular disease, and multi-organ complications both with and without prior surgical or transcatheter palliation. This understanding provides the framework for predicting clinical problems decades after initial intervention and for managing both surveillance strategies and therapeutic decision-making.

(b) *Advanced Imaging and Hemodynamics*

ACHD management significantly relies on advanced cardiovascular imaging. Competence in transthoracic echocardiography including three-dimensional and transesophageal modalities in ACHD is essential for anatomical and functional assessment. Cardiac magnetic resonance (CMR) and computed tomography (CT) are critical for evaluating complex spatial relationships, quantifying ventricular volumes, and monitoring vascular structures and conduits in mostly palliated but also in some non-palliated CHD lesions. In parallel, cardiac catheterization remains essential, both from a diagnostic hemodynamic standpoint and also to understand the indications for transcatheter interventions. Education in ACHD fellowships must be able to interpret invasive hemodynamics, perform shunt and resistance calculations, and assess pulmonary hypertension, thereby incorporating multimodality imaging with hemodynamic physiologic data to guide clinical decision-making.

(c) *Arrhythmias and Electrophysiology*

Arrhythmias are among the most common and clinically significant late complications of congenital heart disease. Education must cover the spectrum of atrial and ventricular arrhythmias seen in various CHD lesions, alongside risk stratification for sudden cardiac death (SCD) in ACHD. Competency includes understanding medical therapy, indications for catheter ablation strategies, and the technical challenges of device implantation in patients with surgically palliated CHD where access can often be challenging. Management of pacemakers, defibrillators, and cardiac resynchronization therapies must be tailored to ACHD by extrapolating from adult cardiovascular guidelines, requiring close collaboration with electrophysiology specialists trained in ACHD.

(d) *Pregnancy, Genetics, and Multisystem Considerations*

ACHD providers must be well-versed in counseling and managing patients before and during pregnancy, where maternal and fetal risks vary by lesion type, ventricular function, and arrhythmia burden. Preconception planning, contraceptive counseling, and multidisciplinary collaboration with maternal-fetal medicine (MFM) are essential components of education in ACHD especially during fellowship. Genetics represents another critical area, as many congenital lesions are syndromic or associated with heritable mutations; thus, clinicians should understand the role of genetic testing as and when needed, family screening, and appropriate counseling. An exceedingly important aspect of ACHD fellowship education is multidisciplinary care since often these patients may require cross collaboration with other specialties including hepatology especially in Fontan survivors.

(e) *Systems of Care, Transition, and Lifelong Management*

Finally, ACHD education extends beyond clinical knowledge to encompass systems-based practice and long-term patient engagement. Structured transition programs help adolescents navigate the shift from pediatric to adult services, a vulnerable period where loss to follow-up is common. Psychosocial issues—including employment, insurance, and mental health—must be addressed alongside medical care. Equally important are quality improvement initiatives, advocacy efforts, and research literacy, which together advance the field and enhance long-term outcomes. Providers must be trained not only as clinicians but also as stewards of systems that deliver sustainable, patient-centered ACHD care.

33.10 Assessment and Professional Development in ACHD

There are several methods for assessment to ensure that competency-based education metrics are being met. Fellows may undergo workplace-based assessments such as mini-clinical exams, direct observation of procedural skills, and case-based discussions. ACHD fellowship education has to ensure that these competencies translate into observable practice behaviors so that the fellows are able independently provide clinical care. Objective testing in annual in-service assessments and mock oral boards have not been standardized in the United States. Case logs and reflective portfolios document exposure to imaging, cath/EP procedures, pregnancy conferences, and transition clinics, benchmarked against published ACGME and ABIM requirements. This multilayered evaluation during the educational journey of an ACHD fellow ensures that fellows graduate with the knowledge, skills, and leadership capacity to provide high-quality, evidence-based care for adults with CHD while advancing the field through scholarship and multidisciplinary collaboration. During their training, fellows are expected to develop research literacy and productivity consistent with the ACGME expectations for scholarly activity [7, 1]. This comprehensive approach equips trainees with the academic, professional, and personal tools essential for success as clinicians, educators, and leaders in ACHD.

33.11 Conclusion

It is estimated that the US ACHD population is now ~2.3 million (≈ 2:1 adult-children; ~1.15 million adults with moderate to complex), yet staffing lags recommendations since there is not enough ACHD. This growing and aging cohort of adults with CHD live longer with repaired/palliated CHD and face lifelong concerns including risk of arrhythmias and SCD, advanced heart failure, need for re-interventions either surgical or transcatheter, and multisystem disease processes. Outcomes improve with structured, team-based training which is essential in ACHD fellowship. ACHD training aligns with ACGME's six core competencies. ACHD fellowship education is unique in its essence since fellows may enter a core ACHD fellowship from either adult CVD or PC fellowships with varying baseline framework, leading to fellowship education that has to be catered to the needs of each individual fellow. ACHD education includes multiple facets including ACHD clinical care in the outpatient or inpatient setting, focus on multimodality imaging, cardiac catheterization with a focus on hemodynamics and indications for interventions, arrhythmias, devices, advanced heart failure management, mechanical circulatory support, cardiac transplantation, cardiac critical care, high-risk pregnancy, transition of care from pediatrics to ACHD, and research and quality improvement. Competence is measured via multiple assessments and case logs with an eventual board certification exam via the ABIM.

References

1. Marelli AJ, et al. Lifetime prevalence of congenital heart disease in the general population from 2000 to 2010. Circulation. 2014;130(9):749–56.
2. Ephrem G. The current state of the board-certified adult congenital heart disease workforce 10 years after initial certification. Am J Cardiol. 2025;255:12–6.
3. Bonanni F, et al. Congenital heart disease after mid-age: from the "grown-up" to the elderly. Diagnostics (Basel). 2025;15(4):481.
4. Marelli AJ, et al. Planning the specialized care of adult congenital heart disease patients: from numbers to guidelines; an epidemiologic approach. Am Heart J. 2009;157(1):1–8.

5. Gurvitz MZ, et al. Variations in adult congenital heart disease training in adult and pediatric cardiology fellowship programs. J Am Coll Cardiol. 2005;46(5):893–8.
6. Warnes CA, et al. Task force 1: the changing profile of congenital heart disease in adult life. J Am Coll Cardiol. 2001;37(5):1170–5.
7. Stout KK, et al. 2018 AHA/ACC Guideline for the management of adults with congenital heart disease: executive summary: a report of the American College of Cardiology/American Heart Association Task Force on Clinical Practice Guidelines. Circulation. 2019;139(14):e637–97.
8. Freeman LJ. Grown up congenital heart (GUCH) disease: a half century of change. Clin Med (Lond). 2008;8(2):169–71.
9. Somerville J. Grown-up congenital heart disease–medical demands look back, look forward 2000. Thorac Cardiovasc Surg. 2001;49(1):21–6.
10. Stout K, et al. Task force 6: pediatric cardiology fellowship training in adult congenital heart disease. SPCTPD/ACC/AAP/AHA Circ. 2015;132(6):e91–8.
11. Nguyen LT, et al. Current and future status of adult congenital training in North America. Am J Cardiol. 2015;115(8):1151–3.
12. Martin GR, et al. The adult congenital and pediatric cardiology section: increasing the opportunities for the congenital heart disease community within the American College of Cardiology. J Am Coll Cardiol. 2012;59(1):84–7.
13. Landzberg MJ, et al. Task force 4: organization of delivery systems for adults with congenital heart disease. J Am Coll Cardiol. 2001;37(5):1187–93.
14. Stoffman JM. Overcoming the barriers to implementation of competence-based medical education in post-graduate medical education: a narrative literature review. Med Educ Online. 2022;27(1):2112012.

Acute Kidney Injury: Future Training and Education

34

Rubina Naqvi

Key Points

- A uniform definition for acute kidney injury (AKI) is lacking, with different definitions from different parts of world.
- The epidemiology of AKI remains diverse because of lack of uniformity in definition and variability in hospital- and community-acquired causes.
- Renal replacement therapy (RRT) in its different modalities is not available in all parts of world.
- There is increasing use of artificial intelligence (AI) in AKI diagnosis and management.
- The World Health Organization (WHO) and international organizations should support education, training, and availability of different modes in management of AKI to improve patient outcomes.

34.1 Acute Kidney Injury (AKI)

Acute kidney injury (AKI) is a serious medical condition resulting from abrupt onset kidney damage. Clinically, AKI is characterized by sudden and sustained decline in urine output/glomerular filtration rate and rise in serum urea and creatinine. This results in certain metabolic and electrolyte disturbances which frequently accompany the scenario. It is invariably an under-recognized condition. It can occur in a variety of clinical settings and is a predictor of adverse outcomes in the short and long term. It is estimated that approximately 13.3 million people develop AKI around the world, this AKI may resolve or turn into chronic kidney disease (CKD), or some patients die with AKI [1].

R. Naqvi (✉)
Sindh Institute of Urology and Transplantation, (SIUT), Karachi, Pakistan

J. Sandars et al. (eds.), *Modern Medical Education*,
https://doi.org/10.1007/978-3-032-27958-3_34

34.2 Definitions

The incidence and prevalence of AKI, which is one of most prominent subjects in nephrology, varies widely world over. The main reason for such wide variation is the definitions used for diagnosis. Previously, when this condition used to call acute renal failure (ARF), it was defined as "rapid fall in the rate of glomerular filtration, occurring over hours or few days," "an abrupt and sustained decline in renal function," "a temporary rise in creatinine to at least 300 μmol/L," "an increase in serum creatinine of >0.5 mg per deciliter over the baseline" (where the baseline was lowest serum creatinine over past 3 months), and "an increase of >50% over the baseline value." Slight alterations in phrasing the words in one of these statements were used to define AKI from all continents in the world. More recently, area experts have designed criteria which can be or should be used universally. The RIFLE criteria were made in May 2002 in a meeting in Vicenza, but this criterion had several short comings and could only be applied in intensive care settings. Another meeting in Amsterdam in September 2005 was he,ld and the AKIN classification was designed, but this had low popularity and had similar shortcomings as the RIFLE criteria. The KDIGO guidelines were laid out in 2012 for the definition of AKI, and this is the most widely used definition at the current time [2].

34.3 Variations in Epidemiology of AKI

AKI has a marked impact on families, societies, and national economies. However, there is a marked diversity in the incidence and prevalence in different parts of world, along with categorization into the hospital-acquired and community-acquired AKI. Knowledge of the diversity in the spectrum of AKI is relevant in developing a global response to diminish the impact of this health condition, especially in resource-poor settings [3].

Over time, it has become clear that in high-income countries, AKI develops primarily in already hospitalized patients, often with multiple preexisting conditions. These patients are categorized as hospital-acquired AKI. However, the AKI population in low- and middle-income countries is generally persons who were previously healthy and AKI categorized as community acquired. Hypovolemic shock, infections, use of over-the-counter medicines and poisons are the predominant causes of AKI in this group [3]. A complex interplay between geographical characteristics, environmental factors, and poverty drives the presentation and outcome of this condition [2].

Countries in tropics where temperature is high year around differ from those in temperate climates, and both of these differ in not only social but economic terms. The use of herbal medicines and herbal tea, many of which are nephrotoxic, are a common practice in many countries falling in tropical region.

In hospitalized patients, hospital-acquired infections, sepsis, exposure to contrast, and surgical trauma are the main contributors of AKI, while in intensive care (ICU) setting, sepsis and multi-organ failure (MOF) are the top causes. The mortality rate also differs in different settings, with the highest in ICU and MOF to lowest in community-acquired causes of AKI, provided underlying cause is timely addressed.

Patients with AKI are at risk of developing recurrent AKI, progressing toward CKD, and by further progressing end up in end-stage renal failure (ESRF), which requires lifelong renal replacement therapy (RRT) in one or other form.

34.4 Diagnosis

The large spectrum of AKI is associated with a diversity of pathophysiological mechanisms. The three broad categories of these mechanisms (prerenal, renal, and post-renal) will require different set of investigations to reach a diagnosis. Diagnosis begins with performing a detailed history and clinical examination before moving toward assigning an appropriate investigation. Traditionally, some hematological and biochemical investigations have generalizability to all three broad categories, while serological markers and histopathology are more specific in renal origin AKI and radiology in post-renal. Over the past few decades, some biomarkers in blood and urine have been listed, but the majority of these are not specific for the above-mentioned categories [4, 5].

Some biomarkers have been reported to predict progression toward CKD after AKI [6] and have shown promise in this very important field where measures can be taken to halt this progression toward an irreversible condition and reducing long-term burden on family and the society at large.

34.5 Trends in AKI Management

The main previous trends have been conservative and renal replacement therapy (RRT). Conservative management includes correction of fluid overload/volume depletion, acidosis, electrolyte imbalance, and hematologic disorders. The main approaches include diuretics/replacement fluids, use of bicarbonate, addressing hyperkalemia with dietary restriction, use of potassium-binding resins, and measures for shift of K^+ to intracellular with use of dextrose, insulin, and beta agonist, addressing anemia with blood transfusions and platelet dysfunction with use of desmopressin. Dietary modifications according to fluid and electrolyte situation is key to conservative management in AKI. In patients who do not respond to conservative management, RRT as intermittent hemodialysis (IHD) or intermittent peritoneal dialysis (IPD), according to the availability of the modality and requirements for the individual patient, can be provided. IPD has been named as "Cinderella" of RRT in AKI patients and has proved efficacy in low-income countries (LIC) and lower-middle-income countries (LMICs).

In addition to the past practices of managing AKI, newer approaches include the refinement of RRT with continuous renal replacement therapy (CRRT), which is 24 h' continuous therapy with use of filters, slow continuous ultrafiltration (SCUF), and sustained low efficiency daily dialysis (SLEDD), which is 6–12 h daily hemodialysis. While IHD mostly removes low molecular weight toxins, SLEDD and CRRT provide an opportunity to remove small and middle molecule weight toxins. Later techniques have also opened an opportunity to provide RRT in critically ill patients who are in intensive care setting; these patients often have low blood pressure and cannot stand IHD where toxins and fluid removal occur at a rapid pace. Hemodynamic stability is more sustained with SLEDD or CRRT. The high cost, trained staff, and other logistics restrict the use of SLEDD or CRRT to limited centers in LMICs and almost completely hinders in LICs. CRRT has also been suggested in AKI patients with brain injury and high intracranial pressure.

The use of biomarkers is likely to become routine, but despite hundreds of publications on the use of urinary and serum biomarkers proving their credibility, they have still not become routine clinical practice. While some will argue that currently identified biomarkers are limited to prognosis and do not guide toward actual management, many of the biomarkers systematically meet the potential milestones in diagnosing and clinical care [4–6].

Mesenchymal stem cell (MSC) therapy could significantly improve the renal function and injured renal tissue and has future clinical use. A meta-analysis published on the use of mesenchymal stem cell (MSC) therapy demonstrated reduced inflammation and regeneration of damaged renal parenchyma in rat models [7].

It is essential to take measures for minimizing further harm and risk of AKI following complete recovery from AKI. During the initial recovery period, early review and frequent follow-up with a nephrologist is recommended. Medication reconciliation and regimen review with consideration of nephrotoxins during recovery and post-AKI is of utmost importance. Identifying discrepancies between the patient's previous medications and recent hospital discharge prescription, to avoid medication error and adverse events, should also be considered. These recommendations are key components of the multimodal approach in the ongoing *Caring for OutPatiEnts after Acute Kidney Injury (COPE-AKI)* clinical trial.

34.6 Role of AI in Early Diagnosis and Prediction

Artificial intelligence (AI) has increasingly being explored for its potential role in modern healthcare, though its application in acute emergencies like AKI still remain uncertain [8]. Machine learning (ML), a subset of AI, has potential of analyzing large volumes of data and can identify the risk of developing AKI, predict its progression, and can recommend individualized treatment plans [9]. Similarly, deep learning (DL), another subset of AI which is inspired by human brain's structure and functions, utilizes neural network and offers powerful tools for complex data. Most described DL architectures are convolutional neural networks (CNNs) designed for image processing and utilized for analysis of renal biopsies and recurrent neural networks (RNNs) used for sequential data modeling [8]. Natural language processing (NLP) which is interaction between computers and human language helps in transformation of available information.

AI might play a role in diagnosing histopathological variation with AI-powered image analysis and identify elusive patterns in renal biopsies that might escape human observation [10]. Even when renal biopsy is considered gold standard for diagnosis in certain disorders causing AKI, the variability among observers can impact the final diagnosis. AI has produced whole slide images (WSIs) via slide digitalization on high throughput, making computer-assisted analysis of histopathology more reliable [11]. DL further involves data preparation and processing and has shown promise in pathology image analysis [12].

A study published during the COVID-19 era used AI and developed a prognostic scoring with ML technique which they found useful in predicting development of AKI in these patients and mortality [13]. Sepsis is a major cause for AKI in both community and hospital acquired, though more prominently in the latter. AI has also shown promising results in early detection of sepsis. Previously used scoring systems for sepsis like sequential organ failure assessment (SOFA) score, systemic inflammatory response syndrome (SIRS), and modified early warning system (MEWS) seem to be left behind with ML models of AI [14]. AI's application in sepsis prediction is still being researched, and the best model type is yet to be formulated. Some have also used DL for doing subphenotypes of AKI associated with sepsis. This approach would direct AI's approach in guiding personalized treatment options for individuals.

The possible presence of bias in AI models can affect the precision of its analyses, actions, and outputs related to patient management. These biases could be selection bias when available data is not representing the overall population affected by AKI, such as when different definitions are used for diagnosis. Algorithmic bias during processing of data can occur and an important aspect are cultural biases [15]. For example, an AI model prepared in the western world will reflect these biases when applied in LICs or LMICs where AKI causes are infections, such as gastroenteritis, malaria, and dengue; animal toxins, such as snake bites, scorpion stings, and bee stings; or pregnancy-related complications [3]. To address these biases, there should be diversified data collection models and standardized measurements for the different values, as well as constant learning mechanisms. While AI in nephrology practice can transform the diagnostic abilities of physicians, it also highlights the need to observe standard ethical practice in keeping privacy of data among healthcare providers and patients at each step [8].

34.7 Future Education and Training in AKI Management

Priorities for future teaching of undergraduates and recently qualified graduates include the need to develop skills in meticulous history taking and physical examination of the patient since these are essential for the early diagnosis of AKI and also its management. Knowledge of the most recent definition of AKI and further categorization of AKI into prerenal, renal, or post renal is also essential.

A wide variety of online learning resources are freely available for health professionals and patients, especially in the age of digitalized cell phones when there is access in LICs. Interactive packages designed for multidisciplinary staff can help their understanding of AKI and fluid and electrolyte imbalance occurring during AKI. Some sites also provide information about those who are at risk of developing AKI and where to go for consultation in case it happens. Web-based learning modules have been designed for patients undergoing major cardiac or orthopedic surgeries and who are at risk of developing AKI in the postoperative period. Postgraduate medical trainees are advised to follow the guidelines provided in such programs. The machine-based algorithms feature different variables which need to be assessed and addressed preoperatively and followed postoperatively [16].

Electronic alerts have become increasingly implemented during patient care and can be considered as an educational method to guide patient diagnosis and management. A recent systematic review concluded that automated AKI alerts when not linked with clinical decision support (CDS) were unable to impact on the rate of RRT or mortality [17]. CDS systems can provide healthcare providers and patients with knowledge and person-specific information at appropriate times.

The International Society of Nephrology (ISN) has launched many programs, such as regular webinars from world-renowned experts to spread worldwide awareness about kidney diseases and their diagnosis and management. There is also a world kidney day on the second Thursday of March every year. ISN also offers fellowship programs where young trainees from the developing world can obtain scholarships for further experience and training at an established nephrology unit and then returning to their home country to uplift nephrology practice at underdeveloped centers.

34.8 Conclusion

An essential first step in understanding the importance of AKI would be the implementation of a universal definition of AKI. Despite early diagnosis, patient outcomes from AKI across the world can only be achieved by addressing the preventable causes in many LIC and LIMC, such as volume loss, snake bites, and infections. Increasing equitable access to newer technologies for diagnosis and management is a global priority. The World Health Organization (WHO) and international societies, such as the International Society of Nephrology, should continue to play their role but also ensure a commitment to provide equity in healthcare, bridging the gap between advanced medical technology and ground realities in different socioeconomic settings, for all AKI patients internationally. Education and training will be a key approach for achieving this vision.

References

1. https://www.theisn.org/more-than-850-million-worldwide-have-some-form-of-kidney-disease-help-raise-awareness/. Accessed 25 July 2025 at 14:10 hours.
2. Kellum JA, Romagnani P, Ashuntantang G, Ronco C, Zarbock A, Anders HJ. Acute kidney injury. Nat Rev Dis Primers. 2021;7(1):52.

3. Naqvi R. Epidemiological trends in community acquired acute kidney injury in Pakistan: 25 years' experience from a tertiary care renal unit. Pak J Med Sci. 2021;37(2):312.
4. Yang H, Chen Y, He J, Li Y, Feng Y. Advances in the diagnosis of early biomarkers for acute kidney injury: a literature review. BMC Nephrol. 2025;26(1):115.
5. Naqvi R, Hossain N, Butt S, Bhellar Z, Fatima E, Imtiaz S, Moosa PG, Abbas K, Jafri SB, Khan S. Efficacy of multiple biomarkers: NGAL, KIM1, Cystatin C and IL18 in predicting pregnancy related acute kidney injury. Pak J Med Sci. 2023;39(1):34.
6. Wen Y, Thiessen-Philbrook H, Moledina DG, Kaufman JS, Reeves WB, Ghahramani N, Ikizler TA, Go AS, Liu KD, Siew ED, Himmelfarb J. Considerations in controlling for urine concentration for biomarkers of kidney disease progression after acute kidney injury. Kidney Int Rep. 2022;7(7):1502–13.
7. Wanyan P, Wang X, Li N, Huang Y, She Y, Zhang L. Mesenchymal stem cells therapy for acute kidney injury: a systematic review with meta-analysis based on rat model. Front Pharmacol. 2023;14:1099056.
8. Jayaraman P, Vasudev I, Bhardwaj A, Nadkarni G, Sakhuja A, Meena P. Artificial intelligence in nephrology: pioneering precision with multimodal intelligence. Indian J Nephrol. 2025;35:470–9.
9. Gellert GA, Rasławska-Socha J, Marcjasz N, Price T, Heyduk A, Mlodawska A, Kuszczyński K, Jędruch A, Orzechowski P. The role of virtual triage in improving clinician experience and satisfaction: a narrative review. Telemed Rep. 2023;4(1):180–91.
10. Jayapandian CP, Chen Y, Janowczyk AR, Palmer MB, Cassol CA, Sekulic M, Hodgin JB, Zee J, Hewitt SM, O'Toole J, Toro P. Development and evaluation of deep learning–based segmentation of histologic structures in the kidney cortex with multiple histologic stains. Kidney Int. 2021;99(1):86–101.
11. Wang S, Yang DM, Rong R, Zhan X, Xiao G. Pathology image analysis using segmentation deep learning algorithms. Am J Pathol. 2019;189(9):1686–98.
12. Weis CA, Bindzus JN, Voigt J, Runz M, Hertjens S, Gaida MM, Popovic ZV, Porubsky S. Assessment of glomerular morphological patterns by deep learning algorithms. J Nephrol. 2022;35(2):417–27.
13. Ponce D, de Andrade LG, Claure-Del Granado R, Ferreiro-Fuentes A, Lombardi R. Development of a prediction score for in-hospital mortality in COVID-19 patients with acute kidney injury: a machine learning approach. Sci Rep. 2021;11(1):24439.
14. Islam MM, Nasrin T, Walther BA, Wu CC, Yang HC, Li YC. Prediction of sepsis patients using machine learning approach: a meta-analysis. Comput Methods Prog Biomed. 2019;170:1–9.
15. Fletcher RR, Nakeshimana A, Olubeko O. Addressing fairness, bias, and appropriate use of artificial intelligence and machine learning in global health. Front Artif Intell. 2021;3:561802.
16. Ko S, Jo C, Chang CB, Lee YS, Moon YW, Youm JW, Han HS, Lee MC, Lee H, Ro DH. A web-based machine-learning algorithm predicting postoperative acute kidney injury after total knee arthroplasty. Knee Surg Sports Traumatol Arthrosc. 2022;30(2):545–54.
17. Lachance P, Villeneuve PM, Rewa OG, Wilson FP, Selby NM, Featherstone RM, Bagshaw SM. Association between e-alert implementation for detection of acute kidney injury and outcomes: a systematic review. Nephrol Dial Transplant. 2017;32(2):265–72.

35 The Future of Solid Organ Transplantation: Postgraduate Education and Training

Abbas Ghazanfar

Key Points

- There are two key elements in solid organ transplantation: organ procurement and preservation, as well as organ transplantation. Any postgraduate education and training program should address both of these elements.
- Machine perfusion is rapidly becoming the gold standard for preserving abdominal and cardiothoracic organs, especially for higher-risk donors.
- With the help of advanced preservation techniques like normothermic machine perfusion (NMP) and normothermic regional perfusion (NRP), more organs from donations after circulatory death (DCD) donors are being successfully transplanted. This is a critical step in addressing the organ shortage.
- Simulation and virtual reality (VR): VR and augmented reality (AR) should be integrated into the curriculum as a standard part. Trainees should be able to practice high-stakes scenarios in a risk-free environment.
- AI and data analytics: Training should incorporate how to use AI and machine learning tools.

Solid organ transplantation has transformed the management of end-stage organ failure with improved quality of life and prolonged life expectancy. It has evolved from an experimental procedure into a life-saving medical practice, marked by advancements in surgical techniques, organ preservation, immunology, and the development of organ donation systems. From the first kidney transplant by Dr. Joseph Murray and his team from Boston in 1954 to the most recent attempts at xenotransplantation, solid organ transplantation has seen many challenges and developments.

A. Ghazanfar (✉)
Department of Renal and Transplant Surgery, St George's University Hospitals NHS Foundation Trust, London, United Kingdom

J. Sandars et al. (eds.), *Modern Medical Education*,
https://doi.org/10.1007/978-3-032-27958-3_35

The future of postgraduate medical education and training is shifting from traditional, time-based models to more flexible, personalized, and technology-driven approaches. The focus is now on ensuring that physicians possess the necessary competencies to meet the evolving needs of patients and the healthcare system.

The field of organ transplantation is undergoing rapid evolution, driven by significant advancements across several key areas. These innovations are designed to address the persistent challenges of organ shortages, improve transplant success rates, and enhance the long-term health and quality of life for recipients. It is therefore essential to maintain these priorities in focus when planning and delivering postgraduate medical education and training related to solid organ transplantation.

There are two key elements in solid organ transplantation: organ procurement and preservation as well as organ transplantation. Any postgraduate education and training program should address both of these elements.

35.1 Organ Procurement and Preservation

The first key element in solid organ transplantation is organ procurement from deceased and living donors. This complex process involves a series of meticulously coordinated steps to ensure the donated organ remains viable for transplantation. This involves surgical steps to safely remove the organs without damage, preserving and transporting them. The basic principles are the same; however, the skill sets for cardiothoracic and abdominal organs differ.

35.1.1 Organ Procurement and Preservation for Cardiothoracic Organs [1, 2]

Organ procurement and preservation for the heart and lungs is a particularly challenging and time-sensitive process due to their high metabolic demands and susceptibility to damage. The success of a heart or lung transplant is heavily dependent on the quality of the donated organ and the preservation techniques used.

The key challenge in cardiothoracic organs is less tolerance to ischemia. The heart is a continuously working muscle. When it is stopped and removed from the body, its cells begin to die due to a lack of oxygen and nutrients. A heart must be transplanted within a very short timeframe —typically 4–6 h —to ensure it functions properly after being reconnected to the recipient's circulatory system. The lungs are also highly delicate and prone to injury. They are constantly exposed to the environment, making them susceptible to infection and inflammation in the donor. The recommended cold ischemic time for lungs is also very short, generally 6–8 h.

Due to these strict time limits, a highly coordinated and efficient system is required for the procurement and preservation of cardiothoracic organs. Currently, the following options are available for preserving and storing cardiothoracic organs in practice.

A. Static Cold Storage (SCS): This is the traditional, and still the most common, method for heart and lung preservation. After the organs are surgically removed from the donor, they are immediately flushed with a cold, specialized preservation solution (cardioplegia for the heart and a lung-specific solution for the lungs). This solution is designed to stop the organs' metabolic activity and protect the cells from damage. The organs are then placed in a sterile bag, which is sealed and put on ice in a cooler for transport. The cold temperature reduces the organs' metabolic rate, slowing oxygen and energy consumption. This buys the transplant team a crucial window of time to transport the organ to the recipient.
B. Machine Perfusion (MP): This is a more advanced and increasingly common method, particularly for high-risk or marginal organs. In normothermic machine perfusion (NMP), this revolutionary technique utilizes a portable machine to maintain the heart or lungs in a near-physiological state outside the body. The heart is connected to a circuit that perfuses it with a warm, oxygenated, nutrient-rich solution, allowing the heart to continue beating during transport. This allows the surgical team to evaluate the heart's function in real time, which is a significant advantage for hearts from donors with a more complex medical history. The lungs are connected to a circuit that ventilates them and perfuses them with a warm, oxygenated solution. This technique can not only extend the preservation time but also improve the function of lungs that might have been initially deemed unsuitable for transplant due to factors like fluid accumulation or injury.

To prolong organ preservation time with the best outcomes, various advancements in cardiothoracic organ procurement and preservation have been made, aiming to address the persistent organ shortage and improve long-term outcomes [3]. The main areas of focus are as follows:

A. Ex Vivo Organ Repair: NMP is the platform for this. Researchers are exploring ways to use the perfusion machine to actively repair a donor organ. This could involve adding therapeutic agents, such as anti-inflammatory drugs or gene therapies, to the perfusion solution to reverse damage or improve the organ's health before transplantation.
B. Long-Term Preservation: The ultimate goal is to "organ bank" hearts and lungs for long periods. Techniques such as subzero preservation and vitrification are being researched to enable the storage of organs for days, weeks, or even months. This would eliminate the time-sensitive nature of current transplant logistics, enabling the best possible match for every patient, regardless of their geographic location.
C. Donation After Circulatory Death (DCD): Historically, most heart and lung transplants came from donors who were brain dead but whose hearts were still beating. With the advent of NMP and other advanced techniques like NRP, there is a growing trend to utilize organs from DCD donors whose hearts have stopped beating. These methods enable the recovery and reanimation of organs, significantly expanding the donor pool.

35.1.2 Organ Procurement and Preservation for Abdominal Organs [4]

The procurement of abdominal organs is a highly coordinated and meticulous surgical procedure, the aim of which is to retrieve high-quality organs for transplants. The steps in abdominal organ preservation are as follows:

(i) Preparation and In Situ Perfusion: Once a deceased donor is confirmed, a surgical team exposes the abdominal organs. A key step is in situ perfusion, in which a cold preservation solution is infused into the organs while they remain in the body. This rapid cooling halts cellular metabolism and flushes out blood, which can be damaging during preservation.
(ii) Organ Dissection and Removal: After the initial flush, the surgical team carefully dissects the organs. The order of removal is crucial and depends on the organs being procured. For example, if both the liver and pancreas are being taken, the portal vein is dissected to preserve the vascular supply to both organs.
(iii) Split Liver Transplantation: A unique aspect of liver procurement is the possibility of a split liver transplant. This is a procedure where a single deceased donor's liver is divided into two parts—a smaller left lobe and a larger right lobe—to be transplanted into two different recipients, typically a child and an adult. This innovative approach helps to increase the number of organs available, especially for paediatric patients.
(iv) Final Assessment and Packing: Once removed, each organ is inspected by the procurement surgeon for quality and integrity. They are then placed in sterile bags, sealed, and packed into a cooler with ice for transport to the recipient's transplant center. The cold temperature maintains the low metabolic state.

The preservation of abdominal organs is primarily defined by the duration they can be maintained and the techniques used to maintain their viability. The following methods are currently in practice:

A. Static Cold Storage (SCS): This is the most common method of preservation for abdominal organs. After being flushed with a preservation solution (such as University of Wisconsin, Celsior, or HTK solution), the organs are placed in sterile plastic bags, sealed, and packed in a cooler with ice for transport.
B. Machine Perfusion (MP): Machine perfusion is rapidly becoming the gold standard for preserving abdominal organs, especially for higher-risk donors.
   (a) Hypothermic Machine Perfusion (HMP): This technique involves continuously pumping a cold, oxygenated solution through the organ. In kidney transplants, HMP has been shown to reduce the rate of delayed graft function (DGF), a common complication in which the transplanted kidney doesn't function immediately and requires dialysis.
   (b) Normothermic Machine Perfusion (NMP) [5]: This is a game-changing technology, particularly for livers from donations after circulatory death

(DCD). DCD organs are exposed to a period of warm ischemia, which can cause significant damage. NMP allows the liver to be perfused with a warm, oxygenated solution, restoring its metabolic activity and giving the transplant team a chance to assess and even repair the organ before transplantation. NMP has been shown to reduce biliary complications and increase the utilization of marginal livers that would have otherwise been discarded.

Future developments in abdominal organ procurement and preservation aim to expand the donor pool and improve outcomes.

(i) Utilization of DCD Donors: With the help of advanced preservation techniques like NMP, more organs from DCD donors are being successfully transplanted. Most recently the use of NRP in DCD donors have resulted in better transplant outcomes. These are critical steps in addressing the organ shortage.
(ii) Organ Reconditioning and Repair: The development of machine perfusion is moving beyond simple preservation to active repair. Researchers are exploring ways to use the perfusion platform to deliver drugs, stem cells, or gene therapies to the organ, potentially reversing damage and improving its long-term function.
(iii) Advanced Imaging and AI [6, 7]: The use of artificial intelligence and advanced imaging techniques during machine perfusion can provide real-time data on an organ's viability, helping surgeons make better decisions about which organs to transplant and reducing the risk of a poor outcome.

35.2 Postgraduate Education and Training in Organ Procurement and Preservation

The focus is shifting from a traditional, surgical-centered model to a holistic, multidisciplinary approach that addresses the entire organ donation ecosystem. Future programs will be defined by their integration of technology, emphasis on a broader skill set, and a commitment to collaborative, immersive learning. Therefore, the curriculum of the future should not just teach about new technologies; it must be built around them. The training should cover the key topics as follows:

A. Hands-on Machine Perfusion Training: Trainees should receive extensive, practical experience with all types of machine perfusion (MP) systems. The training should focus on:

   (a) *Data Interpretation:* Learning to analyze real-time data on oxygen consumption, lactate levels, and bile production to make critical, data-driven decisions about organ viability.
   (b) *Therapeutic Application:* Utilizing the MP platform to deliver therapeutic agents, such as anti-inflammatory drugs, stem cells, or gene therapies, to an organ, thereby actively working to repair damage and improve its function before transplantation.

B. Simulation and Virtual Reality (VR): VR and augmented reality (AR) should be integrated into the curriculum as a standard part. Trainees should be able to practice high-stakes scenarios in a risk-free environment. These should include:

   (a) *Multi-Organ Retrieval Simulation:* Practicing the complex coordination required for multi-organ procurement, including navigating anatomical variations and managing time-sensitive situations.
   (b) *Simulated Family Conversations:* Training professionals to handle complex and emotionally charged conversations with donor families. VR simulations can provide a realistic environment for practicing empathy, active listening, and delivering difficult news—a skill that is paramount but often difficult to teach in a traditional setting.

C. AI and Data Analytics: Training should incorporate how to use AI and machine learning tools for:

   (a) *Optimized Allocation:* Understanding and using AI algorithms that analyze millions of data points to find the best possible donor-recipient match, minimizing rejection risk and improving long-term outcomes.
   (b) *Predictive Viability Assessment:* Learning to interpret AI-generated scores that predict an organ's viability, helping to prevent the discard of usable organs from marginal donors and expanding the donor pool.

D. Donor Management and End-of-Life Care: Training should extend beyond the operating room to the intensive care unit. Professionals must learn advanced techniques for managing potential donors to ensure organs remain healthy and viable. This includes understanding the unique physiological changes that occur with brain death and how to mitigate their impact on organ health.
E. Communication and Ethics: This is a crucial area of focus. Training should address the nuances of communication, moving from simply "asking for consent" to a deeper understanding of compassionate care for the donor family. Education must also tackle the complex ethical and legal questions posed by new technologies like xenotransplantation and the use of organs from donation after circulatory death (DCD) donors.
F. Logistics and Quality Assurance: Future training should emphasize logistics and quality management. This includes mastering organ transport, managing the supply chain for preservation fluids and equipment, and understanding the regulatory frameworks governing organ donation to ensure safety and compliance.

35.3 Organ Transplantation

The procedure of organ transplantation is becoming increasingly challenging. With the growing aging population, recipients are becoming more complex, demanding greater knowledge and skills for perioperative management. Likewise, minimal-access surgery, perioperative rehabilitation, and enhanced recovery are norms in current clinical practice. The key focus of future medical education in transplantation should be to address these issues.

A. Xenotransplantation as a Viable Option [8]: This is no longer science fiction. Recent clinical trials involving the transplantation of genetically modified pig kidneys and hearts into humans have demonstrated remarkable progress. The future will see the approval of the first multi-patient clinical trials. Using advanced gene-editing tools like CRISPR, scientists are making pig organs more compatible with the human immune system by adding human genes and inactivating pig genes that cause rejection and carry the risk of transmitting viruses. This has the potential to provide a virtually unlimited and on-demand supply of organs, dramatically reducing waiting list deaths.
B. Bioengineered Organs [9]: While further off, the ultimate goal is to create patient-specific organs in a lab. These include:

    (a) 3D Bioprinting: Scientists are making significant strides in 3D bioprinting, a process that uses "bio-ink" (a mix of cells and a biocompatible gel) to build functional organs layer by layer. The vision is to print a custom organ from a patient's own cells, thereby eliminating the risk of rejection and the need for immunosuppressive drugs.
    (b) Decellularization: This process involves using a "skeleton" or scaffold of a donated or animal organ and "re-cellularizing" it with a recipient's cells. This creates a natural, functioning organ that the patient's body will not reject.

C. Optimize Matching: Analyze vast datasets to predict the best possible donor-recipient match based on a multitude of factors, going beyond traditional criteria to improve long-term outcomes.
D. Predict Organ Viability: Interpret AI-generated scores and image analysis to make more confident decisions about accepting or discarding a donor organ, particularly those from extended-criteria donors.
E. Immunosuppressive Medications: The current need for lifelong immunosuppressive drugs is a significant burden for transplant recipients, leading to a host of side effects and an increased risk of infection and cancer. The primary focus of current advancements is as follows:

    (a) Targeted Immunosuppression: Researchers are developing more specific immunosuppressive drugs that only target the pathways responsible for rejection, leaving the rest of the immune system intact. This would reduce side effects and improve the patient's quality of life.
    (b) Inducing Immune Tolerance: The ultimate goal is to achieve immune tolerance, a state where the recipient's body accepts the new organ as its own, eliminating the need for drugs. Early clinical trials are showing promising results with cellular therapies, in which donor cells are infused into recipients to "retrain" their immune systems. This could be a proper cure for organ failure.

(c) Personalized Posttransplant Care: AI will help clinicians manage a patient's posttransplant care by predicting the risk of rejection or complications and personalizing medication dosages to achieve the best balance between preventing rejection and minimizing side effects.

35.4 Future of Postgraduate Education and Training in Solid Organ Transplantation

A confluence of technological, ethical, and clinical advancements is redefining the future of postgraduate education and training in solid organ transplantation. The traditional model of a single surgeon performing a procedure is giving way to a new paradigm of team-based, technologically fluent, and ethically aware professionals.

Postgraduate education will move beyond traditional lectures and books, embracing a more dynamic, hands-on, and collaborative approach. Therefore, the focus should be on the following:

A. Team-Based Learning: Training programs should be designed for multidisciplinary teams, including surgeons, intensivists, transplant coordinators, perfusionists, and nurses. This mirrors the real-world environment, ensuring that every team member understands their role within the context of the entire process. The key to this is simulation training.
B. Case-Based and Problem-Based Learning: Instead of rote memorization, the curriculum should be built around real-life case studies and challenges. Trainees should work through complex scenarios—such as an urgent procurement from a DCD donor with an extended warm ischemic time—to develop critical thinking and problem-solving skills.
C. Mentorship and Global Collaboration: Future training should leverage technology to connect trainees with world-renowned experts from across the globe. Online platforms, international masterclasses, and virtual mentorship programs should facilitate the sharing of best practices and a deeper understanding of global donation models.
D. Transplant Coordination as a Core Competency: The role of the transplant coordinator will be elevated in training. Professionals should receive comprehensive education on donor management, logistics, and communication, recognizing the coordinator's central role in the success of a transplant.
E. The Ethics of Xenotransplantation: With the rise of xenotransplantation, training should include a thorough discussion of the ethical issues surrounding the use of animals as organ sources. This includes animal welfare, the risk of cross-species disease transmission (xenozoonosis), and the need for rigorous informed consent from the recipient.
F. Equity and Allocation: The use of AI in organ allocation raises questions about potential bias. Future training should include in-depth discussions of the ethical and legal frameworks governing organ allocation to ensure the process remains

fair and equitable for all patients, regardless of background or socioeconomic status.

G. Bioethics of New Technologies: Professionals should be trained to navigate the complex ethical dilemmas posed by new technologies such as ex vivo organ repair and bioengineered organs. This includes discussions on how to define "death" in the age of advanced life support and the long-term societal implications of these life-changing advancements.
H. Robotic and Minimally Invasive Surgery: While open surgery remains a cornerstone of transplantation, the use of robotic systems like the da Vinci Surgical System is increasing for both organ retrieval (e.g., live donor nephrectomy) and transplantation procedures. Surgeons should be highly skilled in operating these systems to perform complex, minimally invasive procedures with greater precision, reduced blood loss, and faster patient recovery times.
I. AI and Machine Learning (ML) Literacy: The role of AI in transplantation is expanding. Surgeons must understand how to interpret and utilize AI-driven tools.
J. Data Analysis and Informatics: Surgeons must be comfortable with large datasets and health informatics. The ability to interpret and apply data from advanced monitoring systems will be crucial for managing posttransplant care, predicting rejection, and personalizing immunosuppressive regimens.
K. Advanced Communication and Counselling: The complexity of new technologies and therapies, particularly xenotransplantation and experimental procedures, will require surgeons to have exceptional communication skills to counsel patients and their families, ensuring they understand the risks, benefits, and ethical considerations.
L. Team Leadership and Collaboration: The future of transplant surgery is highly multidisciplinary. Surgeons will need to effectively collaborate with a wide range of professionals, including data scientists, bioengineers, immunologists, ethicists, and palliative care specialists.
M. Remote and Tele-Surgery: The combination of AI and robotics with telemedicine could enable surgeons to assist with, or even perform, procedures in remote locations. This will require new skills in remote guidance and operation.

35.5 Conclusion

In summary, future postgraduate education and training in organ procurement and preservation will create a new kind of professional: one who is not only a skilled clinician but also a technological innovator, an ethical leader, and a compassionate communicator, capable of navigating the full spectrum of challenges in modern organ donation. Any postgraduate training program should be designed with these key elements in mind.

References

1. Hess NR, Ziegler LA, Kaczorowski DJ. Heart donation and preservation: historical perspectives, current technologies, and future directions. J Clin Med. 2022;11(19):5762. https://doi.org/10.3390/jcm11195762. PMID: 36233630; PMCID: PMC9571059.
2. Kukreja J, Campo-Canaveral de la Cruz JL, Van Raemdonck D, Cantu E, Date H, D'Ovidio F, Hartwig M, Klapper JA, Kelly RF, Lindstedt S, Rosso L, Schaheen L, Smith M, Whitson B, Saddoughi SA, Cypel M. The 2024 American association for thoracic surgery expert consensus document: current standards in donor lung procurement and preservation. J Thorac Cardiovasc Surg. 2025;169(2):484–504. https://doi.org/10.1016/j.jtcvs.2024.08.052. PMID: 39826938.
3. Siddique A, Parekh KR, Huddleston SJ, Shults A, Locke JE, Keshavamurthy S, Schwartz G, Hartwig MG, Whitson BA. A call to action in thoracic transplant surgical training. J Heart Lung Transplant. 2023;42(11):1627–31. https://doi.org/10.1016/j.healun.2023.05.017. Epub 2023 Jun 1. PMID: 37268052.
4. Hameed AM, Hawthorne WJ, Pleass HC. Advances in organ preservation for transplantation. ANZ J Surg. 2017;87(12):976–80. https://doi.org/10.1111/ans.13713. Epub 2016 Aug 4. PMID: 27490874.
5. Silpe S, Martinez E, Wall A. Normothermic regional perfusion procurement for abdominal organ donors: techniques and troubleshooting. Curr Opin Organ Transplant. 2024;29(3):200–4. https://doi.org/10.1097/MOT.0000000000001140. Epub 2024 Mar 11. PMID: 38465664.
6. Bhat M, Rabindranath M, Chara BS, Simonetto DA. Artificial intelligence, machine learning, and deep learning in liver transplantation. J Hepatol. 2023;78(6):1216–33. https://doi.org/10.1016/j.jhep.2023.01.006. PMID: 37208107.
7. Alamgir A, Hussein H, Abdelaal Y, Abd-Alrazaq A, Househ M. Artificial intelligence in kidney transplantation: a scoping review. Stud Health Technol Inform. 2022;25(294):254–8. https://doi.org/10.3233/SHTI220448. PMID: 35612067.
8. Kamberi S, Meier RPH. Xenotransplantation literature update December 2023-June 2024. Xenotransplantation. 2024;31(5):e12883. https://doi.org/10.1111/xen.12883. PMID: 39276074.
9. Dey M, Ozbolat IT. 3D bioprinting of cells, tissues and organs. Sci Rep. 2020;10(1):14023. https://doi.org/10.1038/s41598-020-70086-y. PMID: 32811864; PMCID: PMC7434768.

Future Training in the Field of Organ Transplantation: How to Transfer Skills and Knowledge to the Postgraduates

36

Muhammad Shahzad Anwar and Mohammad Ahmad

Key Points

- The Halstedian apprenticeship model has traditionally been employed for the surgical training of postgraduate residents.
- The rapidly evolving nature of organ transplantation necessitates that the crude apprenticeship model be replaced with a more sophisticated one.
- Structured fellowship programs, competency-based medical education, multidisciplinary curriculum design, case-based learning, trainee-centered learning, surgical skills workshops, and international training programs are among the proposed techniques.
- Technological advancements such as simulation-based training, virtual reality and augmented reality, artificial intelligence, machine learning, telemedicine and remote training, and robotics are poised to transform organ transplantation training.
- Continuous adaptation in surgical practice and training methodologies is required to optimize the training of future organ transplant surgeons.

36.1 Introduction

Organ transplantation represents one of the most important success stories of modern medicine. It is a highly specialized and complex field which has transformed the management of end-stage organ failure. It is the epitome of a true multidisciplinary approach in medicine, combining surgical skill, critical care management, immunological expertise, and an understanding of ethical and societal considerations.

M. S. Anwar (✉) · M. Ahmad
Department of Urology, Services Institute of Medical Science, Lahore, Pakistan

J. Sandars et al. (eds.), *Modern Medical Education*,
https://doi.org/10.1007/978-3-032-27958-3_36

Organ transplantation is not a new concept. For millennia, human beings have been fascinated by tales of mystical creatures made up of the amalgamation of various animal and human body parts. It has also been documented in the folklore of many ancient civilizations and has also gained fame in the word of science fiction. However, the first verifiable case of a human organ transplant occurred in 1869 when a Swiss surgeon, Jacques-Louis Reverdin, performed the first successful epidermal skin grafting [1]. This was followed by several other successful organ transplants over the years, such as:

- 1905: First corneal transplant [2]
- 1954: First living-related kidney transplant [3]
- 1962: First aortic homograft to replace the aortic valve [4]
- 1962: First kidney transplant between genetically nonrelated patients done using immunosuppression [5]
- 1966: First pancreatic transplant [6]
- 1967: First liver transplant [7]

The history of organ transplantation in Pakistan dates back to 1979 when the first successful kidney transplant was performed where the organ was retrieved from a living related donor. Initially, the case load was low with only 50 cases being performed in a year; however, by the mid-1990s, this number doubled to 100 cases per annum [8]. Similarly, other organ transplants were also started, such as hematopoietic stem cell transplant 1995 [9] and liver transplant in 2003 [10].

Organ transplantation was long considered an experimental procedure and there were numerous failed attempts before cases of successful organ transplantation began to appear in medical literature. However, advancements in surgical techniques, preoperative assessment, postoperative care, immunosuppressive regimens, and organ preservation, over the past seven decades, have significantly improved the success rates and long-term outcomes of organ transplantation. These medical improvements have transformed organ transplantation from an experimental procedure into the standard of care for patients with end-stage organ failure.

The number of organ transplant cases has been steadily increasing over the past several decades. According to The Global Observatory on Donation and Transplantation, 172.409 organs were transplanted in 2023, indicating a 9.5% increase over 2022. This increase in the case load not only increases the demand for organ transplantation infrastructure but also the skilled personnel required to perform these complex procedures. As a result, the training of the next generation of surgeons and health professionals involved in organ transplantation has become paramount.

Unlike other specialties, organ transplantation requires a true multidisciplinary approach involving immunological principles, perioperative management, surgical technique, and ethical considerations. This makes the process of medical education of postgraduate trainees a uniquely challenging ordeal.

While the apprenticeship model has traditionally been the cornerstone of medical education, the increasing complexity and specialization within the organ transplantation field necessitate a shift toward more modern and structured training programs.

This chapter aims to examine the current state of organ transplantation training, identify its limitations, and explore alternative strategies for optimal training of postgraduate trainees in this ever-evolving field.

36.2 The Current State of Organ Transplantation Training

Most surgical disciplines, including organ transplantation, have historically used the Halstedian model for the surgical training of postgraduate residents. This model, developed by William Stewart Halsted, is an apprenticeship-based system designed on the principles of hands-on training. It involves a step-by-step progression from observation to direct assistance, to supervised performance, and eventually independent practice. It relies heavily on experiential learning and direct mentorship of seasoned surgeons and is characterized by long hours in the operating room, exposure to a high volume of diverse cases, and gradual acquisition of surgical expertise.

This model has long been effective in producing highly skilled surgeons due to its emphasis on direct, hands-on experience and immediate feedback from experienced mentors.

36.3 Challenges in Traditional Training Methods

Over the years, the conventional training system has produced excellent surgeons who are well-equipped to deal with the complexities of organ transplantation. These surgeons, in turn, have helped propel the field of organ transplantation into a landmark success for treating end-stage organ failure. However, despite this success, this orthodox model faces increasing limitations, primarily due to the rapidly evolving nature of organ transplantation. There are several factors contributing to these limitations, such as:

- Patient load
- Uneven distribution of transplant cases across centers
- Expertise of the supervisor
- Ethical imperatives to avoid unnecessary risk to patients
- Global disparities in training due to divergent healthcare infrastructures, organ availability, and access to technology
- Multidisciplinary nature of transplantation
- The exponential growth of knowledge in immunology, genetics, and organ preservation

36.4 The Need for Innovation in Organ Transplantation Training

Much like other medical specialties, the field of organ transplantation is evolving rapidly, necessitating reevaluation of the existing training methods. It is the need of the hour that the traditionally employed crude apprenticeship model be replaced with a more structured one that focuses on the integration of novel technologies and educational methodologies. Future organ transplant surgeons must not only have meticulous surgical technique but also a complex understanding of immunology, pharmacology, patient care, and the ethical dilemmas posed by organ transplantation.

36.5 Overview of Future Training Approaches

Advancement in the field of organ transplantation has created a need for more sophisticated surgical training models. Several innovative strategies have been proposed such as structured fellowship programs, competency-based medical education, multidisciplinary curriculum design, case-based learning, specialized skills workshops, and integration of technological advancements. This chapter will explore these emerging training methodologies and evaluate their potential in improving postgraduate organ transplantation training.

36.6 Structured Fellowship Programs

Most fellowship programs, currently, are based on a mentorship model where trainees gain experience by shadowing their senior colleagues. This model has considerable advantages, such as exposure to a wide array of complex cases and direct feedback from experienced surgeons; however, it often lacks standardization and is dependent on the supervisor's availability and willingness to teach the trainees. Additionally, many surgeons rely on their own teaching methods, which might deviate from the established norms. This creates a considerable variability in the training of upcoming surgeons across different centers.

To address this, there is a need to create standardized, structured, accredited fellowship programs with a defined curriculum. These should include exposure to:

- Multiple organ systems (kidney, liver, pancreas, heart, lung)
- Both donor and recipient procedures
- Longitudinal patient follow-up
- Immunology
- Vascular access
- Transplant radiology
- Genetics

This comprehensive approach would ensure that the future transplant surgeons follow standardized transplant protocols and possess a holistic understanding of all the intricacies involved in organ transplantation.

36.7 Competency-Based Medical Education

Shifting from time-based training to competency-based frameworks ensures that trainees progress upon demonstrating mastery rather than simply completing rotations. This approach focuses on the acquisition of specific skills and knowledge required for better patient management rather than simply spending a predetermined amount of time in training programs. The fellows are judged based on the attainment of these proficiencies rather than the time that they have spent in training programs. Some of these competencies include:

1. Knowledge and critical thinking
2. Technical skills
3. Communication skills
4. Teamwork
5. Research
6. Professionalism
7. Pedagogy
8. Advocacy

By the end of the fellowship program, fellows would be expected to acquire these competencies and their constituent learning outcomes and provide promotive, preventive, curative, and rehabilitative patient-centered (or population-centered) care.

36.8 Multidisciplinary Curriculum Design

The multidisciplinary nature of organ transplantation necessitates a curriculum that transcends the traditional silos of surgical training. Conventional surgical training is often monopolar in nature, focusing on the essential surgical skills required for the procedures. It fails to adequately train the potential surgeons in essential specialties that are interconnected with organ transplantation. A comprehensive curriculum should therefore incorporate training modules from these diverse fields, ensuring that the future surgeons are well-versed in the multifaceted aspects of organ transplantation. Based on the recommendations of the Royal College of Physicians of Ireland and Pakistan Kidney and Liver Institute, such a curriculum should include:

- *Organ transplant recipient evaluation*
  Objective: To ensure that the trainee acquires the skills and knowledge to assess and manage organ transplant recipients.
- *Organ donor evaluation*

Objective: To ensure that the trainee acquires the skills and knowledge to evaluate the suitability of the organ donor for transplantation.

- *Tissue typing and crossmatching*
  Objective: To ensure that the trainee is well-versed in methods of blood and tissue typing, crossmatching, and alloantibody measurement, and he/she is able to apply this knowledge in organ transplant setting.
- *Perioperative care of organ transplant recipients and donors*
  Objective: To ensure that the trainee acquires the skills and knowledge to manage organ transplant recipients and donors in the perioperative period.
- *Principles of transplant immunosuppression*
  Objective: To ensure that the trainee has adequate knowledge of transplant immunosuppression regimens for use in organ transplant recipients.
- *Identification and management of organ transplant dysfunction*
  Objective: To ensure that the trainee has the skills and knowledge to identify and manage patients with organ transplant dysfunction.
- *Transplant rejection*
  Objective: To ensure that the trainee has the skills and knowledge to diagnose and treat organ transplant rejection.
- *Infectious complications* of organ transplantation
  Objective: To ensure that the trainee has the skills and knowledge to be able to diagnose and manage infectious complications in organ transplant patients.
- *Malignancy in organ transplantation*
  Objective: To ensure that the trainee has the skills and knowledge to diagnose and manage malignancy in the transplanted organs.
- *Highly sensitized transplant recipient*
  Objective: To ensure that the trainee has the skills and knowledge to manage highly sensitized potential organ transplant recipients.
- *Plasmapheresis*
  Objective: To ensure that the trainee has the necessary skills and knowledge to be able to plan, prescribe, and monitor plasmapheresis in the transplant patients.
- *Pediatric organ transplantation*
  Objective: To ensure that the trainee has acquired the skills and knowledge for the management of pediatric organ transplant patients.
- *Deceased donor organ transplant program*
  Objective: To ensure that the trainee has an understanding of the allocation process for deceased donor organs and is familiar with the organ transplant registry.
- *Ethical considerations in organ transplantation*
  Objective: To ensure that the trainee receives adequate training in dealing with the ethical and societal aspects of organ transplantation.
- *Transplanted organ failure*
  Objective: To ensure that the trainee possesses the skills and knowledge to adequately manage patients with failing transplants.
- *Procedures*
  - *Transplant biopsy*

Objective: To ensure that the trainee acquired the skills necessary to perform transplant organ biopsies.

– *Ultrasound scanning of the transplanted organ*

Objective: To ensure that the trainee is proficient at performing and interpreting ultrasound scanning of transplant organs and ultrasound-guided organ biopsy.

– *Transplant recipient surgery*

Objective: To ensure that the trainee develops proficiency in performing organ transplant recipient surgeries, with a focus on the surgical techniques, recipient safety, and the management of intraoperative complications.

– *Living donor surgery*

Objective: To ensure that the trainee develops proficiency in performing living donor surgery, focusing on surgical techniques, donor safety, and the management of intraoperative and postoperative complications.

– *Vascular access surgery*

Objective: To ensure that the trainee develops proficiency in performing vascular access surgery for hemodialysis, focusing on surgical techniques, patient selection, and the management of intraoperative and postoperative complications.

36.9 Case-Based Learning

Traditional teaching methods rely on didactic lectures and passive information transfer. However, case-based discussions encourage active learning through the analysis of real-world scenarios. It allows the trainees to apply theoretical knowledge to complex clinical problems, helping them to develop critical thinking, problem-solving skills, and clinical decision-making. This approach is effective in the delivery of health professional education and enhancing learning outcomes [11].

36.10 Trainee-Centered Learning

Historically, surgical education has been teacher centered. It involves the teacher taking the lead role and trainees passively absorbing information. However, this method often limits the amount of information and skill that the trainee can absorb. A trainee-centered learning program would make the trainees cocreators in their education process, engaging them in decisions regarding the content, pace, and methodology of their training. This approach is deemed to be more helpful for the students in achieving their educational objectives [12].

36.11 Surgical Skills Workshops

These specialized workshops are conducted in a controlled environment where trainees can practice and refine their surgical skills using cadaveric models, animal specimens, and surgical simulators without the pressure of performing on live patients. Such workshops allow the trainees to work on their shortcomings under the supervision of experienced surgeons without the fear of patient complications and help the mentors to teach freely without the ethical considerations associated with on-patient training.

36.12 International Training Programs

The magnitude of organ transplant cases around the world depends on a number of factors, including disease prevalence, socioeconomic factors, healthcare infrastructure, and cultural and religious attitudes toward transplantation. Hence, there is a disparity in training across different centers. International training programs are essential in bridging these gaps and facilitating an all-around training of young surgeons. These training programs allow trainees to observe and learn different clinical practices across diverse patient populations and healthcare systems. This helps to broaden their perspectives and enhancing their surgical skills.

36.13 Technological Advancements in Training

Over the past few decades, the world of organ transplantation has gone through rapid evolution. This transformation has been driven primarily by technological advancements. These innovations have had a positive impact on surgical techniques and overall patient outcomes. In the field of organ transplantation, these technological innovations are poised to revolutionize the training of postgraduate residents and young surgeons. Some of these technological advancements include simulation-based tools, virtual reality, artificial intelligence, machine learning, telemedicine, and robotics.

36.14 Simulation-Based Training

Simulation-based training is one of the recent technological innovations that has transformed surgical education. The use of high-fidelity models, virtual reality platforms, and anatomically accurate organ replicas allows trainees to practice a wide range of surgical procedures in a controlled and stress-free environment. These simulators provide grossly accurate surgical scenarios mimicking real-life surgery. These allow for an immersive experience for the trainees so that they can be prepared for live surgery beforehand.

The benefits of such surgical simulators include unlimited opportunities for practice along with objective assessment through standardized metrics. These metrics include operative time, surgical accuracy, and error rate. Additionally, this approach minimizes the risk to the patients associated with premature surgical attempts by inexperienced trainees.

36.15 Virtual Reality (VR) and Augmented Reality (AR)

Virtual reality and augmented reality platforms have been widely used in nonmedical fields with positive results. These platforms simulate real-life scenarios and allow the users an immersive and interactive experience

Their use in medical field is an upcoming phenomenon. In surgical training, particularly organ transplantation, such platforms allow the trainees to perform complex procedures in a realistic virtual environment, preparing them for live surgical interventions.

36.16 Artificial Intelligence (AI) in Training

Artificial intelligence is perhaps one of the most groundbreaking and disruptive innovations of recent times. It has rapidly transformed many sectors, including medicine, surgery, and public health. In the context of surgical training, particularly organ transplantation, AI offers unprecedented opportunities. With the help of data analytics, AI can perform an objective skill assessment of trainees and help enhance their surgical training.

The integration of AI algorithms into surgical simulators and surgical robots has greatly increased the ability of these modalities to be of assistance in surgical training. This can be used to analyze a trainee's performance, provide real-time feedback, and identify areas for improvement. Furthermore, it can predict complications and patient outcomes based on intraoperative decision-making and allow real-time warnings. Additionally, AI tools can be used to devise individualized surgical training pathways for upcoming surgeons based on their strengths and weaknesses. Academic research is another area where AI can facilitate trainees by analyzing complex data and predicting patient outcomes.

36.17 Machine Learning for Personalized Training

By analyzing large datasets of organ transplant procedures and the subsequent patient outcomes, machine learning models can be helpful in identifying patterns and correlations. The analyses of such patterns can help devise personalized surgical training pathways and optimize organ transplant training curricula. This would enable the development of adaptive learning modules that would accelerate surgical skill acquisition by the trainees.

36.18 Telemedicine and Remote Training

Advancements in digital communication, especially 5G technology, can prove to be a game-change in organ transplant training. The use of high speed internet can allow seasoned transplant surgeons to mentor their junior counterparts across the globe. They can provide real-time guidance during live procedures, share valuable surgical experience and provide intraoperative feedback to their trainees. Such programs would be especially useful in low-volume, geographically inaccessible, and resource-limited centers.

36.19 Robotics

Robotics has increasingly become an integral part of modern surgery. It offers enhanced visualization, manual dexterity, and improved precision during complex surgeries, especially where deep body cavities are encountered. Having revolutionized surgical practice, robotic systems are now being used for optimizing surgical training. It offers a unique opportunity to young surgeons allowing them to gain proficiency in intricately complex surgical procedures by providing them with unlimited chances of practicing their surgical skills. The trainees can do so without the fear of complications during live surgery. Additionally, the integration of surgical robots with artificial intelligence programs can provide trainees with personalized feedback. This can help devise adaptive training pathways which would be designed to address the individual learning curves and skill gaps of the trainees.

36.20 Emerging Technologies and Their Potential Impact

The rapidly evolving nature of healthcare not only impacts patient care in organ transplantation but also influences the surgical training. This necessitates continuous adaptation of the organ transplantation curriculum by integrating novel tools and updated methodologies. It is pertinent for training programs to apprise their trainees of these recent developments so that they may not be left behind. Some of these emerging trends include:

1. Personalized Medicine and Genetics: Genomic profiling for tailored immunosuppressive therapy
2. Organ Preservation Innovations: Improving graft survival and function
3. 3D Bioprinting: Creating functional tissues and organs
4. Stem Cell Regenerative Medicine: Repairing or replacing damaged tissues
5. Xenotransplantation: Addressing organ shortages

36.21 Conclusion

The field of healthcare is evolving at a rapid pace. Organ transplantation has come long way from a simple epidermal skin graft to complex, multiple solid organ transplants. This meteoric progression also demands continuous adaptation in surgical practice and training methodologies to ensure that the future surgeons are equipped with the requisite skills and knowledge required in organ transplantation. Training of the future transplant surgeons requires a shift from the obsolete time-based apprenticeship model to a competency-based framework. Such a model must include cutting-edge technologies such as artificial intelligence, virtual reality platforms, simulator-based models, and robotics. Furthermore, it is paramount that supervisors and trainers themselves embrace these new technologies before they can be integrated into organ transplantation training modules. This will ensure that the newly trained transplant surgeons are fully equipped to meet the challenges of organ transplantation in the future.

References

1. Nordham KD, Ninokawa S. The history of organ transplantation. Proc (Bayl Univ Med Cent). 2022;35(1):124–8.
2. Röck T, Landenberger J, Bramkamp M, Bartz-Schmidt KU, Röck D. The evolution of corneal transplantation. Ann Transplant. 2017;22:749.
3. Rana A, Gruessner A, Agopian VG, Khalpey Z, Riaz IB, Kaplan B, Halazun KJ, Busuttil RW, Gruessner RW. Survival benefit of solid-organ transplant in the United States. JAMA Surg. 2015;150(3):252–9.
4. Bortolotti U, Vendramin I, Milano AD, Livi U. Milestone operations in heart valve and aortic replacement: anniversaries worth remembering. Aorta. 2023;11(06):203–6.
5. Hatzinger M, Stastny M, Grützmacher P, Sohn M. The history of kidney transplantation. Urologe A. 2016;55(10):1353–9.
6. Casanova D. Pancreas transplantation: 50 years of experience. Cir Esp. 2017;95(5):254–60.
7. Meirelles RF, Salvalaggio P, Rezende MB, Evangelista AS, Guardia BD, Matielo CE, Neves DB, Pandullo FL, Felga GE, Alves JA, Curvelo LA. Liver transplantation: history, outcomes and perspectives. Einstein (Sao Paulo). 2015;13(1):149–52.
8. Qaisar I, Manzoor S, Hashmi M. Legal and ethical issues of organ transplantation in Pakistan a critical appraisal in Sharī 'ah's perspective. MEI. 2020;19(1)
9. Ali N, Iftikhar R, Ayaz Mir M, Bokhari SW, Rehman JU, Zaidi U, Nasir S, Adil SN, Satti T, Nisa Chaudhry QU, Farhan M. Haematopoietic stem cell transplant trends in Pakistan: activity survey from Pakistan bone marrow transplant group. J Transplant. 2023;2023(1):8865364.
10. Syed IA, Khalid A, Khan BA, Aujla UI. The evolution of liver transplant program in Pakistan and the challenges ahead. J Liver Transpl. 2023;12:100187.
11. McLean SF. Case-based learning and its application in medical and health-care fields: a review of worldwide literature. J Med Educat Curri Dev. 2016;3:JMECD-S20377.
12. Yusof YA, Taridi NM, Mustapa M, Shaharuddin S, Hamid MW, Shakrin NN, Rahmat F, Roos NA, Zaidi NA, Lugova H. Student-centred approach in medical education: a review of the teaching-learning activities and the perceptions of educators on the students engagement and performance at the faculty of medicine and defence health, national defence university of Malaysia. Adv Human Biol. 2022;12(2):101–7.

Deafness: A Silent Malady 37

Shabih Zaidi, Noweed Ahmad, Farzana Naqvi, and Patricia Castellanos de Muñoz

Key Points

- Types and causes of deafness can be classified as congenital or acquired, mild to profound, and genetics to illness or injury.
- Medical and technological interventions for deafness include audiology and hearing aids, surgical interventions, and cochlear implants.
- Communication methods are sign language, lip-reading, hearing aids, and assistive technology.
- Educational approaches using modern educational strategies at medical schools, e.g., AI, VR, AR, simulation, and live surgery.
- Public Health and the deaf community.

37.1 Introduction

The WHO has been actively involved in global campaigns for the prevention of deafness and hearing impairment, particularly focusing on children for nearly three decades. It worked on prevention projects for many years and published a highly informative paper outlining the public health approach to preventing deafness and

S. Zaidi (✉)
al-Sadiq International Virtual University, London, UK

N. Ahmad
Department of Otolaryngology – Head and Neck Surgery, Tawam and STMC University Teaching Hospitals, Al Ain, United Arab Emirates

F. Naqvi
Rtd Professor and Head of Genetics, Karachi University, Karachi, Pakistan

P. C. de Muñoz
Audiology, Centro de Audición, CEDAF, Guatemala, Guatemala
e-mail: pdemunoz@cedaf.com.gt

J. Sandars et al. (eds.), *Modern Medical Education*,
https://doi.org/10.1007/978-3-032-27958-3_37

hearing impairment, especially through primary ear and hearing care [1]. Emphasis was placed on noise-induced hearing loss, with two authors (SZ & PC) contributing to the development of guidelines for community noise as part of that project [2].

Hearing loss can vary in severity from mild to profound, with some profoundly deafened individuals experiencing minimal benefit even from the most powerful hearing aids. Such individuals can benefit from cochlear implants, with one author (NA) developing expert guidelines for adult patients.

37.2 Clinical

Hearing impairment is a silent (often insidious) malady. Its impact on human life is well documented and a major cause (along with visual impairment) contributing to the global burden of disease. Its impact, particularly in early childhood, can lead to significant developmental challenges, affecting an individual's awareness of language, including highly disabling speech impairment.

37.2.1 Types of Hearing Impairment

1. Conductive Hearing Loss:

This occurs when sound is not conducted efficiently through the outer ear canal to the eardrum and the middle ear ossicles (malleus, incus, and stapes). The causes can include impacted wax, ear infections (otitis media), effusion in the middle ear (glue ears), or developmental blockages in the ear canal (partial or total atresia).

2. Sensorineural Hearing Loss:

This arises from damage to the inner ear (cochlea) or the auditory nerve pathways to the brain. It can be caused by genetics, noise exposure, aging (presbycusis), or certain illnesses (e.g., typhoid, antibiotic abuse, chemotherapy). Sensorineural hearing loss is often permanent and more challenging to treat than conductive hearing loss.

3. Mixed Hearing Loss:

This is a combination of conductive and sensorineural hearing loss, resulting from issues in both the middle (e.g., chronic otitis media) and inner ear (e.g., noise-induced or age-related hearing loss (presbycusis).

4. Auditory Processing Disorder (APD):

This rare condition affects how the brain processes auditory information, even when hearing ability is normal. Individuals may struggle to distinguish sounds, follow conversations, or understand spoken language in noisy environments.

37.2.2 The Causes of Deafness

They are varied; some are universal, while others are region specific.

Factors contributing to hearing loss in children aged 0–3 years include prenatal factors (15.4%) such as family history of hearing loss and TORCH (toxoplasmosis, others, rubella, cytomegalovirus, and herpes simplex virus) infections, perinatal causes (70.3%) like low birth weight and neonatal asphyxia, and postnatal factors (14.3%) including mechanical ventilation and febrile seizures [3].

Communicable diseases remain prevalent in many Asian, African, and Latin American countries. A common cause of deafness is ototoxicity, often resulting from aminoglycosides and similar antibiotics used to treat tuberculosis and intractable chronic supportive otitis media. Where cholesteatoma complications occur (rare in western countries but common in Asia), ototoxic antibiotics are often employed to prevent life-threatening conditions like meningitis, often resulting in profound sensorineural hearing loss.

Genetic factors, including hereditary and nonhereditary causes, significantly contribute to hearing loss. In many South Asian communities, consanguineous marriages were historically common, but increasing awareness through education and social media has led to a decline in these practices. Intrauterine infections like rubella and cytomegalovirus are important causes as well, and vaccination initiatives have successfully reduced maternal infections that contribute to intrauterine deafness.

It has long been recognized that unidentified hearing loss at birth can adversely affect speech and language development as well as academic achievement and social-emotional development. Historically, moderate-to-severe hearing loss in young children was not detected until well beyond the newborn period, and it was not unusual for diagnosis of mild hearing loss and unilateral hearing loss to be delayed until children reached school age [4].

Congenital hearing loss is frequently associated with a pathological vestibular system. Early identification allows timely intervention with personalized therapies. In current literature, there is still no gold standard test to identify balance disorders in patients with congenital hearing loss [5].

37.2.3 Diagnosis

Early diagnosis is the key to successfully preventing and managing hearing impairment. History taking, clinical examination, and investigations such as audiometry (and sometimes imaging) form the bedrock of any service.

1. Otoscopy.

   This simple procedure excludes many conditions such as atresia, partial atresia, wax buildup, effusions, perforated eardrum, and fungal infections.
2. Tuning Fork Tests.

   These are routinely performed to differentiate the type of hearing loss (e.g., conductive, sensor neural, unilateral, or bilateral). Rinne's and Weber's tests are established methods (but less reliable than audiometry).
3. Audiometry and tympanometry {See Item B}.
4. Additional investigations such as imaging (CT, MRI, MRA) sometimes may be required.

37.3 Audiology

Audiology is a time-tested discipline for hearing loss evaluation. It is experiencing rapid evolution through innovations in technology, emerging knowledge of neuroscience and personalized care. There have been many recent advances such as auditory rehabilitation, genetic management, and artificial intelligence.

The audiological assessment in individuals with suspected or confirmed deafness involves a systematic battery of tests designed to evaluate the integrity of the auditory system and determine the type, degree, and configuration of hearing loss. This assessment is adapted to the patient's age, developmental status, and communication abilities, ensuring both diagnostic accuracy and patient-centered care.

1.1 Case Histories and Clinical Interview

Evaluation begins with a thorough history, which provides context for diagnostic interpretation. For neonates and infants, this includes prenatal and perinatal factors, such as exposure to infections, medications, or birth complications. In children, developmental milestones, history of ear diseases, and familial hearing loss are assessed. Adults are queried about occupational and recreational noise exposure, ear symptoms, and current hearing concerns. This step guides the choice of diagnostic tests and shapes management planning.

1.2 Pure-Tone Audiometry

Pure-tone audiometry is the gold standard for assessing hearing sensitivity. It measures air and bone conduction thresholds across frequencies from 250 to 8000 Hz, classifying hearing loss as conductive, sensor neural, or mixed. Play audiometry and visual reinforcement audiometry (VRA) are employed in children, especially those under 5 years of age, while infants may undergo behavioral testing.

1.3 Speech Audiometry

Speech audiometry assesses functional hearing using speech stimuli. Two core measures are:

Speech Recognition Threshold (SRT): The lowest intensity at which a patient can identify familiar words.
Word Recognition Score (WRS): The percentage of correctly identified words at a comfortable listening level.

Speech audiometry is critical in understanding how hearing loss impacts everyday communication and helps shape rehabilitation strategies.

1.4 Tympanometry and Acoustic Reflex Testing

Tympanometry evaluates middle ear function by measuring the mobility of the tympanic membrane in response to air pressure changes. It diagnoses middle ear effusion, Eustachian tube dysfunction, and tympanic membrane perforations. Acoustic reflex testing complements tympanometry by assessing the stapedius muscle reflex, offering insight into the integrity of the neural pathway.

1.5 Otoacoustic Emissions (OAEs)

OAEs are sounds generated by the cochlea's outer hair cells in response to acoustic stimuli. Their presence indicates normal cochlear function, while their absence suggests damage. OAEs are essential for newborn hearing screening, monitoring ototoxicity, and differentiating cochlear from retrocochlear pathology.

1.6 Auditory Brainstem Response (ABR)

ABR testing measures neural responses from the auditory nerve to the brainstem following sound stimulation. It is indispensable for:

(a) Neonatal hearing screening; especially in high-risk infants.
(b) Diagnosing auditory neuropathy spectrum disorder (ANSD), etc.
(c) Assessing individuals unable to provide reliable behavioral responses.

1.7 High-Frequency and Extended High-Frequency Audiometry

High-frequency audiometry (9000–20,000 Hz) detects early cochlear damage, especially from ototoxic medications or occupational noise exposure. It identifies subclinical changes before they manifest in conventional audiometry.

2. Management and Rehabilitation Approaches

Once hearing loss is diagnosed, individualized management plans are developed. These include hearing aids, cochlear implants, auditory training, and counselling and multidisciplinary management.

2.1.1 Early Intervention: Pediatric Populations

Early detection and intervention are crucial for language and cognitive development. Universal Newborn Hearing Screening (UNHS) programs, identification by 1 month, diagnosis by 3 months, and intervention by 6 months—the "1–3-6" model. Such a screening with early intervention is crucial for alleviating the developmental impacts of hearing loss (e.g., speech impairment).

2.1.2 Hearing Aids

Infants with permanent hearing loss benefit from behind-the-ear (BTE) hearing aids fitted using real-ear measurements. Verification through behavioral testing ensures appropriate amplification.

2.1.3 Cochlear Implants

For children with severe-to-profound sensorineural hearing loss who derive limited benefit from hearing aids, cochlear implants are effective. Early implantation, ideally before 12 months of age, often leads to normal speech perception and development and significant improvements in quality of life. Cochlear implants play a crucial role in restoring speech perception and intelligibility in postlingual deaf adults, i.e., hearing loss that occurs after a person has already acquired speech and language.

Clinical studies consistently show that adults who lost their hearing after developing language skills experience significant improvement in speech discrimination and intelligibility scores following cochlear implantation. Many postlingually deaf cochlear implant users can communicate without lip-reading and can even use the telephone after implantation [6]. Outcomes are generally positive regardless of the duration of auditory deprivation, although factors such as age at implantation and cognitive processing speed may influence the level of speech recovery.

Cochlear implants are considered a safe and effective intervention for postlingual deaf adults, with low complication rates and high user satisfaction, even in the very elderly (e.g., 103-year-old patient surgery by NA) [7]. The technology enables aural communication and greatly improves the quality of life by restoring the ability to perceive speech.

37.3.1 Modern Auditory Rehabilitation

Auditory rehabilitation has become increasingly personalized. Smart hearing aids and cochlear implants are equipped with adaptive algorithms that automatically adjust to the user's environment. Hybrid electroacoustic stimulation benefits those with partial hearing loss. For children, auditory-verbal therapy, interactive apps, and caregiver training are vital for language development. For adults and the elderly, auditory-cognitive training supports better speech understanding and may mitigate cognitive decline. Brain-computer interfaces are being tested as future solutions for profound deafness, though their use raises important ethical considerations.

37.3.2 Futuristic Audiology

Technological progress has dramatically enhanced the precision and accessibility of audiological diagnostics. High-frequency audiometry, ooacoustic emissions (OAEs), and electrocochleography (ECochG) now allow clinicians to detect hearing deficits that were previously overlooked. AI-based algorithms support diagnosis by analyzing audiometric data, reducing variability, and enhancing accuracy. Mobile audiometry tools and tele-audiology are also expanding reach to remote and underserved populations. For pediatric patients, automated auditory brainstem response (AABR) and real-time feedback improve early detection. All these approaches are bound to increase in the coming years, particularly as artificial intelligence grows further as a diagnostic tool and precision medicine manifests over in the future management of deafness.

37.3.3 Age-Related Hearing Loss (Presbycusis)

Presbycusis is common among older adults and has been linked to social isolation and dementia. Early screening is critical and can be facilitated through mobile tools. Interventions should include bilateral hearing aids, assistive listening devices, and auditory-cognitive rehabilitation. Simplified interfaces, caregiver support, and integration with geriatric care improve adherence and outcomes [6]. Advances in cochlear implant technology are helping the young as well as older patients, with excellent results [8].

37.3.4 Noise-Induced Hearing Loss (NIHL)

Noise can cause several harms to human health. Noise-induced hearing loss is a recognized health issue. Exposure to persistent noise at or above 85 dBA can cause hearing loss. The time of exposure leading to hearing loss is inversely proportional to the intensity of noise in decibels. NIHL is a major cause of hearing loss, tinnitus, insomnia, and even suicidal tendency in the developing countries, where there are no legal restrictions on excessive noise or the time of day or night it is produced. Since many Asian, African, and Latin American countries have mainly outdoor lives, NIHL contributes hugely to the global burden diseases caused by hearing deficiencies.

37.3.5 Genetic Insight

Hereditary causes play a significant role in causing deafness, adding huge volumes to the global burden of disease [9]. Genetic discoveries have enhanced our understanding of both syndromic and non-syndromic hearing loss. Mutations in GJB2, OTOF, and MYO7A are frequently implicated. Next-generation sequencing is becoming part of newborn screening programs. Genetic counselling helps families understand inheritance and recurrence risks. Gene therapy using viral vectors is in early clinical trials and shows promise for restoring hearing in monogenic disorders.

The subject is discussed at length in subsequent paragraphs.

37.3.6 Artificial Intelligence in Audiology

AI is redefining audiological care by offering decision support, automating diagnostics, and improving hearing aid performance. Machine learning models analyze audiometric patterns, predict hearing loss progression, and personalize interventions. Mobile apps allow users to self-screen and manage their hearing health. Despite its benefits, AI raises concerns about its ethical use, data privacy, equity, and clinical oversight. Models must be trained on diverse populations to avoid biased outcomes [10].

37.4 Genetics of Hearing Loss

Genetic factors have played a central role in the etiology of hearing loss and deafness. In children, the genetic causes are responsible for 50% to 60% of such loss. The genetic mechanisms underlying hearing are diverse, impacting various cellular processes essential for normal auditory function. Mutations in specific genes can disrupt critical biological pathways within the inner cell.

The genetic landscape of hearing loss is vast, with over 120 independent genes identified. Among these, the GJB2 gene, which encodes Connexion 26, stands out as the most common genetic cause of deafness. Mutations in GJB2 are responsible for up to 50% of non-syndromic sensor neural hearing loss. The prevalence of this gene makes GJB2 a primary target to initiate genetic testing. Several other genes that are implicated in loss are:

SLC26A4 (encoding Pending).
MYO7A (encoding Myosin VIIA).

OTOF (otoferlin, also known as DFNB9).
CDH23, PCDH15, USH2A (associated with Usher syndrome).
GJB6 (gap junction protein gene).
POU3F4 (X-linked non-syndromic hearing loss).
STRC (encodes stereoclin).

37.4.1 Inheritance Patterns

Autosomal recessive inheritance is the most prevalent, responsible for about 77–88% of all cases, of which GJB2 gene is particularly significant. For autosomal recessive inheritance, both parents are heterozygous carriers with a 25% probability to have an affected child.

Autosomal dominant inheritance accounts for a smaller proportion of hearing loss, causing 10–20% of all cases and about 19–22% of non-syndromic hearing loss. Over 30 genes have been implicated in autosomal dominant non-syndromic hearing loss. Unlike autosomal recessive, not a single gene accounts for a large proportion of cases.

X-linked inheritance is less common and accounts for about 1–2% of all cases. Five genes are currently known to cause X-linked non-syndromic hearing loss. Mitochondrial inheritance pattern is characterized by maternal inheritance, i.e., males and females could be affected but can only inherit the mutated gene from the mother. Specific MTDNA mutations such as A1555G (1494C > T and 961delT within the 12S rRNA) are known causes of deafness.

37.4.2 Non-syndromic and Syndromic Hearing Loss

This form of hearing loss is not associated with other medical conditions. It accounts for approximately 70–80% of genetic hearing loss cases. Mutations in more than 100 genes have been associated with non-syndromic deafness. The most commonly implicated gene is GJB2, which encodes the protein Connexin 26, essential for normal auditory function. Other important genes include GJB6, SLC26A4, and MYO15A.

37.4.3 Syndromic Hearing Loss

Hearing loss occurs in conjunction with other symptoms and medical conditions. Syndromic forms of deafness are less common but can be more informative for genetic diagnosis, e.g., Usher syndrome, Pendred syndrome, and Alport syndrome.

With advancements in genetic testing and sequencing technologies, it is now possible to identify specific gene mutations responsible for hearing loss, facilitating targeted interventions and family planning.

37.4.4 Current and Futuristic Therapies

Significant genetic research and therapeutic technologies are making advancements in the treatment and diagnosis of hearing loss.

1. Singer sequencing analyzes specific gene variants (GJB2) and (GJB6).
2. Next-generation sequencing (NGS) panels; focus on simultaneous analysis of multiple genes associated with common, less common, and non-syndromic forms.
3. Whole exome sequencing/whole genome sequencing; involves a large number of genes, identifying novel variants; they can detect both single-nucleotide variants and copy number variants.

37.4.5 Gene Therapy

Gene therapy is the ultimate answer for the treatment of any genetic disease. The adenosine-associated virus is being used for incorporating a corrected copy of the mutant gene to the inner ear. Initial encouraging results are noted in autosomal recessive deafness caused by a mutation in the OTOF gene. Therapies for other hearing loss genes are currently in various stages of development.

37.4.6 Gene Editing

CRISPR/Cas9 gene editing technology represents a revolutionary advance, operating as a two-part molecular tool: the Cas9 enzyme acts as molecular scissors, cutting DNA at specific points [11], while a guide RNA (gRNA) directs the Cas9 enzyme to the precise location in the genome that requires editing. This system allows for precise modifications to the DNA of living organisms, enabling the correction of genetic hearing defects.

37.4.7 RNA Therapies

Beyond DNA-level gene editing, RNA therapies represent another promising frontier in treating hearing loss [12]. They offer huge potential in the futuristic medicine.

37.4.8 Genetic Screening and Counselling

Rapidly developing genetic technologies are introducing procedures such as pregenetic screening or intrauterine evaluation for genetic hearing loss, providing parents the opportunity to consider termination of pregnancy to avoid lifelong challenges.

Innovative strategies are emerging in genetics to correct or replace unhealthy genes that may lead to hearing loss. Viral vectors are being explored for delivering functional copies of mutated genes or rescue pathways.

Researchers have recently developed a genetic "barcoding" method to trace how stem cells in embryos develop into neurons and inner ear cells. By labelling early stem cells in mice, they can follow their development and map the formation of the inner ear, revealing that hearing-critical cells arise from two main types of stem cells. This insight could lead to new therapies for hearing loss, offering a detailed "family tree" of nervous system development and reducing the need for animal testing.

37.4.9 Pharmacological Approaches: Precision Medicine

Research is underway to identify compounds that can protect hair cells in the inner ear from damage caused by ototoxic drugs, loud noises, or aging. Identifying molecules that regulate protective cellular pathways may lead to therapies for at-risk populations.

37.4.10 Summary of Future Strategies

Genetic discoveries have enhanced our understanding of both syndromic and nonsyndromic hearing loss. Next-generation sequencing is becoming part of newborn screening programs. The newborn screening aims to identify infants with hearing loss within the first month, ensuring a diagnosis by 3 months, which is crucial for alleviating the developmental impacts of hearing loss. Genetic counselling helps families understand inheritance and recurrence risks. Gene therapy using viral vectors is in early clinical trials and shows promise for restoring hearing in monogenic disorders.

37.5 Education

Teaching medical graduates and postgraduates through didactic lectures is becoming less common. Educational strategies have evolved since the introduction of problem-based learning (PBL) at McMaster University in the 1960s, followed by Maastricht University and New Mexico, leading to an influx of innovative teaching methods. Recent developments like competency-based education (CBE) have further enhanced global teaching and learning quality. At the postgraduate level, surgical simulation labs, VR, AR, hands-on workshops, and practical sessions in operating rooms are now major methods of surgical training. It is believed that the existing ENT provision should be reconsidered to help students achieve a basic level of competence in managing common ENT conditions. This can be achieved by ENT teaching in additional contexts, including general practice, e-learning, and simulation workshops [13].

Microlearning and mobile learning using flashcards (e.g., Anki) and question banks are all but replacing the time-honored methods of long didactic lectures, voluminous books, and outdated texts. AI has just entered the field of healthcare and education. Its ethical use along with the human mind is bound to increase the collective wisdom in resolving many future issues.

37.6 Public Health Initiatives and Engaging the Deaf Community

Public health strategies play a vital role in preventing hearing loss. Awareness campaigns that educate the public about the risks of noise exposure, ototoxic medications, and the importance of early intervention can help reduce the incidence of acquired hearing loss. Promoting hearing conservation programs, particularly in occupational settings, can further mitigate risk factors.

Hereditary causes of hearing loss are numerous, and addressing them through genetic counselling and evolving technologies could significantly diminish the global prevalence of deafness.

Equally important is the active involvement of the deaf community. This is a unique community that generally dislikes pity or unhelpful intrusion. Many individuals suffer in silence, as communication barriers can lead to frustration and mental health challenges. Engaging with empathy and developing tailored support programs—focusing on improving communication, understanding personal and financial issues, and promoting mental well-being—can make a substantial difference in their quality of life [14].

37.7 Conclusion

Deafness and hearing loss stem from congenital or acquired causes. Some are preventable; others are manageable through medical, surgical, or rehabilitative care. Universal newborn hearing screening, mandated in many countries, enables early detection of congenital loss. Early intervention—hearing aids, surgical treatment, cochlear implants, and rehabilitation—significantly improves long-term outcomes. Research increasingly tailors interventions to genetic profiles and gene editing. Audiology is becoming data driven and patient centered, with advances in diagnostics, rehabilitation, genetics, and AI. Improved surgical techniques have improved outcomes as cochlear implants continue to become more accessible. As technologies advance, they will transform the detection, management, and prevention of hearing loss. Otolaryngology has always been an important subject in medical curricula. The future is even brighter as competence-based education, interprofessional education, innovative educational workshops, AR, VR, simulation labs, and telesurgical workshops will improve the knowledge and skills of health professionals managing hearing impairment and deafness.

References

1. Deafness: World Health Organization (WHO) – https://www.who.int.
2. Smith AW. WHO activities for the prevention of deafness and hearing impairment in children. Scand Audiol. 2001;30(2):93–100.
3. Lieu JEC, Kenna M, Anne S, Davidson L, et al. Hearing Loss in Children. JAMA. 2020;324(21):2195–205. https://doi.org/10.1001/jama.2020.17647.
4. American Academy of Paediatrics, Joint Committee on Infant Hearing. Year 2019 position statement: principles and guidelines for early hearing detection and intervention programs. Paediatrics. 2019;144(2):e20192765.
5. Genovese E, et al. Paediatric vestibular disorders—a focused diagnostic approach for best management outcomes. Congenital deafness and vestibular disorders: a systematic literature review. Front Neurol. 2024;15:1463234. https://doi.org/10.3389/fneur.2024.1463234.
6. Lin FR, Albert M. Hearing loss and dementia—who is listening? Aging MentHealth. 2021;25(6):975–81.
7. https://www.entandaudiologynews.com/news/post/world-s-oldest-recipient-of-a-cochlear-implant. Accessed 16 Aug 2025.
8. Patel S, Lee J. Cochlear implant advancements and future trends. Oto Neurotol. 2024;45(2):e50–6.
9. Shearer AE, Hildebrand MS, Smith RJH. Hereditary hearing loss, and deafness overview. In: GeneReviews®; 2023.
10. Miller C, et al. Machine learning in audiological diagnosis: a systematic review. J Am Acad Audiol. 2023;34(3):213–24.
11. Geyin X-HW, Sun Y. Recent advances in CRISPR-Cas system for the treatment of genetic hearing loss. Am J Stem Cells. 2023;12(3):37–50.
12. Xue Y, et al. RNA base editing therapy cures hearing loss induced by OTOF gene mutation. Mol Ther. 2023;31(12):3522–30.
13. Patel B, Saeed SR, Smith S. The provision of ENT teaching in the undergraduate medical curriculum: a review and recommendations. J Otolaryngol Cambridge University Press. 2021;135(7):610–5.
14. Septiana NZ, Rahmawati NR, Rahayu DS, Hanggara GS. Empowering the deaf community: enhancing healthcare access and mental health support. J Public Health. 2025;47(2):e234–5. https://doi.org/10.1093/pubmed/fdae212. Published:16 August 2024.

Creating a Genetics-Literate Healthcare Workforce: The Road to Precision Medicine

38

Fatima Gardezi, Salman Kirmani, Umn Ahmed Kirmani, and Zakaria Muhammad Asghar

Key Points

- Gaps in genetics literacy arise from systemic shortcomings in teaching and training rather than individual learner deficits.
- Genomics education remains outdated by isolating content in pre-clinical years instead of integrating it across the curriculum.
- LMICs face amplified disparities because genomics is viewed as a luxury despite high burdens of genetic disease.
- Evidence-based analyses highlight the urgent need to strengthen genomic literacy and modernise educational delivery.
- Innovative methods, AI-driven simulations, and aligned national policies are essential to build a genomics-literate workforce for precision healthcare.

38.1 Introduction

Over the past few decades, genomics has evolved into a branch of science that impacts routine clinical decision-making. The interpretation of personal genomic data is becoming the foundation of patient care. This has led to more efficient health systems that use genomic information in all aspects of prevention and care, from choosing targeted therapies, planning out reproductive options for couples at risk, and creating benchmarks for cancer treatment, to how we control the spread of infectious vectors. Genomic medicine is no longer a future aspiration but rather a necessity in day-to-day clinical practice.

F. Gardezi · U. A. Kirmani · Z. M. Asghar
Dow University of Health Sciences, Karachi, Pakistan

S. Kirmani (✉)
Aga Khan University, Karachi, Pakistan
e-mail: salman.kirmani@aku.edu

J. Sandars et al. (eds.), *Modern Medical Education*,
https://doi.org/10.1007/978-3-032-27958-3_38

Despite these advantages, clinical genomics generally remains neglected in medical curricula worldwide, with students and young medical graduates currently not being given the necessary skills to use genetic information in the diagnosis and management of their patients [1, 2]. Without fully implementing genomics training in medical schools, we are seeing gross inequities in patient outcomes, due in part to a healthcare workforce that is uncomfortable in applying genomic knowledge in the clinical setting.

This chapter will delve into four topics: (1) why every new doctor should have a basic understanding of genomics; (2) where the biggest gaps in teaching and training are; (3) what skills future doctors actually need (from the science itself to ethics and communication), and finally (4) how to deliver the knowledge in ways that work for various healthcare systems, especially those lacking resources. The goal is to create a roadmap on how to incorporate relevant genomics competencies in the medical curriculum, so that the coming generations of physicians find innovative ways to improve human health, from individualized medicine for every patient to utilizing a precision public health approach for the prevention of disease.

38.2 Why Genomics?

38.2.1 Genomics in Modern Medicine

Genomics holds the promise to improve outcomes in every medical specialty, whether it is targeted therapy selection in oncology, cardiology, neurology, reproductive health, etc. In oncology, DNA sequencing of a tumor to reveal its mutation profile can help doctors directly target those changes. Pharmacogenomics, where genetic testing for DNA variants that alter drug metabolism, allows for better drug selection and dosing, improving efficacy and reducing the risk of side effects. In reproductive health, early detection of genetic anomalies can allow for early interventions and prevention of life-long suffering. Genome sequencing has also proven invaluable in tracking, controlling and limiting communicable diseases, such as what we witnessed during the COVID-19 pandemic.

These applications are not limited to specialist clinics. As noted in the report "From Helices to Health," doctors in all specialties including primary care, emergency medicine, and surgical specialties are increasingly encountering scenarios where genomic information influences their decisions [1]. Without a solid grounding in genomics, these opportunities can be missed which leads to slower diagnoses, less precise treatments, and avoidable gaps in patient care.

38.2.2 Need for Genomic Literacy Across All Physicians

As awareness about the utility of genetic testing is increasing among the lay public, patients will generally discuss genetic testing with their family doctor or a general practitioner, rather than an expert in the field of genetics. This is because of the global shortage of clinical geneticists even in well-resourced settings, making it essential that every medical graduate needs to know the basics of the clinical applications of genomics. They need to know when and how to order genetic testing, which test to choose, how to interpret the results, and most importantly, how those results influence the management of their patients and family members. Without these abilities, doctors risk missing the chance to use genetic information in ways that could dramatically improve health outcomes. Building genomics into undergraduate medical education is one of the most effective ways to make sure future doctors are ready for these challenges.

38.2.3 What Current Doctors Think

A survey titled "Physician Perception on Genomics" found most doctors agreeing on the importance of fresh graduates having core genomics knowledge [2]. Not surprisingly, many of the physicians surveyed acknowledged their own training as inadequate. This leads to a lack of confidence in ordering genetic tests, interpreting results, or explaining findings to patients. This lack of confidence was not limited to any specific field of medicine but was across all specialties, suggesting the issue lies in the education system rather than in individual learning. A need was also expressed for more case-based teaching techniques in tandem with on-hand actual clinical scenarios. This would lead to a more effective approach to bridge the gap between medical education and the practical skills required for a genomics-driven healthcare environment.

38.2.4 Better Patient Care and Ethical Practices

Beyond the boundary of technical competence lies the domain of ethical and moral challenges associated with genomic information. The Association of Professors of Human and Medical Genomics (APHMG) released a report in 2022, pointing to common clinical issues such as explaining uncertain or incidental findings, addressing implications for family members, and ensuring informed consent [3]. Without preparation and adequate pretest counseling, genetic findings can have negative consequences for the patient and their family. The healthcare professional should be fully trained in explaining all the possible scenarios to the patient and ensure patients give informed consent before any genomic testing. There are also broader ethical considerations such as data privacy, genetic discrimination, and the responsible use of genomic databases. For this reason, genomic education should also include skills to communicate sensitively with the patient and respect their privacy and individuality.

38.2.5 Parallel from Dentistry

Recent advances in dental school curricula offer a useful example of how genomics can be successfully integrated into professional training [4]. In several progressive colleges, dental students now receive targeted training in assessing genetic risk for oral diseases and tailoring treatment accordingly. Early evidence shows this improves both student confidence and patient outcomes. To exploit the full potential of genomics, medical schools should ensure that all medical graduates, and not just geneticists, have this foundational literacy to aid them in becoming better healthcare providers.

38.3 Current Gaps

38.3.1 LMICs Furthest Behind

Genomics is transforming healthcare in wealthier countries, but many low- and middle-income countries (LMICs) are still finding it hard to bring this field into mainstream medical education [5]. This is due to limited resources, competing health priorities, and unique challenges of each setting. Gaps in the implementation of genomics are the result of missing national plans, limited local research, and medical curricula that often overlook health issues specific to the region [6]. In settings where even basic health facilities are not available, genomics may seem to be an unnecessary luxury. Unfortunately, this utilitarian approach only worsens disparities in the quality of medical education in poorly resourced settings and consequently worsens health outcomes even further.

38.3.2 Multiple Challenges in LMICs

While high-income countries have integrated genomics into their healthcare policies, LMICs have failed to develop a coherent strategy, with few qualified trainers and rudimentary genomic infrastructure. A review on strategies for genomic medical education in LMICs highlights that many LMIC's lack even a basic framework [5]. All this while countries like the UK and US have invested in long-term research projects and implementation strategies, such as the UK Biobank, Genomics England, and the All of Us program. High-income settings typically have access to genetic sequencing facilities, highly qualified educators, and established referral networks, accelerating the integration of genomics into mainstream medicine. In many LMICs, there are few trained educators, limited access to laboratory facilities, and little government investment in genomic programs. These challenges have formed a wide gap in genomic knowledge compared to better-resourced countries, creating physicians who are not confident in fully exploiting its full potential. This weakens the entire healthcare system, where most patients are denied the benefits of precision medicine. Even when the patients are offered genetic testing, the lack of adequately trained clinicians may lead to the test results being misinterpreted, with catastrophic consequences.

Challenges encountered in LMICs are summarized in Table 38.1.

38.3.3 Catch 22 Situation

Without trained professionals, you cannot have a high-quality curriculum, and without a good curriculum, you cannot have trained professionals. This conundrum is being faced in many parts of the world, leaving medical graduates unprepared to embrace novel diagnostic and therapeutic strategies.

Table 38.1 Challenges encountered in LMICs in delivering genomics medical education

Barrier	Description	Impact
No formal genomics curriculum	Many medical schools lack a dedicated genomics module	Students are unable to build a solid foundation
Shortage of trained faculty	Few educators have specialized genomics training	Limited quality of training and education
Lack of laboratories and testing facilities	Regardless of theory being taught, there are few resources for practical training	Students miss out on hands-on skills and practice
Lack of contextual content	Teaching materials are often imported from high-income countries	Fails to address genetic disorders specific to that population
No national policy	Governments do not have adequate budgets for genomics education	The progress relies on isolated and short-term projects

Without intervention, these challenges lead to serious consequences. A study on changes in genetic literacy found that without structured education, physicians' knowledge of genomics declines over time [7]. This growing gap means that doctors in LMICs risk falling further behind their counterparts in wealthier nations. This unpreparedness on the part of healthcare practitioners will have serious consequences on medical outcomes. It can mean patients never get offered a genetic test that might explain their symptoms or families waiting far too long for a diagnosis of an inherited condition. This is currently being played out in countries with high levels of consanguinity, where autosomal recessive conditions such as thalassemia and cystic fibrosis have become major public health concerns.

During the COVID-19 pandemic, many countries without genomic tracking delayed their response, leading to preventable deaths and wasteful use of resources. The result is a cycle where lack of education limits implementation. This in turn limits the perceived value of genomics in national health priorities.

38.3.4 The Need for a National Policy

Some countries have shown that national commitment can accelerate genomics education [8]. For example, Brazil's "DNA do Brasil" project merged large-scale sequencing with investments in workforce training. This helped medical professionals interpret and apply the data in clinical care. Similarly, Greece's National Genomics Initiative combined educational programs alongside its research projects, which prepared medical professionals for the successful integration of genomic medicine into practice. These examples show that progress is possible when education, infrastructure, and policy development happen in tandem. They also demonstrate that genomics initiatives don't need to start with a complete system reboot. Investments in training and facilities can bring about great changes.

Low- and middle-income countries (LMICs) can look to the UK's approach of integrating genomics education into clinical practice. Educator preparation, structured curricula, and region-specific implementation plans have been introduced to make genomics accessible to all areas of the country. Although LMICs may face greater resource constraints, the key principle remains the same; policy and education must move forward together. Even small-scale measures, such as piloting regional training hubs or developing open-access learning materials, can help build the workforce needed to apply genomics knowledge in clinical care. Resource constraints notwithstanding, policies need to be geared toward structured curriculum development and infrastructure expansion. Policy-linked educational efforts are more likely to achieve lasting impact, regardless of the resources available [5]. For it to succeed, efforts must be broad based, involving all stakeholders from governments, academia, and practitioners. If these steps are not taken, the healthcare void will continue to widen between high-income countries and LMICs. Closing the gap will take a joint effort from governments, universities, and healthcare organizations. Different strategies will have to be discussed to fit the specific circumstances of each LMIC.

38.4 Genomics Essentials in Medical Curricula

38.4.1 Defining the Core Competencies

Due to the field of genomics being so vast, it is very difficult to precisely outline the essential competencies that every medical practitioner should be well-versed in. Furthermore, not every medical student will pursue clinical practice. Therefore, the necessary fields of study within genomics should prepare students for roles in all domains: clinical, research, laboratory, public health, etc. Hence, organizations such as the Association of Professors of Human Medical Genetics (APHMG) work continuously to outline the topics within genomics which every medical student should be taught, to keep up with the ever evolving and advancing field of genomics. In the latest education report by the APHMG (2022), they clearly outlined the "Core Competencies for Undergraduate Medical Education in Genetics and Genomics" [3], shown in Table 38.2.

Table 38.2 Core competencies for undergraduate medical education in genetics and genomics

Medical knowledge	Medical genetics
Genome organization/gene regulation	Genetics and genomic testing
Genetic variation	Cancer genetics
Population genetics	Reproductive and prenatal genetics
Inheritance	Treatment and management
Cytogenetics and molecular genetics	Practice-based learning and improvement
Biochemical genetics	Interpersonal and communication skills
Patient care	Systems-based practice
Professionalism	

38.4.2 Core Competencies for Undergraduate Medical Education in Genetics and Genomics

These competencies cover a vast base, from clinical application of genetics to perspectives in community medicine and pharmacogenetics, providing a comprehensive curriculum to be followed throughout all years of medical education.

Moreover, supplementation should be provided for current medical practitioners, alongside addressing incoming generations of healthcare providers. Such material should be thorough enough to cover current gaps previously mentioned, however, easily digestible, applicable, and relevant. A great example of this is the open-access web page hosted by the National Human Genome Research Institute (NHGRI), which displays a library of educational resources, videos, infographics, presentations, etc. all relevant to the field of genomics [9]. In addition, resources are arranged at various levels and difficulties, from infographics that are applicable to the general population and an entire section dedicated to genomics literacy among medical practitioners.

38.5 Teaching Methodologies for Genomics

38.5.1 Stepping Away from Traditional Approaches

Modernization of genomics education is not only limited to the content of the curriculum, but the way it is taught in medical institutions is just as important to this reform. The traditional way to teach genomics has been as a standalone subject in the preclinical years, which often becomes extremely dry and tedious for students. The most efficient way to ensure that competencies mentioned in Table 38.2 are met is to integrate them into every relevant module, keeping the students engaged and highlighting its relevance to the practice of medicine. In addition, lecture heavy formats are not sufficient; students need teaching methods that are relevant and mirror how genomics is utilized in clinical life. Table 38.3 summarizes various pedagogical techniques that can be employed in different settings to deliver genomics content effectively.

38.5.2 Promoting Critical Thinking

The field of genomics itself challenges you to keep up with new knowledge, and delivering this knowledge in innovative ways requires educators to keep up with new teaching tools and technologies as well. Thus, it is imperative to consider reforms to the way knowledge is delivered, when educating the present and coming generations of medical practitioners. Points to highlight are inclusion of CBLs, PBLs, and patient stories. Simulating clinical scenarios and drawing from real patient recounts instills empathy and helps bridge the gap between textbook science and human experience. Moreover, the use of sequenced genome data to reinforce genetics, especially from a clinical aspect, could be highly beneficial. It trains clinicians to consider the bigger picture and become more comfortable and familiar with genomic data.

Table 38.3 Teaching methodologies for genomics

Teaching method	Practical example
Flipped classroom	Assign a student or students a topic and have them present and teach the class, opening an opportunity to teach the topic, suited to the way they understood it
Problem-based/ case-based learning	Solidify the concept of a topic, simulating a clinical scenario, where a patient presents to a hospital. The students work together to research and diagnose the patient, along with explaining the pathogenesis of the diagnosis
E-learning	Supplement classroom learning with video lectures, infographics, and presentations that students can opt to watch in their own time, to reinforce concepts
Practical use of genotypes	Students learn concepts of practical genomics, using their own sequenced genotypes, or those available in a public domain, exposing students to the application of genetic testing in clinical and research settings
Electing champions	Employ certified specialists in the field to review and modify current curriculums at medical institutions, as well as educate teachers and lecturers, ensuring content is being taught in the most effective manner
Use of artificial intelligence in clinical simulation	AI chatbots, specifically developed to act as and simulate patient interactions

38.5.3 Innovation and the Use of Technology and AI

With the revolution of artificial intelligence, it is imperative that it is integrated into medical education. AI has been used in clinical training through virtual patients [10]; chatbots have been developed to simulate real patient interactions, customized to patients with different disorders, their family members, and at different levels of understanding. This method of exposure and teaching is a vital inclusion to modern curricula as it provides students with an opportunity to practice and prepare for real interactions, easing the transition from classroom to clinic. Moreover, clinical genomics is a particularly hard area for students to get comfortable with, due to the multitude of rare cases, each with their own signs and symptoms. Virtual patients provide an avenue to prepare trainees to better cater to such patients and their families. Embracing these novel approaches prevents rote memorization of facts about genes and syndromes and promotes critical thinking about the pathophysiology of disease and potential diagnostic and therapeutic approaches.

38.5.4 Conclusion

Genomics is now certainly at the front and center of medicine, and the contemporary physician is underprepared to utilize this knowledge effectively. A concerted effort is needed to ensure that we create a genomics-literate healthcare workforce ready to take on the challenges that lie ahead. Medical curricula worldwide are letting health systems down by not providing current and relevant knowledge in this field, and the gaps are the widest in LMICs, further exacerbating the health disparities between them and better-resourced countries. We have thoughtfully laid out a roadmap which can be used by medical educators globally, to start delivering genomics education to medical students efficiently and effectively. We have identified various genomics education resources that can be used by students and teachers alike. The genomics revolution in healthcare will fail to be as transformative as it promises to be unless we make a concerted effort toward ensuring that medical graduates embrace this new knowledge and develop skills to be lifelong learners in this field.

References

1. Salari K, Karczewski KJ, Hudgins L, Ormond KE. From helices to health: undergraduate medical education in genetics and genomics. Am J Hum Genet. 2015;97(2):172–83. https://doi.org/10.1016/j.ajhg.2015.06.014.
2. Stanek EJ, Sanders CL, Taber KA, Khalid M, Patel J, Agapito MA. Physician perception of the importance of medical genetics and genomics in medical education and clinical practice. Genet Med. 2019;21(8):1879–89. https://doi.org/10.1038/s41436-018-0431-5.
3. Bennett RL, et al. Core competencies in genetics for medical students: recommendations of the Association of Professors of Human and Medical Genetics (APHMG). Genet Med. 2022;24(11):2167–78. https://doi.org/10.1016/j.gim.2022.08.005.
4. Mokeem SA, et al. Genomics in dental education: preparing future dentists for precision oral healthcare. J Dent Educ. 2023;87(5):549–58. https://doi.org/10.1002/jdd.13156.
5. Abou Tayoun AN, Rehm HL, Faulkner N. Strategies for genomic medicine education in low- and middle-income countries. NPJ Genom Med. 2022;7(1):52. https://doi.org/10.1038/s41525-022-00327-9.
6. Tindana P, et al. Grand challenges in global health genomics. Nat Genet. 2020;52(6):537–45. https://doi.org/10.1038/s41588-020-0633-9.
7. Manolio TA, et al. Understanding changes in genetic literacy over time. Genet Med. 2019;21(6):1444–51. https://doi.org/10.1038/s41436-018-0298-5.
8. Mullen AB, et al. A roadmap for large-scale genomic initiatives in emerging economies. Lancet Glob Health. 2021;9(5):e589–96. https://doi.org/10.1016/S2214-109X(21)00035-5.
9. National Human Genome Research Institute. Genomics educational resources. Available from: https://www.genome.gov/About-Genomics/Educational-Resources.
10. Kononowicz A, Woodham L, Edelbring S, Stathakarou N, Davies D, Saxena N, Tudor Car L, Carlstedt-Duke J, Car J, Zary N. Virtual patient simulations in health professions education: systematic review and meta-analysis by the digital health education collaboration. J Med Internet Res. 2019;21(7):e14676. https://doi.org/10.2196/14676.

39 The Digital Scalpel: Robotic Surgery and the Evolution of Innovative Surgical Training

Syed Jaffry

Key Points

- Robotic-assisted surgery (RAS) has transformed minimally invasive surgery with precision, visualization, and ergonomics.
- Traditional apprenticeship training is insufficient for RAS; simulation-based education is essential.
- Psychomotor adaptation, team dynamics, and cognitive load management are critical in robotic training.
- Future innovations include AI, AR/VR, advanced haptics, and hyperrealistic simulation.
- Ethical concerns around data, liability, and surgeon deskilling must be addressed.

39.1 Introduction

39.1.1 A Paradigm Shift in the Operating Room: Beyond the Hand of Man

The operating theater has historically been a sanctum of manual skill, defined by the direct, tactile connection between the surgeon's hand and the patient's anatomy. Mastery was cultivated through years of mentorship, guided by the principles of

S. Jaffry (✉)
University College Hospital, Blackrock Health and Bons Secours Hospital, Galway, Ireland

ERASMUS S.MO.C, Rotterdam, The Netherlands

RCSI, Dublin, Ireland

JPMA, Karachi, Pakistan

Irish Medical Council, Dublin, Ireland
e-mail: jaffry@urology.ie

J. Sandars et al. (eds.), *Modern Medical Education*,
https://doi.org/10.1007/978-3-032-27958-3_39

Halstedian apprenticeship, where embodied knowledge was transferred from one generation to the next [12]. This environment was characterized by the immediate feedback of tissue resistance, the three-dimensional perception of anatomy, and the intimate physical presence of the surgical team.

This centuries-old paradigm is undergoing a profound and accelerated revolution. Robotic-assisted surgery (RAS), once a futuristic concept, is now an established pillar of minimally invasive care. Platforms like the da Vinci Surgical System have transitioned from rare novelties to standard tools in numerous surgical specialties, from urology and gynecology to general and cardiothoracic surgery. These systems offer capabilities that border on the revolutionary: enhanced dexterity within confined anatomical spaces, high-definition three-dimensional magnification, intrinsic tremor filtration, and access to regions previously approachable only through large, invasive incisions [6].

However, this technological leap transcends the simple adoption of a new device. It necessitates an equally profound metamorphosis in the very fabric of surgical education. The venerable "see one, do one, teach one" model, while still foundational for instilling surgical principles, is demonstrably inadequate and ethically untenable for the initial acquisition of complex robotic proficiencies [17]. The confluence of high capital investment, operational costs, and, most importantly, paramount patient safety concerns mandates the development of robust, standardized, and simulation-intensive training pathways. These pathways must be rigorously completed before a surgeon ever assumes control of a console in a live operating environment.

This chapter will delve into the transformative impact of RAS on contemporary surgical practice. It will dissect the unique cognitive and psychomotor demands it imposes, survey the current state of structured robotic surgical education, and, most critically, explore the horizon of cutting-edge technologies and methodologies poised to redefine how we train the surgeons of tomorrow. The future of surgery is inextricably linked to the future of its education, and both are being irrevocably reshaped by the digital scalpel.

39.2 Robotic Surgery

39.2.1 Beyond Mechanical Arms: A New Surgical Paradigm

A critical initial clarification is essential: contemporary surgical robots are not autonomous entities. They are best understood as sophisticated telemanipulators, complex systems designed to amplify a surgeon's skill and extend their capabilities through a digital interface [2]. The surgeon remains the unequivocal director of the procedure, with their movements translated through intricate hardware and software. An examination of the core components illuminates this new paradigm:

1. The Surgeon Console
   This ergonomic command center isolates the surgeon from the distractions of the operating room. Seated comfortably, the operator views the surgical field through

a high-definition stereoscopic display that provides a true sense of depth and immersion. Their fingers manipulate master controllers that track hand, wrist, and finger movements with high fidelity. An array of foot pedals governs ancillary functions such as camera positioning, energy activation, and instrument clutching—the crucial act of repositioning the master controls without moving the patient-side instruments.

2. The Patient-Side Cart
   Positioned adjacent to the operating table, this unit typically comprises three or four robotic arms. One arm manipulates the endoscope, providing the visual feed, while the others deploy proprietary wristed instruments that enter the patient's body through small keyhole incisions or ports. These arms are slaves to the commands issued from the surgeon's console.
3. The Vision System
   This is the cornerstone of the robotic advantage. The system processes an ultra-high-definition (often 4 K or beyond) video signal from a dual-channel endoscope, integrating the two feeds to create a magnified, immersive, and stereoscopic view for the console surgeon. Advanced image processing, such as fluorescence imaging (e.g., Firefly™ technology), is increasingly integrated to visualize critical structures like vasculature and bile ducts or to assess tissue perfusion [4].
4. The Transformative Advantages
   - Enhanced Dexterity and Precision:
     Robotic instruments feature "EndoWrist" technology that affords seven degrees of freedom of movement—mimicking the human wrist but exceeding its natural range of motion within confined spaces. This enables complex maneuvers like suturing, dissection, and knot-tying in anatomically challenging areas (e.g., the deep pelvis or mediastinum) with unparalleled precision. Integrated tremor filtration further enhances microsurgical capabilities by eliminating minute hand tremors.
   - Superior Visualization:
     The immersive, magnified (often 10× or greater) 3D view provides an unparalleled level of anatomical detail. Surgeons can discern tissue planes, minute nerves, and microvasculature with a clarity that far surpasses the two-dimensional view of traditional laparoscopy and even rivals or exceeds the direct view in some open procedures.
   - Improved Ergonomics:
     Operating from a seated, ergonomically designed console significantly reduces the physical strain associated with prolonged standing in awkward positions during open or laparoscopic surgery. This ergonomic benefit can mitigate surgeon fatigue, potentially reducing errors and extending the functional lifespan of surgical careers [14].
   - Minimally Invasive Mastery:
     RAS has been a principal driver in expanding the scope and complexity of minimally invasive surgery (MIS). Procedures once considered prohibitively difficult or risky laparoscopically—such as radical prostatectomy, complex

hysterectomy, intricate colorectal resections requiring total mesorectal excision, and mitral valve repair—are now routinely performed robotically. The patient benefits are well-documented and include reduced blood loss, less postoperative pain, shorter hospital stays, and faster recovery times [11].

- Potential for Telesurgery:
  While still constrained by significant regulatory, latency (signal delay), and infrastructural hurdles, the core technology underpinning RAS enables the theoretical possibility of remote surgery. Pioneering experiments, such as the Lindbergh operation [8], have demonstrated the technical feasibility of a surgeon operating on a patient located across the Atlantic Ocean, pointing toward a future where geographic barriers to expert care may be diminished.
  Evolving Ecosystem: While Intuitive Surgical's da Vinci system maintains market dominance, the landscape is rapidly diversifying. Competitors like Medtronic's Hugo™ RAS, CMR Surgical's Versius®, and Asensus Surgical's Senhance® system are entering the market with different form factors (e.g., modular carts, open console designs) and potentially lower cost structures, driving innovation and increasing accessibility. Furthermore, specialized robotic systems for microsurgery, neurosurgery, and orthopedics are continually emerging, signaling a broader technological shift across the surgical disciplines.

39.3 The Training Imperative

39.3.1 Cultivating a Distinct Surgical Skillset

Achieving proficiency in robotic surgery is not analogous to learning a new laparoscopic technique or adapting open surgical skills. It demands the cultivation of a fundamentally distinct psychomotor and cognitive skillset, one that is decoupled from the surgeon's direct physical interaction with the patient [15]. This decoupling presents unique challenges:

- *Console Proficiency* (Psychomotor Remapping):
  - *Hand-Eye Coordination Dissociation*: Surgeons must adapt to manipulating instruments they cannot see or directly feel with their hands, relying entirely on visual feedback from the console monitor. Their hands move controllers in one spatial plane, while the instruments move within the patient's body in another, requiring significant neural adaptation and the development of new visuomotor pathways.
  - *Foot Pedal Mastery*: The requirement to control camera movement, energy activation, and instrument swapping simultaneously with intricate hand movements adds a layer of complexity largely absent in traditional surgery. This demands sophisticated bimanual and pedal coordination, akin to playing a complex musical instrument.

  - *Clutching Strategy*: Efficiently repositioning the master controllers (clutching) to maintain optimal ergonomics and instrument range without moving the patient-side instruments is a unique robotic skill. It requires advanced spatial awareness and deliberate practice to execute seamlessly without disrupting surgical flow.
- *Spatial Cognition and Depth Perception*: Surgeons must learn to translate the magnified, immersive 3D view into an accurate understanding of the actual spatial relationships within the patient's body. They must constantly mentally scale the view and maintain anatomical orientation, a task complicated when instruments frequently move in and out of the fixed field of view.
- *Haptic Translation (The Missing Sense):* A significant challenge with current mainstream robotic systems is the lack of true haptic feedback (force feedback). Surgeons cannot feel tissue resistance, tension on sutures, or the subtle "give" when dissecting anatomical planes. They must learn to rely entirely on visual cues—such as tissue deformation, vessel pulsation, and instrument bending—to infer tactile information. This represents a considerable sensory deficit compared to both open and laparoscopic surgery [9].
- *Cognitive Load Management*: The immersive console environment, while beneficial for focus, can inadvertently create a form of tunnel vision. The console surgeon must actively maintain situational awareness beyond the magnified field, integrating auditory and verbal information from the bedside assistant, nurses, and anesthesiologist. Managing the cognitive load of instrument control, visual processing, team communication, and higher-order clinical decision-making is intensified.
- *Team Dynamics and Orchestration*: RAS fundamentally reconfigures OR team roles and communication patterns. The physical separation of the console surgeon from the patient and the rest of the team necessitates a paradigm of effective, clear, and proactive communication. The role of the bedside assistant—responsible for instrument changes, suction, retraction, introducing sutures, and managing emergencies—becomes more critical than ever. Roles and responsibilities must be meticulously defined, practiced, and rehearsed to ensure safety and efficiency [3].
- *Technical Troubleshooting and System Literacy*: A foundational understanding of the robotic system's mechanics, software, and potential failure modes is essential. Surgeons must be able to recognize errors (e.g., arm collisions, instrument failures, vision system glitches), initiate safe troubleshooting protocols, and know when and how to convert to laparoscopic or open surgery swiftly and safely.

The high stakes—encompassing patient safety, the cost of system downtime, and the potential for catastrophic error due to unfamiliarity—render it ethically and practically indefensible to use the live patient as the primary training ground for initial RAS skills acquisition. A structured, simulation-based curriculum is not a luxury; it is an absolute necessity for safe implementation.

39.4 The Present Landscape

39.4.1 Foundational Training Modalities and Structured Pathways

In response to these unique demands, professional societies (e.g., SAGES's Fundamental Use of Surgical Energy™ (FUSE) and FRS programs, AUA, AAGL) and robotic platform manufacturers have collaboratively developed structured training and credentialing pathways. Contemporary training typically follows a multimodal, progressive approach, moving from low-risk to higher-fidelity environments [13]:

1. *Comprehensive Didactic Learning*
   - *Content*:
     This foundational phase includes an in-depth understanding of system components, setup, draping, instrumentation (types, functions, limitations), and docking strategies. It also covers the principles of energy devices specific to the platform, tissue interaction physics, and procedure-specific knowledge (anatomy, surgical steps, potential pitfalls, complication management). A critical component is formal team training and communication protocols, often incorporating principles of crew resource management (CRM).
   - *Format*:
     Delivered through online modules, webinars, manufacturer-led courses, and dedicated didactic sessions within residency or fellowship programs. Knowledge is often assessed through pre- and post-testing.
2. *Virtual Reality (VR) Simulation Training*

The Bedrock of Skill Acquisition:
   - Purpose:
     VR simulators provide a safe, controlled, repeatable, and objective environment to master fundamental psychomotor skills before any interaction with tissue. They are proven to significantly reduce the learning curve on the actual system [7].
   - Platforms and Content:
     Dedicated simulators (e.g., da Vinci Skills Simulator, Mimic dV-Trainer, RobotiX Mentor) offer a curriculum that progresses from basic skills (camera targeting, instrument clutching, needle targeting, energy application) to suturing and knot-tying modules and finally to procedural modules that simulate key steps of specific operations (e.g., bladder neck dissection in prostatectomy).
   - Objective Performance Metrics (OPM) and Proficiency-Based Progression (PBP):
     This is a cornerstone of modern training. VR simulators continuously track and quantify performance using metrics such as time to completion, economy

of motion (path length of instrument tips), instrument collisions, excessive force, and errors. Trainees must meet validated performance benchmarks before advancing, ensuring a standardized base level of proficiency (PBP) rather than simply logging time [1].

3. *Dry Lab Training: Bridging the Digital and Physical*
   - Purpose:
     Dry labs provide hands-on experience with actual robotic instruments and a console (or replica) in a non-biological setting. The focus is on system setup, instrument handling, basic maneuvers, and crucially, suturing and knot-tying using real needle drivers and suture on synthetic models, which provides valuable tactile feedback on needle driving and knot security.
   - Team Training:
     This environment is ideal for practicing OR team dynamics, communication, docking sequences, and managing simulated emergencies (e.g., instrument failure, bleeding scenarios) in a low-pressure, low-cost setting.
4. *Wet Lab Training: Introducing Tissue Realism*
   - Purpose:
     This high-fidelity phase provides experience with real tissue handling properties—cutting, dissection, sealing, and bleeding control—using the actual robotic system.
   - Models:
     This typically involves animal tissue (e.g., porcine models) or human cadavers. While animal models offer live tissue response, they present ethical, cost, and logistical challenges. Cadavers provide unparalleled anatomical accuracy but lack the bleeding and pliability of living tissue. Both are essential but resource-intensive components of training, requiring proctoring by experienced robotic surgeons.
5. *Structured Clinical Proctoring and Mentorship*

The Bridge to Independence:

- Purpose:
  This is the critical transition to live surgery, conducted under the close supervision of an expert proctor to ensure patient safety. It involves a phased approach, where the trainee begins with discrete portions of a procedure (e.g., docking, closure) and gradually progresses to performing the entire operation.
- Competency Assessment:
  Proctors use validated assessment tools like the Global Evaluative Assessment of Robotic Skills (GEARS) to evaluate technical proficiency, decision-making, and communication. Specific outcome metrics like console time and blood loss are also tracked. This phase is supported by ongoing mentorship, including case discussion and video review.

39.5 The Future Horizon

39.5.1 Innovative Technologies Reshaping Surgical Training

The current modalities, while effective, are merely the foundation. The future of surgical training lies in the convergence of several disruptive technologies that promise to make learning more immersive, intelligent, personalized, and accessible:

1. Advanced Haptics and Multisensory Feedback:
   Next-generation systems are integrating sophisticated haptic actuators to provide realistic kinesthetic and tactile feedback, allowing surgeons to feel tissue resistance and suture tension. This will dramatically reduce the cognitive load of visual interpretation and close the critical sensory gap [10]. Future simulators will also integrate auditory and even olfactory feedback to enhance realism and situational awareness.
2. Artificial Intelligence (AI) and Machine Learning (ML):
   - Intelligent Tutoring Systems (ITS): AI-driven simulators will act as personalized coaches, analyzing performance in real time to identify deficiencies and dynamically adapt training scenarios to address individual weaknesses.
   - Automated Performance Assessment: AI algorithms will move beyond basic metrics to perform nuanced analysis of surgical technique (e.g., instrument smoothness, suture accuracy), comparing a trainee's performance against vast anonymized datasets of expert surgeons to provide granular feedback.
   - Predictive Analytics: By analyzing longitudinal performance data, AI can predict a trainee's readiness for the OR or their likelihood of struggling with specific procedural steps, enabling proactive, personalized interventions.
   - Surgical Data Science: Aggregating and anonymizing data from thousands of procedures will allow AI to identify the "digital fingerprints" of surgical expertise, helping to define optimal techniques and create new evidence-based standards for performance [5].
3. Augmented Reality (AR), Mixed Reality (MR), and VR Convergence:
   - Intraoperative Guidance: The ability to overlay critical anatomical structures (e.g., nerves, tumors), planned resection planes, or real-time perfusion data directly onto the surgeon's console view will act as a powerful navigational aid, enhancing safety in both training and live surgery.
   - Hybrid Simulation: Combining physical anatomical models with dynamic AR/MR overlays will create training experiences with high tactile fidelity and dynamic visual feedback (e.g., a model that "bleeds" when an AR-highlighted vessel is cut).
   - Remote Proctoring and Telementoring: Experts will be able to remotely view a trainee's console feed and overlay annotations or virtual guiding hands within the trainee's AR/MR headset view, enabling real-time guidance from anywhere in the world and democratizing access to expertise.

4. Hyperrealistic Simulation and Bio-integration:
    - 3D Bioprinting and Engineered Tissues: The creation of vascularized, multi-layered tissue constructs with realistic mechanical properties will allow for rehearsal of complex dissection and anastomosis on models that bleed and respond physiologically.
    - Patient-Specific Rehearsal (PSR): Using a patient's own preoperative imaging to generate a highly accurate, interactive VR/MR simulation of their unique anatomy will allow surgeons to meticulously plan and rehearse complex cases beforehand, potentially improving outcomes [16].
5. Cognitive Training and Neuroergonomics:
   Integrating eye-tracking to assess situational awareness and physiological monitoring (EEG, EDA, HRV) to measure cognitive load and stress will provide insights into the surgeon's mental state. This data can be used to optimize cognitive performance, train stress resilience, and design better interfaces that reduce mental fatigue.

39.6 Building the Future Curriculum

39.6.1 Integration, Accessibility, and Competency

Implementing these innovations requires a fundamental redesign of surgical curricula around core principles:

- Mandatory Mastery Learning: PBP must become the nonnegotiable standard for advancement at every stage.
- Longitudinal and Lifelong Learning: Simulation must be woven throughout a surgeon's career, from residency through continuing professional development (CPD), to combat skill decay and facilitate lifelong learning.
- Integrated Team Training: Curricula must explicitly train the entire OR team together using shared simulation scenarios to build shared mental models and optimize communication.
- Data-Driven Credentialing: Objective performance data from simulators and live procedures (where feasible) should inform credentialing and privileging decisions, moving beyond subjective case numbers.
- Global Accessibility: Innovation must address cost barriers through cloud-based solutions, shared regional training centers, and tele-simulation to ensure equitable global access to high-quality training.

39.7 Ethical Considerations, Human Factors, and the Surgeon's Role as Technology Advances: Critical Questions Demand Ongoing Vigilance

- Deskilling:
  Curricula must ensure surgeons retain fundamental open and laparoscopic skills to safely convert when technology fails or when it is the best approach for the patient.
- Bias in AI:
  Vigilance is required to prevent algorithmic bias in AI assessment tools based on gender, ethnicity, or training institution.
- Data Privacy:
  Clear policies must govern the ownership, security, and use of the vast amounts of sensitive performance data generated by simulators and AI systems.
- Liability:
  Legal frameworks must evolve to address questions of liability when AI-driven guidance systems are involved in patient care.
- The Surgeon-Machine Interface:
  Technology must be designed to enhance, not replace, the surgeon's critical judgment, decision-making, and compassion. The surgeon must remain the captain of the ship.

39.8 Conclusion

39.8.1 Forging the Adaptable, Technologically Adept Surgeon of Tomorrow

Robotic surgery is more than a new set of tools; it is a fundamental shift in the surgical paradigm, altering sensory input, motor control, and team interaction. Preparing for this reality demands an equally transformative approach to surgical education. The convergence of simulation, AI, AR/VR, and cognitive science holds the promise of creating safer, more efficient, and more effective training.

The ultimate goal is not to train mere operators of machinery but to cultivate adaptable, resilient, and highly skilled clinicians who can seamlessly integrate technology to enhance their innate abilities. It is to ensure that the digital scalpel serves to make procedures safer and more effective for patients while preserving the irreplaceable human elements of judgment, ethics, and empathy. By proactively embracing innovation within a structured, competency-based, and ethically sound framework, the surgical community can ensure it is ready to meet the demands of the future operating room.

References

1. Aggarwal R, Grantcharov TP, Eriksen JR, Blirup D, Kristiansen VB, Funch-Jensen P, Darzi A. An evidence-based virtual reality training program for novice laparoscopic surgeons. Ann Surg. 2010;252(2):316–22.
2. Ballantyne GH, Moll F. The da Vinci telerobotic surgical system: the virtual operative field and telepresence surgery. Surg Clin N Am. 2003;83(6):1293–304.
3. Catchpole KR, Giddings AE, Wilkinson M, Hirst G, Dale T, de Leval MR. Improving patient safety by identifying latent failures in successful operations. Surgery. 2008;144(1):83–9.
4. Dip F, Roy M, Lo Menzo E, Simpfendorfer C, Szomstein S, Rosenthal RJ. The use of near-infrared imaging and fluorescent angiography during robotic rectal resection. J Robot Surg. 2016;10(1):37–41.
5. Hashimoto DA, Rosman G, Rus D, Meireles OR. Artificial intelligence in surgery: promises and perils. Ann Surg. 2018;268(1):70–6.
6. Herron DM, Marohn M. A consensus document on robotic surgery. Surg Endosc. 2008;22(2):313–25.
7. Lendvay TS, Brand TC, White L, Kowalewski TM, Hannaford B. Virtual reality robotic surgery simulation curriculum to teach robotic suturing: a randomized controlled trial. J Urol. 2013;189(3):906–12.
8. Marescaux J, Leroy J, Gagner M, Rubino F, Mutter D, Vix M, et al. Transatlantic robot-assisted telesurgery. Nature. 2001;413(6854):379–80.
9. Okamura AM. Haptic feedback in robot-assisted minimally invasive surgery. Curr Opin Urol. 2009;19(1):102–7.
10. Pacchierotti C, Sinclair S, Solazzi M, Frisoli A, Hayward V, Prattichizzo D. Wearable haptic systems for the fingertip and the hand: taxonomy, review, and perspectives. IEEE Trans Haptics. 2017;10(4):580–600.
11. Pugin F, Bucher P, Morel P, Hagen ME. History of robotic surgery: from AESOP® and ZEUS® to da Vinci®. J Visc Surg. 2011;148(5):e3–8.
12. Satava RM. The future of surgical simulation and surgical robotics. Bull Am Coll Surg. 2005;90(11):9–13.
13. Thomaier L, Orlando M, Abernethy M, Paka C, Chen CC. Development of a robotic surgery training curriculum: the medical student experience. J Robot Surg. 2017;11(4):427–32.
14. van der Schatte Olivier RH, Van't Hullenaar CD, Ruurda JP, Broeders IA. Ergonomics in robot-assisted surgery: a review. Surg Endosc. 2008;22(4):969–77.
15. Yohannes P, Rotariu P, Pinto P, Smith AD, Lee BR. Comparison of robotic versus laparoscopic skills: is there a difference in the learning curve? Urology. 2002;60(1):39–45.
16. Zein NN, Hanouneh IA, Bishop PD, Samaan M, Eghtesad B, Quintini C, et al. Three-dimensional print of a liver for preoperative planning in living donor liver transplantation. Liver Transpl. 2013;19(12):1304–10.
17. Zevin B, Levy JS, Satava RM, Grantcharov TP. A consensus-based framework for design, validation, and implementation of simulation-based training curricula in surgery. J Am Coll Surg. 2012;215(4):580–6.

40 Advances in Head and Neck Surgery (A Training Perspective)

Mohammed Yousaf Mian and Shiraz Syed

Key Points

- Traditional apprenticeship training is limited by variability, patient safety concerns, and reduced exposure.
- Simulation and VR provide safe, repeatable environments to build technical and cognitive skills.
- AI and robotics allow personalized learning, precise planning, and advanced skill assessment.
- Major barriers include cost, infrastructure, and limited faculty resources.
- Future training will likely use blended models with simulation, AI, and gamification for improved competency.

40.1 Introduction

In the modern world, cancer is a growing cause of mortality, with head and neck cancer being the sixth most common cancer worldwide. Importantly, this is not exclusive to the modern population, as historical data from the Cancer Research in Ancient Bodies (CRAB) Database shows occurrences of cancer in head and neck regions, particularly in the skull base. As the burden of disease increases, so too does the need for advanced, structured training to meet the growing complexity of care. There is greater emphasis on subspecialization to address increasing complexity of patient presentations. A key consideration in H&N surgical training is the distinction between benign and malignant disease management. Training in benign conditions—such as thyroid nodules, salivary gland disorders, and benign laryngeal

M. Y. Mian (✉) · S. Y. Syed
Otolaryngology, Sandwell and West Birmingham NHS Trust, Birmingham, UK
e-mail: shiraz.syed@nhs.net

J. Sandars et al. (eds.), *Modern Medical Education*,
https://doi.org/10.1007/978-3-032-27958-3_40

pathology—provides an essential foundation in surgical anatomy, perioperative care, and patient communication. In contrast, malignant H&N surgery, involving oncological resections and complex reconstructions, requires proficiency in multidisciplinary collaboration and advanced surgical techniques [1].

There has been remarkable shift in paradigm in head and neck surgery training over recent decades. Apprenticeship model has been used traditionally and widely, which is described as "see one, do one, teach one." Under this model, trainee surgeons have relied on direct observation of surgeries under supervision [2]. However, recent changes in complexity of procedures, growing concerns regarding patient safety, variable clinical exposure, and changes in working hours have warranted the integration of more structured and evidence-based surgical training strategy.

An important addition to conventional surgical training is simulation-based education, which has recently emerged as a safer, repeatable, and standardized platform to acquire necessary skills without putting patient safety at risk. In a systematic review in the United Kingdom (UK) in 2017, 64 simulator models in otolaryngology were identified. It showed that current evidence base for effectiveness of many simulators is limited. However, integration of simulation surgical learning is being increasingly recognized. It is thus important that current simulators demonstrate high validation and fidelity to ensure safe and effective learning [3]. Another meta-analysis done in Canada in 2017 by Lui and Hoy demonstrated that virtual reality (VR)-based mastoidectomy surgical training significantly improved surgical performances of trainees as compared to those who received conventional instructions. The authors found a standardized mean difference (SMD) of 0.87 showing VR group performed better than non-VR group ($p < 0.006$), even though there was moderate variability between the studies ($I^2 = 64.3\%$) [4].

These developments have demonstrated a broader trend in surgical training—a move from variable and opportunistic training to a structured, competency-based learning supported by validated tools. This chapter explores major advances in head and neck surgical training and will examine emerging educational technologies available for trainees. It aims to provide an overarching overview of changing landscape in modern surgical training to meet twenty-first-century demands.

40.2 Traditional Training Paradigms

The traditional apprenticeship model has emphasized on experiential learning under supervision in the operating room. Several limitations have become evident in context of modern surgical training methods.

This model is limited in its unstructured and nonobjective performance criteria. The feedback provided to trainees is usually informal and progression is variable. A study done by Bhatti and Ahmed in the Department of Otolaryngology, Head and Neck Surgery, Johns Hopkins University School of Medicine, in 2015, has shown that there is room for development of structured competency-based and learner-based training in otolaryngology. Author used deliberate practice, defined milestone, and formative feedback which showed improvement on efficiency and quality in surgical skill acquisition [5]. Apprenticeship model provides valuable real-time hand on clinical experience with exposure and mentorship; however, it is limited in consistent competency development, and thus, better objective means to educate surgical trainees will enhance reliability and quality of training.

40.3 Simulation-Based Surgical Education

Modern surgical education has offered structured simulation-based training with its reproducibility and consistency to build technical proficiency. It allows repeated, standardized practice without risks to patients. In head and neck surgery, there are significant challenges owing to complex anatomy and narrow operative corridors. Simulation tools provide essential key opportunities for deliberate practice and skill refinement. VR-based simulation technologies are an important innovation which can enhance existing surgical skills without putting patients at risk which is traditionally associated with surgical training on live patients. A systematic review by Hudise et al. in 2024 showed that VR simulation in otolaryngology enhances spatial awareness, hand-eye coordination, and surgical confidence in trainees [6]. Simulation-based surgical training tools have provided immense opportunity to train; however, it is also important to critically evaluate their education value, design, and real-world adaptability. A randomized controlled trial by Arnesen et al. in 2022 assessed performance of 24 medical students in University of Copenhagen in mastoidectomy training. They were randomized two groups (multiple anatomically distinct cases vs single repeated case) within a VR-based simulation training environment. Later, all participants' performances were assessed using both a new VR case and realistic 3D-printed temporal bone model. There was no significant difference in the performance level between both groups. This suggested that repetition using a single standardized case may be sufficient for early surgical training. Furthermore, it also showed that VR-based skill acquisition is transferable to real-world physical model supporting the use of a validated tool to support surgical training [7].

40.4 Artificial Intelligence (AI), Robotic, and Image-Guided Surgical Training

AI is poised to play a transformative role in the future training of head and neck surgeons by enhancing both the educational process and clinical preparedness. One of the most significant applications lies in AI-powered simulation platforms, including virtual and augmented reality systems, which allow trainees to practice complex surgical procedures in a risk-free, immersive environment. These platforms can provide real-time, objective feedback based on motion tracking and performance metrics, enabling the identification of skill gaps and targeted improvement. Moreover, AI enables personalized learning pathways by adapting educational content to individual trainee needs, optimizing learning efficiency. In surgical planning, AI can assist in analyzing radiological data, predicting tumor margins, and simulating surgical outcomes, thus familiarizing trainees with advanced decision-making tools. Natural language processing further supports training by curating up-to-date literature and enabling voice-activated access to clinical knowledge. As AI becomes integrated into diagnostic and prognostic tools, it is essential for trainees to develop competencies in interpreting and incorporating AI-generated insights into patient management. Despite its benefits, the integration of AI must be approached with attention to ethical considerations, data bias, and equitable access. Overall, AI offers the potential to elevate the standard of training in head and neck surgery, promoting higher competency, improved patient outcomes, and a more adoptive learning environment [8].

Simulation-based training is becoming an established component of surgical education, the next development in integrating robotic platforms, and image-guided navigation systems into surgical learning environment. The new tools provide novel opportunity to upgrade precision, safety, and trainee confidence. An area of growing interest is incorporation of extended reality (XR) and augmented reality (AR) to support robotic-assisted head and neck surgical procedures. In a systematic review and metanalysis by Bickford et al. in 2025 in the United States of America, the authors analyzed 15 studies comparing performances of novice users in robotic surgery who were trained with XR simulators vs traditional physical simulators. They showed that users of XR had better time to complete performances. The study suggested that XR and other VR simulators provide better precise learning opportunity with opportunity to learn in dynamic variable environments which lacks in conventional physical models [9]. With further advancement in AR technology, trainees will likely benefit in achieving accurate surgical margins during complex head and neck malignancy resection. Yang et al. [11] have proposed integrating AR to project tumor margins onto the surgical site. Trainees in head and neck surgery will learn to perform precise resection by enabling them to visualize subsurface tumor location during head and neck cancer resection [10]. While robotics in head and neck surgical training opens doors to a new learning, it does not come without its limitations. A study by Lechien et al. in 2024 highlighted significant barriers in use of robotics in head and neck surgery. Out of limitations, most common reported was access limitations which was followed by high cost and lack of structured training opportunities. Furthermore, currently, there is an additional barrier of acquiring and maintaining robotic systems in resource-limited hospitals. There are also lack of standardized training pathways in robotic surgery in head and neck which may lead to inadequate attainment of competencies for early-career trainees [11].

In summary, robotics and image-guided technology are transforming head and neck surgical education. Current evidence shows value of adopting these available opportunities while also emphasizing on structured competency-based training pathways and integration of real-world and simulation-based learning tools. Robotics is poised to revolutionize the training of head and neck surgeons by offering highly realistic, precision-based simulation environments that replicate complex surgical procedures with remarkable accuracy. Through robotic-assisted surgical platforms, trainees can gain hands-on experience with delicate anatomy, refine motor skills, and receive real-time feedback without putting patients at risk. Advanced robotic systems simulate complex surgical scenarios involving tumors, vascular structures, and nerve pathways, thereby helping trainees develop competence and confidence. Integration with AR and AI will further enhance robotic training by enabling personalized learning, error detection, and performance tracking.

40.5 Challenges and Barriers to Implementation

A significant challenge of simulation-based training in head and neck surgery lies at institutional level. Large numbers of training programs lack an objective structured curriculum for simulation-based skill acquisition. This leads to inconsistent and underutilized use of such opportunities. Furthermore, there is also lack of administrative and infrastructure support. A multinational qualitative study by Hosny et al. included 37 participants (17 experts and 20 resident surgical trainees) and identified financial cost as a significant barrier to uptake of simulation-based surgical program. The authors also raised concerns regarding accessibility and possible translation of simulation learning to actual surgical skill on a live patient [12]. Furthermore, there are more challenges related to limited faculty time availability to support simulation training. In a study by Acton et al. in 2015, authors showed that faculty resources to implement simulation training had to bear hidden demands such as increased preparation, debriefing, and assessment time. These responsibilities were beyond regular duties. The study highlighted the importance of protected faculty resources in effective simulation-based surgical training program [13].

In summary, there are clear benefits of simulation-based training for skill developments; however, its success depends on adequate fundings, institutional support, dedicated faculty time, and structured training programs.

40.6 Future Directions in Head and Neck Surgical Education

Looking ahead in possible ways in head and neck surgical training, the integration of AI, competency-based gamification offers incredible potential. Gamified learning such as digital reward, leaderboards, and question banks allowing multiple participants online, even remotely, is showing to appear within medical education. A systematic review by Huang et al. in 2024 highlighted use of gamification in medical education to encourage deeper learning and increase in motivation [14]. A similar method employment in otolaryngology has promising relevance, for example, using integrated VR-based gamification in the airway can enhance learner engagement and reinforce in surgical airway skill acquisition without losing clinical relevance.

Similarly, AI-driven surgical education can provide personalized bespoke feedback which can be tailored down to individual surgical trainee needs. There is also added advantage of real-time performance feedback and automated assessment of surgical technique. Individualized training and objective skill assessment are critical to head and neck surgical training, and AI-driven simulation-based learning can address both issues effectively [15].

40.7 Conclusion

There is a shift in paradigm in head and neck surgical training where apprenticeship-based training is moving toward competency-based simulation-enhanced curricula. Introduction of high-quality VR improves procedure-specific performance with evidence of high skill acquisition. There is evidence to show that AI/XR, robotics, and image-based platforms add objective metrics, superior operative planning, and personalized surgical learning experience. The implementation is limited by cost, infrastructure, and dedicated faculty time. An evidence-based blended pathway including benign and malignant disease surgical learning in head and neck disease provides opportunity to deliver consistent competence and improved patient outcomes.

References

1. Hunt K, Kirkpatrick C, Campbell R, Willoughby J. Cancer research in ancient bodies (CRAB) database. Paleo-Oncology Research Organization: https://www.cancerantiquity.org/crabdatabase; 2017.
2. Franzese CB, Stringer SP. The evolution of surgical training: perspectives on educational models from the past to the future. Otolaryngol Clin N Am. 2007;40(6):1227–35.
3. Musbahi O, Aydin A, Al Omran Y, Skilbeck CJ, Ahmed K. Current status of simulation in otolaryngology: a systematic review. J Surg Educ. 2017;74(2):203–15.
4. Lui JT, Hoy MY. Evaluating the effect of virtual reality temporal bone simulation on mastoidectomy performance: a meta-analysis. Otolaryngol Head Neck Surg. 2017;156(6):1018–24.
5. Bhatti NI, Ahmed A. Improving skills development in residency using a deliberate-practice and learner-centered model. Laryngoscope. 2015;125:S1–S14.
6. Hudise JY, Mojiri ME, Shawish AM, Majrashi KA, Ayoub AY, Alshammakhi AM, et al. The role of virtual reality in advancing surgical training in otolaryngology: a systematic review. Cureus. 2024;16(10)
7. Arnesen KA, Frithioff A, Sørensen MS, Andersen SAW, Frendø M. Mastoidectomy training: is anatomical variation needed? A randomized, controlled trial on performance and skills transfer from virtual reality to a three-dimensional printed model. Otol Neurotol. 2022;43(8):900–7.
8. Ayoub NF, Rameau A, Brenner MJ, Bur AM, Ator GA, Briggs SE, et al. American Academy of Otolaryngology–Head and Neck Surgery (AAO-HNS) report on artificial intelligence. Otolaryngol Head Neck Surg. 2025;172(2):734–43.
9. Bickford M, Alruwaili F, Ragab S, Rothenberg H, Abedin-Nasab M. Impact of extended reality on robot-assisted surgery training: a systematic review and meta-analysis. J Robot Surg. 2025;19(1):412.
10. Yang Q, Li F, Xu J, Liu Z, Sridhar S, Jin W, et al. Deformable registration framework for augmented reality-based surgical guidance in head and neck tumor resection. arXiv preprint arXiv:250308802. 2025.
11. Lechien JR, Hamdan A-L, Fakhry N, Vaira LA, Iannella G, Gengler IM, et al. Perception of young European otolaryngologists toward transoral robotic surgery in head and neck oncology and surgery. J Clin Med. 2024;13(11):3055.

12. Hosny SG, Johnston MJ, Pucher PH, Erridge S, Darzi A. Barriers to the implementation and uptake of simulation-based training programs in general surgery: a multinational qualitative study. J Surg Res. 2017;220:419–26. e2.
13. Acton RD, Chipman JG, Lunden M, Schmitz CC. Unanticipated teaching demands rise with simulation training: strategies for managing faculty workload. J Surg Educ. 2015;72(3):522–9.
14. Huang WD, Loid V, Sung JS. Reflecting on gamified learning in medical education: a systematic literature review grounded in the structure of observed learning outcomes (SOLO) taxonomy 2012–2022. BMC Med Educ. 2024;24(1):20.
15. Rubalcava N, Guetter C, Kapani N, Martinez Quinones P. How artificial intelligence is expected to transform surgical training. American College of Surgeons; 2023.

Preparing for Future Pandemics 41

Farzana Mahdi, Sonia Jaiswal, Sucheta Dandekar, and Nirmala Rege

Key Points

- Strengthen early warning systems to prevent escalation of any outbreak.
- Ensure a fair and just health access including an equitable global distribution of vaccines.
- Adopt an integrated approach to address human, animal, and environmental health, thereby preventing pathogen spillover and climate-related diseases.
- Foster transparent governance and multisectoral partnerships, and counter miscommunication to enhance trust within the communities.
- Provide continuous support to healthcare workers through innovative education and sustained physical, mental, and financial assistance.

41.1 Definition of Pandemics and the Way Forward

Terms like endemic, outbreak, epidemic, and pandemic refer to infections that are related to their rate of occurrence in various geographical areas. Endemic occurs at an expected rate in a population. Outbreak occurs at an unexpected rate among people in a new area, epidemics spread to a larger area, while pandemics spread globally [1]. World Health Organization (WHO) explains pandemics as "large scale infections causing significant morbidity and mortality that fracture the socioeconomic and political frameworks of wide geographical areas [2]."

Pandemics have occurred throughout world history with high morbidity and mortality rates and continue to threaten and devastate the global population even today. The Black Death emerged in the year 1347 and was one of the deadliest pandemics. Spanish flu emerged in the year 1918 and Zika virus was discovered in the

F. Mahdi (✉) · S. Jaiswal · S. Dandekar · N. Rege
Era's Lucknow Medical College and Hospital, Lucknow, India

J. Sandars et al. (eds.), *Modern Medical Education*,
https://doi.org/10.1007/978-3-032-27958-3_41

year 1947; both pandemics had high morbidity and mortality rates. The recent COVID-19 was a major pandemic and caused significant deaths in many countries.

A thoughtfully curated methodical system involves multiple processes that can mitigate challenges such as healthcare pressure, economic crisis, food system disruption, and many more. This system should ideally prioritize surveillance, identify the disease as early as possible, and work out ways of quarantining the affected population. It is important to align stakeholder roles with their expertise and responsibilities. At the same time, efforts must be made to prevent healthcare burnout through thoughtful workload distribution and support systems. Essential components include good clinical practice, reliable and ethical clinical trials for cost-effective vaccines, and above all good governance so that the right resources reach the right population cohorts [3]. Building upon the foundations of pandemic preparedness, the discussion will focus on the key areas requiring immediate attention in global health security planning.

41.2 Strengthening Surveillance: Steps Toward a Collaborative Global Response

To reduce vulnerability to infectious hazards, a new integrated approach to surveillance is needed. The following steps outlined by the World Health Organization (WHO) explains how public health systems can move toward collaborative, future-ready surveillance [4]:

1. *Recognize Community-Level Importance*: Early detection begins within communities. Therefore, strengthening local surveillance capacity is essential for timely reporting and response.
2. *Promote Cross-Sector Collaboration*: Infectious disease threats require coordination across sectors—health, environment, agriculture and technology—to ensure a unified response.
3. *Integrate Traditional and New Approaches*: Combine proven surveillance strategies with modern tools such as real-time data platforms, digital technologies, and genomic analysis.
4. *Strengthen Links Between Surveillance and Health Systems*: Surveillance efforts must be better connected to health systems to ensure that data leads to prompt and meaningful action.
5. *Invest in Sustainable Infrastructure*: Long-term investment is required at all levels, from community to global, to support infrastructure, workforce training, and technology.
6. *Foster Trust and Local Capacity*: Local communities must be empowered and supported to recognize, report, and respond to health risks [4]. Trust-building and transparency are key.
7. *Engage Expert Advice and Independent Oversight*: Inputs from a diverse group of experts help shape more effective and inclusive preparedness strategies.

8. *Commitment to Global Coordination and Leadership*: High-level political commitment is needed to sustain momentum and ensure coordinated global surveillance systems are maintained and strengthened.

Early warning systems using artificial intelligence (AI) have gained prominence as they use digital technology to continuously monitor and analyze extensive data. These systems can easily detect anomalous trends thereby raising warning signs without needing human intervention. Such techno-powered systems can be extremely helpful in countries where there is a shortage of manpower [5].

The organizations and countries should collaborate and share their disease tracking information to detect threats in a timely and accurate manner as global information sharing enhances surveillance effectively. Human, animal, and environmental health are deeply connected, and a coordinated action across these domains is essential for preventing and responding to future epidemics [6].

Effective surveillance does raise the alarm, but without an adequate health infrastructure, it is difficult to mitigate the threats. Therefore, health system strengthening is a critical priority.

41.3 Health System Strengthening to Tackle Unforeseen Circumstances

Medical care in most countries is typically designed to face routine and common conditions but not built for unforeseen circumstances. During the recent COVID-19 pandemic, the vulnerabilities of many health systems were exposed with inadequate infrastructure, insufficient healthcare workers, as well as shortage of hospital supplies and medicines leading to high morbidity and mortality. Many studies have highlighted expansion of healthcare facilities by not only establishing new centers, reconfiguring the existing departments and converting public places into temporary healthcare facilities. This helped in effective healthcare capacity building and development [7].

41.4 Preparing and Protecting the Health Workforce

The experience reveals that the human resource recruitment during a pandemic faces several hurdles and challenges as many volunteers may lack basic training and expertise needed to handle the pandemic crisis [8]. The following are the recommendations to ensure preparation in terms of managing the healthcare workforces:

1. *Develop a Flexible Staffing Reserve*
    - Establish and maintain a trained pool of reserve healthcare professionals, including retired personnel, volunteers, and trainees, who can be quickly mobilized in emergencies.
    - Create protocols for interinstitutional staff sharing during crises.

2. *Strengthen Safety Infrastructure for Health Workers*

   - Ensure early access to vaccinations, personal protective equipment (PPE), and infection prevention training.
   - Identify high-risk groups and implement tailored protective policies, including alternate work arrangements.

3. *Invest in Retention Strategies*

   - Introduce long-term retention plans such as mental health support, job security, and transparent communication to maintain morale and reduce burnout.
   - Foster familiarity with emergency procedures and infection control as part of routine training.

4. *Prioritize Mental Health and Well-Being*

   - Set up structured psychological support systems including counselling, peer support groups, and debriefing sessions.
   - Recognize staff contributions publicly and promote a culture of appreciation.

5. *Reform Compensation Models*

   - Implement flexible and transparent payment structures that allow for performance-based incentives, hazard pay, and timely disbursements during emergencies.
   - Reduce disparities and ensure fairness in compensation across all cadres.

6. *Improve Workload Management*

   - Introduce shift regulations and rest protocols to prevent exhaustion.
   - Avoid assigning staff to unfamiliar roles without adequate training and support.

7. *Strengthen Communication Channels*

   - Maintain regular and honest communication between management, frontline workers, and public health authorities.
   - Encourage feedback loops to understand staff concerns and needs in real-time [8].

Well-prepared healthcare workers provide a platform for the implementation of advanced therapeutic and prevention strategies. Strengthening healthcare capacity requires substantial and sustained finance, thus making it an important component of pandemic preparedness.

41.5 Financial Planning

Countries with adequate financial resources were in a better position to respond to the recent COVID-19 pandemic as they had an established system for rapid fund allocation and utilization. This allowed them to act promptly and implement public health measures [9]. In contrast, under-resourced countries struggled with financial management and were heavily dependent on external support for managing the crisis. Certain measures such as the establishment of dedicated emergency health funds that can be utilized during health crisis will be helpful. There is also a need to strengthen the public financial management system to ensure transparency in budget allocation and utilization in such situations. Initiatives such as pandemic bonds or insurance and strengthening public-private collaborations for resource mobilization can mitigate the societal and economic impact of future pandemics [9].

41.6 Preventive and Therapeutic Readiness: Dual Strategies to Combat Crisis

The WHO, Global Alliance for Vaccines and Immunization (GAVI), and Coalition for Epidemic Preparedness Innovations (CEPI) coled the COVAX facility to promote fair distribution of COVID-19 vaccines [10]. Hoarding of vaccines, inequitable distribution, and high manufacturing cost were the challenges faced by this initiative.

Amid global efforts for fair distribution of vaccines, swift advancement of mRNA vaccine technology emerged as a landmark achievement. There have been many intriguing research program on mRNA vaccines in the past, but they gained a lot of importance after COVID-19. Further substantial evidence regarding the safety and efficacy of mRNA vaccines has emerged as they are not only used in infectious diseases but may work well in cancer therapy. Large-scale manufacturing of mRNA vaccines is on the rise as it is easy, safe, and efficacious; hence, its role to combat future pandemics has been widely researched and accepted. However, adverse effects must also be researched. Mini-injector capsules and intranasal routes can also be considered as alternate routes of administration of vaccines. Research on mRNA has opened up a plethora of possibilities in medicine. The establishment of well-equipped continuous manufacturing units worldwide, with accurate and thorough guidelines for manufacture, will offer promising solutions [10]. As the field evolves, clearer manufacturing standards and better facilities are expected to emerge. mRNA technology stands at the forefront of a new phase in medicine, alongside nuclear vaccines are also gaining importance in terms of their stability and potential in long-term disease prevention. The pandemic underscored the importance of a robust infrastructure for a fair access to therapeutics such as antiviral drugs and monoclonal antibodies and immunomodulatory therapies; therefore, strengthening supply chains, swift regulatory approvals with investment in research and development will ensure a well- rounded response.

41.7 Public Health Communication and Community Engagement for Effective Health Crisis Management

Public health emergencies can be effectively managed using risk communication which can be broadly categorized into three types—inadequate, ideal, and infodemic. The WHO, International Federation of Red Cross and Red Crescent Societies (IFRC), and UN Children's Fund (UNICEF) in their analysis entitled "Risk Communication and Community Engagement (RCCE) Action Plan Guidance COVID-19 Preparedness and Response (2020)" [11] emphasize on how different types of communication affect community response and resilience.

The analysis identifies several key gaps in current communication practices (Table 41.1). Top-down messaging often overlooked local risks, cultural differences, and governance systems, leading to mistrust, confusion, and disengagement. Communities received information from multiple sources, sometimes conflicting, which complicated decision-making. Moreover, existing models of participatory communication were rarely adapted to diverse sociocultural contexts, limiting their practical application.

To improve risk communication in future pandemics, a shift toward more inclusive, context-sensitive strategies is recommended. These should empower communities as active stakeholders in risk planning and response. Communication must go beyond information delivery to include empathy, emotional recognition, and trust-building. Local voices should be incorporated in both the design and dissemination of messages to enhance credibility and relevance. Key recommendations include:

- *Adopting community-centered communication models* that prioritize dialogue and participation.
- *Building trust* by acknowledging public emotions and fostering transparency.
- *Tailoring messages* to local sociocultural realities.
- *Improving coordination* across information sources to reduce confusion.
- *Empowering communities* through capacity-building and involvement in decision-making.

Table 41.1 Gaps identified in risk communication and how to address them [11]

Gaps in current practice	How to address them
Overreliance on messaging	Shift to participatory, interactive models that engage communities early
Lack of contextual sensitivity	Develop adaptable communication frameworks based on local needs
Fragmented, unclear information	Streamline and coordinate messaging across all platforms and institutions
Limited application of participatory models	Expand research and implementation of culturally adaptable participatory models
Community confusion from multiple information sources	Train local leaders and influencers to act as trusted messengers
Disconnection from emotional and social realities	Include behavioral science, anthropology, and social work experts in communication planning

There is a need for further research and investment into adaptable communication frameworks that respect the diversity of local communities while providing consistent, scientifically sound information [11]. Strengthening these approaches is essential for fostering resilience, ensuring equitable responses, and enhancing public trust during future health crises (Table 41.1).

41.8 Reinforcing Policy, Governance, and Legal Frameworks to Support Resilient Health Systems

Pandemics cause large and complex issues that cannot be handled alone by a single organization or country. International cooperation and collaboration, therefore, becomes essential to manage the crisis. Policy, governance, and legal frameworks establish the rules, regulations, and protocols that guide governments and institutions to respond to health emergencies. Good governance would mean that there is minimal confusion and efficient decision-making, thereby promoting transparency and responsible conduct. Governance works at three levels: local, national, and global. Transparent and effective governance will ensure that the roles and responsibilities are delegated at each level. For example, local testing and isolation centers are set up by district officials. At the national level, rolling out of vaccines and issuing lockdown orders are taken care of by the ministries and national agencies. Globally, the WHO, World Bank, and UN agencies can work toward sharing of vaccines and global surveillance. Policies can dictate terms on how the resources and medical supplies are manufactured and distributed equitably. Policies must address the needs of vulnerable population, who can be people with disabilities or even the elderly. Legal frameworks should be established and validated with expert deliberations to foster effective collaboration between different government agencies and stakeholders. Legal frameworks can also strike a balance between the need for public health measures and human rights. It is therefore recommended that regular legal and policy audits are done [12]. Recently, on May 20, 2025, the WHO accord was signed by the 78th World Health Assembly to strengthen global pandemic preparedness. The treaty was a landmark event, and the purpose was to foster cooperation and collaboration among countries for pandemic preparedness. The accord is guided by principles of accountability, equity, respect, and solidarity. The agreement proposed a common platform for rapid sharing of pathogen data. An intergovernmental team has been formed to complete the development of PABS (pathogen access benefit sharing system). The WHO has also established partnership with the Food and Agriculture Organization (FAO), the World Organization for Animal Health (WOAH), and the UN Environment Program (UNEP) [12] to work on common grounds to understand human, animal, and environmental health. A joint plan of action includes collaboration with various governments to build infrastructure and assure funds to respond to health threats from humans, animals, and environment. The WHO is the secretariat for OHHLEP (One Health High Level Expert Committee), which gives practice guidelines for surveillance and spillover diseases.

41.9 The Importance of Integrating Social Determinants: Bridging Inequities and Promoting Social Justice

Institutional structures must incorporate principles of equity and ethical decision-making.

Social determinants of health and ethical considerations should play a crucial role toward pandemic management at various levels. One of the key aspects is identifying high-risk groups and also people who may share common characteristics but do not interact with each other. Addressing ethical issues may build a certain level of trust among the public and will thereby help with compliance of infection control measures. Pandemics can magnify problems such as poverty, overcrowded houses, and limited access to clean water with little or no healthcare facilities. Priority support should be given to migrant workers, people with unstable jobs, or those who live in rural areas and are at a greater risk. There should be equitable allocation of ICU beds and medication.

Equity and ethics should be a part of the development and implementation of health interventions. Autonomy, transparency, and informed consent in areas of testing, quarantine, and digitalization of personal data is essential. Furthermore, cultural beliefs and local practices must also be taken into careful consideration. Involvement of ethicists, community leaders, and public representatives can foster credibility and accountability. Ethical and equity considerations should be integrated into government reports and national health strategies [13]. Careful consideration of diversity, equity, and inclusivity can help build resilient systems by nurturing adaptability and a sense of belonging within communities.

41.10 Innovations: A Key to the Education of Health Professionals

Reduced participation in preclinical, para-clinical, and clinical student instruction, clinical procedure training, restricted clinical exposure, and reduced participation in mentoring for all students were the gaps found during the COVID-19 pandemic, which had a profound impact on the education and training of healthcare professionals [14].

Virtual platforms have played a vital role in clinical teaching during the recent COVID-19 pandemic. These digital spaces have prepared students by not only giving them effective theoretical knowledge but also training them in hygiene practices, patient care skills, ethics, and professionalism. Students could participate in webinars and teleconferences; maintaining contact with peers and teachers through platforms such as Zoom, Teams, and Google meet [14]. Virtual assessments through online proctoring and simulation-based technology were some innovative methods for assessment.

The use of virtual platforms has been cost-effective and flexible but there was limited hands-on experience and repeated internet issues [14]. However, further innovations in the form of blended learning, virtual simulation, telemedicine, remote research opportunities, and faculty development in digital teaching methods can counter these limitations.

Information technology in the form of data augmentation, simulation, and artificial intelligence are bringing about a transformation in the healthcare system. Institutes need a longitudinal model involving sustained and continuous learning experiences over an extended period rather than short isolated sessions to foster lasting relationships between learners, educators, and patients [14].

41.11 Strengthening Psychological Support for Holistic and Resilient Healthcare Delivery

The social and psychological effects of COVID-19 are complex and long-lasting. Hence, it is necessary to strengthen and prioritize the emotional, psychological, and social well-being of health professionals. A crucial step for building community resilience is providing psychological support as an early intervention for people experiencing traumatic or catastrophic events. Psychological first aid (PFA) has been further endorsed through deliberations by an expert committee and has been integrated as tenets for mental health and psychological support. These tenets when employed may reduce stress during disasters and address preparedness for future threats. PFA training should be an integral part of the Competency-Based Medical Education (CBME) curriculum for medical students. Mandatory certifications for students will help them to be better prepared for future healthcare emergencies. Long-term training schedules on the other hand will effectively contribute toward community resilience [15].

41.12 Conclusion

The emerging and re-emergence of infectious diseases has shown, time and again, how unprepared systems can suffer disastrous consequences. The adoption of a comprehensive, multisectoral approach that not only responds to outbreaks but strengthens our ability to prevent them is vital. Central to this is a well-supported, resilient healthcare workforce with equitable access to resources and protection.

Real-time surveillance, accurate health reporting, and a globally connected monitoring system are key components of an effective response. These must be backed by sustained investments and efficient resource mobilization to ensure readiness. Equally critical is the continued development of affordable vaccines and a steady supply of essential therapeutics, ensuring no population is left behind.

Preparation for future pandemics demands far more than technical solutions. It requires inclusive policies that reflect cultural contexts, uphold ethical standards, and correct gaps in previous response frameworks. Strengthening health systems alone is not enough; we must also embrace the multisectoral health approach which recognizes a relation between human, animal, and environmental health. This includes stronger links between disease surveillance, climate adaptation, and ecological protection.

Ultimately, tackling future threats will depend on our willingness to collaborate across disciplines, sectors, and borders. A shared commitment to science, equity, and collective responsibility will shape a healthier, more prepared, and more humane global future.

References

1. Mascie Taylor N, Moji K. Pandemics. J Peace Nuclear Disarmament. 2021;4(sup1):47–59.
2. Madhav N, Oppenheim B, Gallivan M, Mulembakani P, Rubin E, Wolfe N. Pandemics: risks, impacts, and mitigation. In: Disease control priorities: improving health and reducing poverty. 3rd ed. Washington, DC: The International Bank for Reconstruction and Development/The World Bank; 2017. p. 315–45.
3. Kamalrathne T, Amaratunga D, Haigh R, Kodituwakku L, Rupasinghe C. Epidemic and pandemic preparedness and response in a multi-hazard context: COVID-19 pandemic as a point of reference. Int J Environ Res Public Health. 2024;21(9):1238. p. 1–24.
4. World Health Organization. Future surveillance for epidemic and pandemic diseases: a 2023 perspective. World Health Organization; 2023. p. 1–116.
5. Chiu KH, Sridhar S, Yuen KY. Preparation for the next pandemic: challenges in strengthening surveillance. Emerg Microbes Infect. 2023;12(2):2240441. https://doi.org/10.1080/22221751.2023.2240441. PMID: 37474466; PMCID: PMC10478602.
6. Carroll D, Morzaria S, Briand S, Johnson CK, Morens D, Sumption K, Tomori O, Wacharphaueasadee S. Preventing the next pandemic: the power of a global viral surveillance network. BMJ. 2021;372:n485.
7. Sadeghkhani O, Mehdi Alamdarloo P, Mahmoodi Mehr MA, Shokri Kazem Abadi E, Tabatabaei Far SS, Delavari S. Resilience model of public health sector during unknown pandemics: a grounded theory approach for COVID-19 in Iran. BMC Public Health. 2025;25(1):1271.
8. Frenk J, Chen LC, Chandran L, Groff EO, King R, Meleis A, Fineberg HV. Challenges and opportunities for educating health professionals after the COVID-19 pandemic. Lancet. 2022;400(10362):1539–56.
9. Aarestrup FM, Bonten M, Koopmans M. Pandemics–One Health preparedness for the next. Lancet Reg Health Eur. 2021;9:100210.
10. Chavda VP, Soni S, Vora LK, Soni S, Khadela A, Ajabiya J. mRNA-based vaccines and therapeutics for COVID-19 and future pandemics. Vaccines. 2022;10(12):2150.
11. Khan S, Mishra J, Ahmed N, Onyige CD, Lin KE, Siew R, Lim BH. Risk communication and community engagement during COVID-19. Int J Disaster Risk Reduct. 2022;74:102903. https://doi.org/10.1016/j.ijdrr.2022.102903. Epub 2022 Mar 16. PMID: 35313476; PMCID: PMC8925315.

12. Taylor RCR. The global governance of pandemics. Sociol Health Illness. 2021;43(6):1540–53. https://doi.org/10.1111/1467-9566.13293. Epub 2021 Jul 19. PMID: 34286858; PMCID: PMC8441821.
13. Hoven H, Dragano N, Angerer P, Apfelbacher C, Backhaus I, Hoffmann B, Icks A, Wilm S, Fangerau H, Söhner F. Striving for health equity: the importance of social determinants of health and ethical considerations in pandemic preparedness planning. Int J Public Health. 2022;67:1604542. https://doi.org/10.3389/ijph.2022.1604542. PMID: 35450128; PMCID: PMC9017774.
14. Boutros P, Kassem N, Nieder J, Jaramillo C, von Petersdorff J, Walsh FJ, Bärnighausen T, Barteit S. Education and training adaptations for health workers during the COVID-19 pandemic: a scoping review of lessons learned and innovations. Healthcare (Basel). 2023;11(21):2902. https://doi.org/10.3390/healthcare11212902. PMID: 37958046; PMCID: PMC10649637.
15. Simon MA, Al-Ghailani AS. Preparedness for future pandemics: utilizing psychological first aid in disaster mental health-care training. J Nat Sci Med. 2024;7(2):140–3.

Index

J. Sandars et al. (eds.), *Modern Medical Education*, https://doi.org/10.1007/978-3-032-27958-3

B

D

J

K

L

GPSR Compliance

The European Union's (EU) General Product Safety Regulation (GPSR) is a set of rules that requires consumer products to be safe and our obligations to ensure this.

If you have any concerns about our products, you can contact us on ProductSafety@springernature.com

In case Publisher is established outside the EU, the EU authorized representative is:

Springer Nature Customer Service Center GmbH
Europaplatz 3
69115 Heidelberg, Germany

Batch number: 10493408

Printed by Printforce, the Netherlands